Evidence-Based Clinical Practice in Otolaryngology

Guest Editor

TIMOTHY L. SMITH, MD, MPH, FACS

OTOLARYNGOLOGIC CLINICS OF NORTH AMERICA

www.oto.theclinics.com

October 2012 • Volume 45 • Number 5

SAUNDERS an imprint of ELSEVIER, Inc.

W.B. SAUNDERS COMPANY

A Division of Elsevier Inc.

1600 John F. Kennedy Boulevard • Suite 1800 • Philadelphia, Pennsylvania 19103-2899

http://www.theclinics.com

OTOLARYNGOLOGIC CLINICS OF NORTH AMERICA Volume 45, Number 5
October 2012 ISSN 0030-6665, ISBN-13: 978-1-4557-4923-2

Editor: Joanne Husovski
Development Editor: Donald Mumford

Otolaryngologic Clinics of North America (ISSN 0030-6665) is published bimonthly by Elsevier, Inc., 360 Park Avenue South, New York, NY 10010-1710. Months of issue are February, April, June, August, October, and December. Business and Editorial Offices: 1600 John F. Kennedy Blvd., Suite 1800, Philadelphia, PA 19103-2899. Customer Service Office: 6277 Sea Harbor Drive, Orlando, FL 32887-4800. Periodicals postage paid at New York, NY and additional mailing offices. Subscription prices is $335.00 per year (US individuals), $628.00 per year (US institutions), $161.00 per year (US student/resident), $442.00 per year (Canadian individuals), $789.00 per year (Canadian institutions), $496.00 per year (international individuals), $789.00 per year (international institutions), $248.00 per year (international & Canadian student/resident). Foreign air speed delivery is included in all *Clinics*' subscription prices. All prices are subject to change without notice. **POSTMASTER:** Send address changes to *Otolaryngologic Clinics of North America*, Elsevier Health Sciences Division, Subscription Customer Service, 3251 Riverport Lane, Maryland Heights, MO 63043. **Telephone: 1-800-654-2452 (U.S. and Canada); 314-447-8871 (outside U.S. and Canada). Fax: 314-447-8029. E-mail: journalscustomerservice-usa@elsevier.com (for print support); journalsonlinesupport-usa@elsevier.com (for online support).**

Reprints. For copies of 100 or more of articles in this publication, please contact the Commercial Reprints Department, Elsevier Inc., 360 Park Avenue South, New York, NY 10010-1710. Tel.: 212-633-3812; Fax: 212-462-1935; E-mail: reprints@elsevier.com.

Otolaryngologic Clinics of North America is also published in Spanish by McGraw-Hill Interamericana Editores S.A., P.O. Box 5-237, 06500 Mexico D.F., Mexico.

Otolaryngologic Clinics of North America is covered in *MEDLINE/PubMed (Index Medicus), Current Contents/Clinical Medicine, Excerpta Medica, BIOSIS, Science Citation Index,* and *ISI/BIOMED.*

Printed and bound by CPI Group (UK) Ltd, Croydon, CR0 4YY

Transferred to Digital Print 2012

Contributors

GUEST EDITOR

TIMOTHY L. SMITH, MD, MPH, FACS
Professor; Director, Clinical Research; Director, Oregon Sinus Center at OHSU; Rhinology and Endoscopic Sinus-Skull Base Surgery, Department of Otolaryngology–Head and Neck Surgery, Oregon Health & Science University, Portland, Oregon

AUTHORS

M.L. BARNES, FRCS-ORL(ED), MD
Specialist Registrar, Ninewells Hospital & Medical School, Dundee, United Kingdom

PETE S. BATRA, MD, FACS
Associate Professor, Co-Director, Department of Otolaryngology–Head and Neck Surgery; Comprehensive Skull Base Program, University of Texas Southwestern Medical Center, Dallas, Texas

SCOTT E. BEVANS, MD
Otolaryngology-Head and Neck Surgery, Madigan Healthcare System, Tacoma, Washington

DANIEL E. CANNON, MD
Otolaryngology Resident, Department of Otolaryngology and Communication Sciences, Medical College of Wisconsin, Milwaukee, Wisconsin

JAIME I. CHANG, MD
Otolaryngology-Head and Neck Surgery, Virginia Mason Medical Center, Seattle, Washington

JUSTIN K. CHAU, MD
Clinical Assistant Professor, Section of Otolaryngology, Department of Surgery, University of Calgary, Calgary, Alberta, Canada

JOHN J.W. CHO, MD
Fellow, Paparella Ear Head & Neck Institute, Minneapolis, Minnesota

JOHN M. DELGAUDIO, MD
Professor and Vice Chair, Residency Program Director, Chief of Rhinology and Sinus Surgery, Department of Otolaryngology, Emory University, Atlanta, Georgia

DIETER K. FRITZ, MD
Resident, Section of Otolaryngology, Department of Surgery, University of Calgary, Calgary, Alberta, Canada

MITCHELL R. GORE
Fellow, Department of Otolaryngology-Head and Neck Surgery, University of North Carolina at Chapel Hill, Chapel Hill, North Carolina

NEIL D. GROSS, MD, FACS
Associate Professor, Department of Otolaryngology/Head and Neck Surgery, Oregon Health and Science University, Portland, Oregon

DANA M. HARTL, MD, PhD
Specialist, Department of Head and Neck Oncology, Institut Gustave Roussy, Villejuif, France

RICHARD J. HARVEY, MD
Associate Professor, University of New South Wales & St Vincent's Hospitals and Macquarie University, Darlinghurst, Sydney, New South Wales, Australia

STACEY L. ISHMAN, MD, MPH
Director, Center for Snoring & Sleep Surgery; Assistant Professor, Division of Pulmonary and Critical Care Medicine, Departments of Otolaryngology–Head and Neck Surgery, Pediatrics & Internal Medicine, Johns Hopkins School of Medicine, Baltimore, Maryland

SELENA LIAO, MD
Department of Otolaryngology-Head and Neck Surgery, Oregon Health and Sciences University, Portland, Oregon

MICHAEL LUPA, MD
Rhinology Fellow Emory, Department of Otolaryngology, Emory University, Atlanta, Georgia

RODRIGO MARTINEZ-MONEDERO, MD, PhD
Department of Otolaryngology-Head and Neck Surgery, Johns Hopkins Hospital, Johns Hopkins University School of Medicine, Baltimore, Maryland

ALBERT L. MERATI, MD, FACS
Professor and Chief of Laryngology, Department of Otolaryngology/Head and Neck Surgery, University of Washington, Seattle, Washington

STEPHANIE MISONO, MD, MPH
Assistant Professor, Department of Otolaryngology/Head and Neck Surgery, University of Minnesota, Minneapolis, Minnesota

VIKASH K. MODI, MD, FAAP
Assistant Professor, Department of Otolaryngology-Head & Neck Surgery, Pediatric Otolaryngology-Head & Neck Surgery, Weill Cornell Medical College, New York, New York

MARCUS M. MONROE, MD
Department of Otolaryngology/Head and Neck Surgery, Oregon Health and Science University, Portland, Oregon

ANH T. NGUYEN-HUYNH, MD, PhD
Assistant Professor, Department of Otolaryngology-Head and Neck Surgery, Oregon Health & Science University, Portland, Oregon

JOHN K. NIPARKO, MD
George T. Nager Professor, Department of Otolaryngology-Head and Neck Surgery, Johns Hopkins Hospital, Johns Hopkins University School of Medicine, Baltimore, Maryland

KARIN P.Q. OOMEN, MD, PhD
Fellow, Department of Otolaryngology-Head & Neck Surgery, Pediatric Otolaryngology-Head & Neck Surgery, Weill Cornell Medical College, New York, New York

ROUNAK B. RAWAL
Medical Student, Department of Otolaryngology-Head and Neck Surgery, University of North Carolina at Chapel Hill, Chapel Hill, North Carolina

JOHN S. RHEE, MD, MPH
Professor and Chairman, Department of Otolaryngology and Communication Sciences, Medical College of Wisconsin, Milwaukee, Wisconsin

LUKE RUDMIK, MD
Rhinology and Endoscopic Sinus - Skull Base Surgery, Division of Otolaryngology–Head and Neck Surgery, Department of Surgery, University of Calgary, Calgary, Alberta, Canada

RODNEY J. SCHLOSSER, MD, FAAOA
Professor, Otolaryngology-Head and Neck Surgery, Medical University of South Carolina and Ralph H. Johnson VA Medical Center, Charleston, South Carolina

SETH R. SCHWARTZ, MD, MPH
Otolaryngology-Head and Neck Surgery, Virginia Mason Medical Center, Seattle, Washington

YEVGENIY R. SEMENOV, MA
Department of Otolaryngology-Head and Neck Surgery, Johns Hopkins Hospital, Johns Hopkins University School of Medicine, Baltimore, Maryland

MAISIE SHINDO, MD
Professor, Department of Otolaryngology-Head and Neck Surgery, Oregon Health and Sciences University, Portland, Oregon

TIMOTHY L. SMITH, MD, MPH
Professor; Director, Clinical Research; Director, Oregon Sinus Center at OHSU; Rhinology and Endoscopic Sinus-Skull Base Surgery, Department of Otolaryngology–Head and Neck Surgery, Oregon Health & Science University, Portland, Oregon

P.M. SPIELMANN, FRCS-ORL(Ed)
Specialist Registrar, Ninewells Hospital & Medical School, Dundee, United Kingdom

MICHAEL G. STEWART, MD, MPH
Professor and Chairman, Vice Dean, Associate Dean of Clinical Affairs, Department of Otolaryngology-Head & Neck Surgery, Weill Cornell Medical College, New York, New York

P.S. WHITE, FRACS, FRCS(Ed), MBChB
Consultant Rhinologist, Ninewells Hospital & Medical School, Dundee, United Kingdom

SARAH K. WISE, MD, MSCR, FAAOA
Assistant Professor, Otolaryngology-Head and Neck Surgery, Emory University, Atlanta, Georgia

ADAM M. ZANATION, MD
Assistant Professor, Department of Otolaryngology-Head and Neck Surgery, University of North Carolina at Chapel Hill, Chapel Hill, North Carolina

Contents

Balloon catheter dilation (BCD) is a treatment paradigm for surgical manage-ment of paranasal sinus inflammatory disease. There are few robust clinical trials evaluating the efficacy of balloon technology in chronic rhinosinusitis (CRS). The available database largely comprises retrospective, uncontrolled studies with insufficiently characterized patient cohorts and a lack of com-parator groups. Thus, the current evidence base is unable to elucidate the role and indications for BCD in the management of medically refractory CRS. Future studies should include selected control groups, preferably with randomization and validated outcome measures, to determine the effi-cacy of balloon technology compared with endoscopic sinus surgery.

This article provides a contemporary management protocol for adult epi-staxis admissions, evidence based where possible, and otherwise based on the authors' own experience.

Postoperative care following endoscopic sinus surgery (ESS) for medically refractory chronic rhinosinusitis (CRS) is believed to be important to opti-mize clinical outcomes. There is no standardized approach to postopera-tive care and, because of the numerous reported strategies, there remains a debate as to what constitutes the optimal postoperative care protocol. This article reviews the evidence and describes an evidence-based ap-proach for postoperative care following ESS for medically refractory CRS.

The cause of nasal obstruction can often be attributed to pathologic con-ditions of the nasal valve. The key physical examination finding in nasal valve compromise is inspiratory collapse of the nasal sidewall. Validated subjective and objective measures evaluating nasal obstruction exist, al-though with weak correlation. Functional rhinoplasty encompasses the surgical techniques used to address obstruction occurring in this area. These techniques aim to increase the size of the nasal valve opening and/or strengthen the lateral nasal wall and nasal ala, preventing dynamic collapse. Much of the supporting evidence for functional rhinoplasty con-sists of observational studies that are universally favorable.

In this article, the authors review the current evidence regarding the public health and economic impact of allergic rhinitis. Diagnostic methods for allergic disease are discussed as well as certain nuances of allergy skin testing protocols. In addition, the evidence supporting sublingual immunotherapy (SLIT) for allergic rhinitis is reviewed, with subsequent attention to certain subgroups, such as adults and children, seasonal versus perennial allergens, and SLIT efficacy for individual antigens. The authors consider the evidence supporting appropriate SLIT dosing as well as the existing data on SLIT safety.

Diagnosis of sleep-disordered breathing (SDB) is most accurately obtained with a nocturnal polysomnogram. However, limitations on availability make alternative screening tools necessary. Nocturnal oximetry studies or nap polysomnography can be useful if positive; however, further testing is necessary to if these tests are negative. History and physical examination have insufficient sensitivity and specificity for definitive diagnosis of pediatric OSA. Adenotonsillectomy remains first-line therapy for pediatric SDB and obstructive sleep apnea (OSA). Additional study of limited therapies for mild OSA are necessary to determine if these are reasonable primary methods of treatment or if they should be reserved for children with persistent OSA.

Tonsillectomy is one of the most common surgical procedures performed in children in the United States. Indications and recommendations for perioperative management are multiple and may vary among clinicians. Although tonsillectomy is a safe procedure, it can be associated with morbidity. Several techniques have been developed to reduce perioperative complications, but evidence of this reduction is lacking. This article provides clinicians with evidence-based guidance on perioperative clinical decision making and surgical technique for tonsillectomy.

Current evidence on the etiologies and presentation, evaluation, and management of unilateral vocal fold paralysis (UVFP) is reviewed. Cross-sectional imaging is appropriate in the work-up of idiopathic UVFP, but routine use of serology is not well supported. With laryngeal electromyography, predictors of poor prognosis for functionally meaningful recovery include fibrillation potentials, positive sharp waves, and absent/reduced voluntary motor unit potentials, but optimal timing remains unclear. Voice therapy may be helpful. Injection and laryngeal framework surgery (medialization thyroplasty) improve vocal quality. The vocal impact of laryngeal reinnervation is comparable with that of medialization. Some patients may benefit from multiple procedures.

This article reviews the evidence for the evaluation and management for patients with dysphonia. The evidence behind laryngoscopy, laryngostroboscopy, laryngeal imaging, laryngeal electromyography, and disease-specific questionnaires are reviewed. The evidence for management of some of the common conditions leading to dysphonia is also reviewed. This article reviews the evidence for voice therapy for various voice pathologies; medical management of dysphonia, including antibiotics, steroids, and antireflux therapy; and surgical management of glottic insufficiency and some benign laryngeal masses.

Successful outcomes of endoscopic approaches to benign sinonasal tumors have launched interest in expanding its use for sinonasal malignancy. Because of the heterogeneity and rarity of sinonasal malignancy, evidence for clinical outcomes of endoscopic approaches versus traditional craniofacial resection is low. Using the Oxford Center for Evidence-based Medicine guidelines, we present the existing evidence comparing both techniques for a variety of sinonasal malignancies.

The main issue in the management of glottic squamous cell carcinoma, as for all cancers, is adequate disease control while optimizing functional outcomes and minimizing morbidity. This is true for early-stage disease as for advanced tumors. This article evaluates the current evidence for the diagnostic and pretherapeutic workup for glottic squamous cell carcinoma and the evidence concerning different treatment options for glottic carcinoma, from early-stage to advanced-stage disease.

This review provides an overview of current guideline recommendations for the clinical evaluation and surgical management of well-differentiated thyroid cancer, and further examines the evidence for controversial topics such as the minimum degree of primary resection, the role of elective central neck dissection, and the extent of lateral neck dissection. Well-differentiated thyroid cancer comprises the majority of thyroid cancers, about 90%, and includes both papillary and follicular carcinomas. Despite convergence of the medical community in establishing treatment guidelines under the American Thyroid Association, there still remain many areas of disagreement.

This article provides a critical review of the evidence surrounding the management of the clinical node negative patient with early-stage oral cavity squamous cell carcinoma.

OTOLARYNGOLOGIC CLINICS OF NORTH AMERICA

RELATED INTEREST

Evidence-based medicine in otolaryngology, part 1:
The multiple faces of evidence-based medicine,
Jennifer J. Shin, Gregory W. Randolph, Steven D. Rauch.
In: Otolaryngology – Head and Neck Surgery, Volume 142, Issue 5, May 2010,
Pages 637–646.

DOWNLOAD Free App!

Review Articles
THE CLINICS

NOW AVAILABLE FOR YOUR iPhone and iPad

Preface

Clinical Decision-Making Based on Evidence

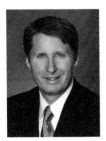

Timothy L. Smith, MD, MPH, FACS
Guest Editor

The concept of evidence-based medicine has flourished in recent years and it seems that clinicians, more than ever, crave evidence from the medical literature to inform their clinical care decision-making. While it is heartening that great volumes of evidence may exist, it is a daunting task to assimilate, critically review, prioritize, grade, and operationalize this crucial information. This volume of *Otolaryngologic Clinics* attempts to do just that.

This book examines evidence-based practices on topics of critical importance to otolaryngologists–head and neck surgeons. The evidence has been gathered and is presented by leaders in their respective fields. I invite you to review their findings and recommendations and use them to the benefit of our patients.

DEDICATION

This issue is dedicated to the loving memory of my grandmother, Lila Wright (1920-2011), who taught me that sometimes you just have to do what feels right.

Timothy L. Smith, MD, MPH, FACS
Professor
Director, Clinical Research
Director, Oregon Sinus Center at OHSU
Department of Otolaryngology-Head and Neck Surgery
Oregon Health & Science University
3181 South West Sam Jackson Park Road, Suite 250
Portland, OR 97239, USA

E-mail address:
smithtim@ohsu.edu

Otolaryngol Clin N Am 45 (2012) xiii
http://dx.doi.org/10.1016/j.otc.2012.06.017
0030-6665/12/$ – see front matter © 2012 Published by Elsevier Inc.

oto.theclinics.com

Evidence-Based Practice
Management of Vertigo

Anh T. Nguyen-Huynh, MD, PhD

KEYWORDS

- Vertigo • Dizziness • Evidence-based otolaryngology • Vestibular
- Benign paroxysmal positional vertigo • Otolaryngologic symptoms

KEY POINTS

The following points list the level of evidence as based on Oxford Center for Evidence-Based Medicine.

- Benign paroxysmal positional vertigo (BPPV) is the most common diagnosis of vertigo (level 4).
- Dix-Hallpike maneuver is the diagnostic test for posterior canal BPPV (level 1).
- Supine roll test is the diagnostic test for lateral canal BPPV (level 2).
- Epley maneuver is the first-line treatment for posterior canal BPPV (level 1).
- Posterior semicircular canal occlusion is an effective treatment for recalcitrant posterior canal BPPV (level 4).
- Lateral canal BPPV can be treated with a variety of repositioning maneuvers (level 2).

  OCEBM Levels of Evidence Working Group.[a] "The Oxford 2011 Levels of Evidence." Oxford Center for Evidence-Based Medicine. http://www.cebm.net/index.aspx?o=5653.

  [a] OCEBM Levels of Evidence Working Group—Jeremy Howick, Iain Chalmers (James Lind Library), Paul Glasziou, Trish Greenhalgh, Carl Heneghan, Alessandro Liberati, Ivan Moschetti, Bob Phillips, Hazel Thornton, Olive Goddard, and Mary Hodgkinson.

PROBLEM OVERVIEW
Vertigo

Vertigo is a symptom, not a disease. Effective diagnosis and management of vertigo begin with understanding what the symptom may represent. A survey of the members of the American Otological Society and the American Neurotology Society revealed that 75% of respondents agreed or agreed strongly that the definition of vertigo in clinical practice should be more precise.[1] Whereas 45% of respondents

This work was supported by grants KL2RR024141 and 5R33DC008632 from the National Institutes of Health. The author has no financial interest to disclose.
Department of Otolaryngology-Head and Neck Surgery, Oregon Health & Science University, 3181 Sam Jackson Park Road PV01, Portland, OR 97239, USA
E-mail address: nguyanh@ohsu.edu

Otolaryngol Clin N Am 45 (2012) 925–940
http://dx.doi.org/10.1016/j.otc.2012.06.001
0030-6665/12/$ – see front matter © 2012 Elsevier Inc. All rights reserved.

favored restricting vertigo to describe a sensation of spinning or turning only, 40% of respondent favored including any sensation of movement in the definition of vertigo. Since acute inner ear pathology typically produces a spinning sensation, the more restrictive definition of vertigo renders it a more specific clue for a possible otologic vestibular disorder. A narrow focus on spinning may not be sensitive to chronic or milder inner ear pathology, however, where sensation of movement other than spinning might be elicited. Even though a consensus has not been reached on the precise definition of vertigo, it is reasonable to infer from the survey results that the overwhelming majority of otologists would recognize vertigo as distinct from other flavors of dizziness, such as presyncopal lightheadedness, disequilibrium, or other unsettling sensations.[2]

Epidemiologic surveys showed that 20% to 30% of the population may have experienced vertigo or dizziness in their lifetime.[3–6] A German national telephone health survey followed by structured neurotologic interview identified the lifetime prevalence of vestibular vertigo to be 7.8%, with an annual incidence of 1.5%.[7] In the United States, 1.7% of ambulatory medical care visits recorded vertigo or dizziness among the chief complaints.[8] Vertigo or dizziness also accounted for 2.5% of presentations to US emergency department in the years 1995 to 2004.[9]

Vertigo is a symptom in a wide range of disorders (**Table 1**). The article focuses on the evidence basis for the management of benign paroxysmal positional vertigo (BPPV), the most common diagnosis of vertigo in both primary care and subspecialty settings.[10,11]

Benign paroxysmal positional vertigo

BPPV is a disorder of the inner ear characterized by episodes of vertigo triggered by changes in head position.[12] BPPV is thought to be caused by the presence of endolymphatic debris in 1 or more semicircular canals. Direct evidence of such debris or canaliths has been demonstrated for posterior canal BPPV.[13] The presence of debris in lateral canal BPPV has not been demonstrated directly. However, treatment of posterior canal BPPV by repositioning the debris can lead to lateral canal BPPV. By inference, lateral canal BPPV can also be caused by endolymphatic debris.[14,15]

A population-based study estimates BPPV has a life-time prevalence of 2.4% and accounts for 8% of the individuals with moderate-to-severe dizziness or vertigo.[16]

Posterior canal BPPV account for about 90% of the cases, and lateral canal BPPV accounts for about 8% of the cases, according to a review of 10 series with a total of 3342 patients.[17] In rare instances, the anterior canal or multiple canals might be involved.[18]

Table 1
Basic differential diagnosis of vertigo

Otological Conditions	Neurological Conditions	Others
Benign paroxysmal positional vertigo	Migraine-associated vertigo	Postural hypotension
Vestibular neuritis/labyrinthitis	Vertebrobasillar insufficiency	Medication side effects
Meniere disease	Demyelinating diseases	Anxiety or panic disorder
Superior semicircular canal dehiscence	CNS lesions	Cervical vertigo

Adapted from Bhattacharyya N, Baugh RF, Orvidas L, et al. Clinical practice guideline: benign paroxysmal positional vertigo. Otolaryngol Head Neck Surg 2008;139:S57.

EVIDENCE-BASED CLINICAL ASSESSMENT
Diagnosis of Posterior Canal BPPV

The diagnosis of BPPV affecting the posterior semicircular canal is established by a history of episodic vertigo with changes in head position and the presence of characteristic nystagmus provoked by the Dix-Hallpike test according to a guideline from the American Academy of Otolaryngology-Head and Neck Surgery.[12]

The Dix-Hallpike test[19] (**Fig. 1**) is generally considered the gold standard test for the diagnosis of posterior canal BPPV in that it is the most common diagnostic criterion required for entry into clinical trials and for inclusion of such trials in meta-analyses.[20,21] The Dix-Hallpike test is not truly 100% sensitive, however, since BPPV is an intermittent condition, and variations in examiners' technique and experience might affect the test outcome. The sensitivity of the Dix-Hallpike test has been estimated at 48% to 88% according to a structured review of published literature.[22] The same review found that estimates for specificity are lacking. In the primary care setting, the Dix-Hallpike test reportedly has a negative predictive value of 52% for the diagnosis of BPPV.[10] In a different series of 95 patients diagnosed and treated for posterior canal BPPV in a specialty clinic, 11 patients did not have a positive Dix-Hallpike on initial examination, and 28 presented with an atypical history that did not suggest BPPV.[23] Given these considerations, the Dix-Hallpike test should be routinely performed if possible in the evaluation of vertigo/dizziness. Whereas a positive test should be considered sufficient for the diagnosis of BPPV in the clinical setting, a negative test should not rule out BPPV completely. Repeated testing in separate occasions may be necessary to avoid missing the diagnosis. Failure to diagnose BPPV may lead to costly diagnostic work-up.[24]

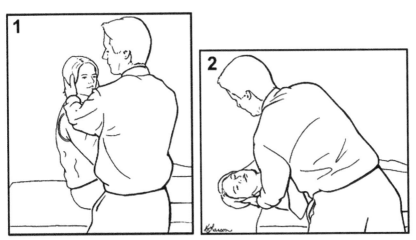

Fig. 1. The Dix-Hallpike test for the diagnosis of posterior canal BPPV. The patient begins by sitting up right with head is turned 45° toward the side to be tested (1). The patient is then laid back to supine position with head still turned and slightly extended (2). In a positive test, torsional nystagmus with the upper pole of the eyes beating toward the dependent ear appears within a few seconds and disappears in less than a minute. A positive Dix-Hallpike test indicates the presence of posterior canal BPPV in the dependent ear. (*Adapted from* Fife TD, Iverson DJ, Lempert T, et al. Practice parameter: therapies for benign paroxysmal positional vertigo (an evidence-based review): report of the Quality Standards Subcommittee of the American Academy of Neurology. Neurology 2008;70:2068; with permission.)

Diagnosis of Lateral Canal BPPV

The diagnosis of BPPV affecting the lateral semicircular canal is established with a history of episodic vertigo with changes in head position and the presence of horizontal nystagmus provoked by the supine roll test according to a guideline from the American Academy of Otolaryngology-Head and Neck Surgery.[12]

The supine roll test (**Fig. 2**) is performed by rotating the patient's head from neutral to one side while the patient is lying supine.[25] After waiting for any nystagmus or vertigo to subside, the test is performed to the opposite side. In a positive test, horizontal nystagmus is observed, either beating toward the dependent ear (geotropic) or beating away from the dependent ear (apogeotropic) on both sides. For geotropic nystagmus, the side associated with the stronger nystagmus is likely the affected ear.[26,27] For apogeotropic nystagmus, the side associated with the weaker nystagmus is the likely the affected ear.[28] Geotropic nystagmus is more common and suggests that the canaliths are located in the long arm of the lateral canal far from the cupula. Apogeotropic nystagmus is less common and suggests that the canaliths are located very close to the cupula or possibly embedded in it. In a review of 9 series with a total of 257 patients with lateral canal BPPV, geotropic nystagmus accounted for about 70% of the cases, and apogeotropic nystagmus accounted for about 30% of the cases.[17]

The supine roll test is the most commonly accepted criterion for the diagnosis of lateral canal BPPV in clinical trials.[29–31] There is no literature on the sensitivity or specificity of this test in the diagnosis of lateral canal BPPV, partly because clinical history alone is often not sufficient for diagnosis, and there is no other gold-standard test to which the supine roll test can be compared.

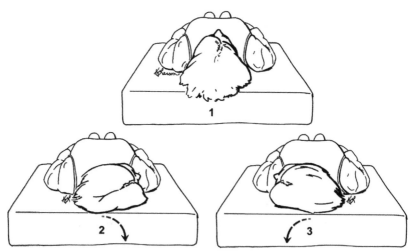

Fig. 2. The supine roll test for the diagnosis of lateral canal BPPV. The patient begins by lying supine with head in neutral position (1). The head is turned to the right side (2) with observation of nystagmus and then turned back to neutral (1). Then the head is turned to the left side (3). The direction of nystagmus in each position is geotropic if it beats toward the lower ear or ageotropic if it beats toward to upper ear. For geotropic nystagmus, the side associated with the stronger nystagmus is likely the affected ear. For ageotropic nystagmus, the side associated with the weaker nystagmus is the likely the affected ear. (*Adapted from* Fife TD, Iverson DJ, Lempert T, et al. Practice parameter: therapies for benign paroxysmal positional vertigo (an evidence-based review): report of the Quality Standards Subcommittee of the American Academy of Neurology. Neurology 2008;70:2071; with permission.)

Limitations of Diagnostic Maneuvers for BPPV

Patients with the following physical limitations may not be good candidate for Dix-Hallpike or supine head roll test: cervical stenosis, severe kyphoscoliosis, limited cervical range of motion, Down syndrome, severe rheumatoid arthritis, cervical radiculopathies, Paget disease, ankylosing spondylitis, low back dysfunction, spinal cord injuries, and morbid obesity.[12] A power-driven, multiaxial positioning chair[32] may facilitate testing of such patients. Alternatives to the Dix-Hallpike test for the diagnosis of posterior canal BPPV have not been well established.[33]

EVIDENCE-BASED MEDICAL AND SURGICAL MANAGEMENT
Natural Remission of Vertigo in BPPV

BPPV is termed benign because it is a naturally resolving condition. In 70 patients with posterior canal BPPV who were observed without treatment, the average time to resolution of vertigo was 39 days, but it took up to 6 months in the extreme.[34] In 16 patients with geotropic variant of lateral canal BPPV who were observed without treatment, the average time to resolution of vertigo was 16 days, and all were free of vertigo in 2.5 months.[34] In 14 patients with apogeotropic variant of lateral canal BPPV, the average time to resolution of vertigo was 13 days, and maximum time was 35 days.[35] Despite its favorable prognosis, BPPV is not an entirely benign condition, especially in the elderly, in whom it is often unrecognized and can lead to falls.[36]

Repositioning Maneuvers for Posterior Canal BPPV

There are 2 effective particle repositioning methods for treatment of posterior canal BPPV: the Epley maneuver[37] (**Fig. 3**) and the Semont maneuver (**Fig. 4**).[38] Both are designed to move the endolymphatic debris from the posterior semicircular canal into the vestibule, where it does not cause vertigo. The Epley maneuver has been extensively studied and is recommended as the first-line treatment of posterior canal BPPV in guidelines from both the American Academy of Otolaryngology-Head and Neck Surgery and the American Academy of Neurology.[12,25]

A Cochrane systematic review[20] included 5 randomized control trials[15,39–42] of the Epley maneuver versus placebo, other active treatment, or no treatment for a total of 292 adults diagnosed with posterior canal BPPV. Updated in 2010, the review excluded other randomized controlled trials (RCTs) with inadequate concealment of randomization or inadequate masking of outcome assessors. Outcome measures included resolution of vertigo and conversion of a positive Dix-Hallpike test to a negative Dix-Hallpike test. The pooled data showed a statistically significant effect in favor of the Epley maneuver over controls. An odds ratio (OR) of 4.2 (95% confidence interval [CI], 2.0–9.1) was found in favor of treatment for resolution of vertigo. An OR of 5.1 (95% CI, 2.3–11.4) was found in favor of treatment for conversion of Dix-Hallpike test result.

In addition to the Cochrane review, 5 other meta-analyses also supported the effectiveness of the Epley maneuver for the treatment of posterior canal BPPV.[21,43–46] There were no serious adverse effects of treatment reported in clinical trials. Minor side effects such as nausea, vomiting, fainting, and conversion of posterior canal BPPV to BPPV involving other canals occurred in a 12% of treated patients.[25] The rate of canal switching after treatment of posterior canal BPPV has been reported in the range of 6% to 7%.[14,15]

Almost all RCTs of the Epley maneuver have been conducted in specialty clinics. The only RCT of the Epley maneuver conducted in primary care setting[42] did not show a statistically significant benefit for the Epley maneuver in term of symptom resolution and reported lower Dix-Hallpike conversion rate than other RCTs.[12] Whether the

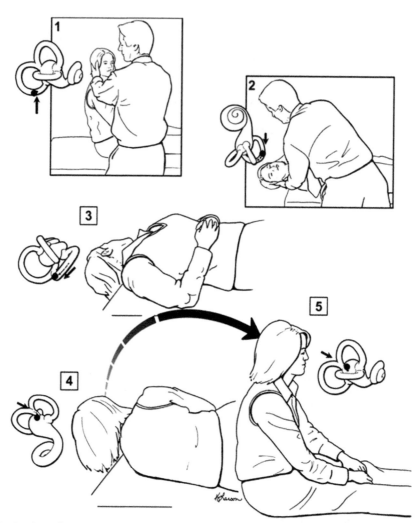

Fig. 3. The Epley maneuver for treatment of posterior canal BPPV. Steps (1) and (2) of the Epley maneuver are the steps of a positive Dix-Hallpike test. After holding for 20 seconds in position 2, the head is turned 90° toward the unaffected side (3). After holding for 20 seconds in position 3, the head is turned again 90° in the same direction to a nearly face-down position with the body also turned to accommodate the head movement (4). After holding for 20 seconds in position 4, the patient is brought to a sitting up position (5). The movement of the otolith material within the labyrinth is depicted with each step, showing how otoliths are moved from the semicircular canal to the vestibule. (*Adapted from* Fife TD, Iverson DJ, Lempert T, et al. Practice parameter: therapies for benign paroxysmal positional vertigo (an evidence-based review): report of the Quality Standards Subcommittee of the American Academy of Neurology. Neurology 2008;70:2069; with permission.)

differences are due to differences in patient populations, reporting of symptoms, or performance of the maneuver is not clear.

There are variations to the Epley maneuver[37] in clinical trials as well as in clinical practice. For example, several RCTs did not include mastoid vibration, which was originally recommended.[15,39–41] Some RCTs maintained upright posture and limit

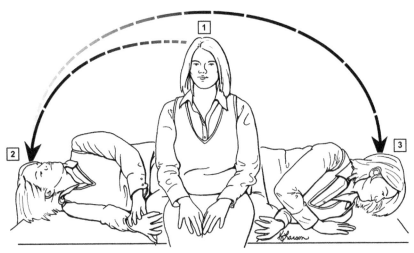

Fig. 4. The Semont maneuver for treatment of posterior canal BPPV. The patient begins by sitting upright (1). For a right posterior canal BPPV, the patient's head is turned 45° toward the left side, and then the patient is rapidly moved to the side-lying position as depicted in position 2. After holding for 30 seconds in position 2, the patient is then moved quickly to the opposite side-lying position (3) without head turning or pausing in the middle. (*Adapted from* Fife TD, Iverson DJ, Lempert T, et al. Practice parameter: therapies for benign paroxysmal positional vertigo (an evidence-based review): report of the Quality Standards Subcommittee of the American Academy of Neurology. Neurology 2008;70:2070; with permission.)

cervical motion after treatment,[39,40] whereas others did not.[15,41] A meta-analysis showed postural restriction after Epley maneuver had no effect on outcome.[47] There were also differences in the number of Epley maneuvers performed in the same visit, ranging from 1 to 5. Since the success rates among different RCTs overlap, it is likely that these variations have little effect on the end results.[20]

The Semont maneuver has not been as extensively studied as the Epley maneuver, but the available evidence also supports its effectiveness in treatment of posterior canal BPPV. In 1 RCT involving 342 patients, the Semont maneuver achieved resolution of vertigo in 79% and 87% of treated patients at 1 hour and 24 hours after treatment, respectively, whereas no sham maneuver-treated patient had resolution of vertigo at such times.[48] Other prospective studies also demonstrated the effectiveness of the Semont maneuver over sham maneuver,[49] over no treatment,[50] and over Brandt-Darroff exercises.[51] There is no high-quality clinical trial comparing the Semont and Epley maneuvers.

Surgical Treatment for Posterior Canal BPPV

In extreme circumstances, patients with intractable posterior canal BPPV that shows no sign of spontaneous remission or response to repositioning maneuvers may require or seek surgical treatment options. In one option, the singular nerve, which selectively supplies the posterior semicircular canal, is identified and divided to prevent aberrant signal generated in the canal from reaching the central nervous system (CNS).[52,53] In another option, the posterior semicircular canal is exposed in the mastoid bone, fenestrated, and occluded to prevent the canal from generating aberrant signal.[54]

Table 2 summarizes the outcome of 6 retrospective case series of singular nerve neurectomy. Ninety-six percent of patients were completely cured of BPPV in the

Table 2
Outcome of singular nerve section for BPPV

Study	Cases	Cure of BPPV	Follow-up	Postoperative Audio	↓ Hearing >10 dB	Postoperative ENG/VNG	↓ Caloric or Absent
Epley,[52] 1980	11	10	2–20 mo	11	5	1?	1
Meyerhoff,[69] 1985	18	15	≧6 mo	18	3	?	?
Silverstein and White,[53] 1990	58	46	6 mo–18 y	56	5	34	14
Fernandes,[70] 1993	7	6	?	7	2	?	?
Gacek and Gacek,[71] 2002	252	244	>1 mo	252	9	?	?
Pournaras et al,[72] 2008	8	8	1 mo–9 y	8	1	?	?
Total	344	329/344 (95.6%)		342/344 (99.4%)	25/342 (7.3%)	35/344 (13.9%)	15/35 (42.9%)

? indicates that the relevant information was not reported. In the case of Epley 1980, 1 patient was reported to have severe vestibular loss postoperatively, but it was not specified how many patients had postoperative ENG/VNG.

Table 3
Outcome of posterior semicircular canal plugging for BPPV

Study	Cases	Cure of BPPV	Follow-up	Postoperative Audio	↓ Hearing >10 dB	Postoperative ENG/VNG	↓ Caloric or Absent
PaceBalzan and Rutka,[73] 1991	5	5	12–36 mo	5	1	5	3
Hawthorne and el-Naggar,[74] 1994	15	15	14–40 mo	15	1	8	3
Zappia,[75] 1996	8	8	3 wk–3 mo	8	0	1	0
Pulec,[76] 1997	17	17	1–13 mo	17	0	17	0
Walsh et al,[77] 1999	13	13	29–119 mo	13	1	13	2
Agrawal and Parnes,[78] 2001	44	44	6 mo–12 y	40	2	?	?
Shaia et al,[79] 2006	20	20	6–64 mo	20	1	?	?
Kisilevsky et al,[80] 2009	32	32	2–205 mo	32	4	23	7
Total	154	154/154 (100%)		150/154 (97.4%)	10/150 (6.7%)	67/154 (43.5%)	15/67 (22.4%)

? indicates that the relevant information was not reported.

affected canal. Seven percent sustained various degrees of postoperative hearing loss greater than 10 dB pure tone average. In a limited number of patients, in whom postoperative electronystagmograms (ENGs) or videonystagmograms (VNG) were obtained, 43% showed absent or reduced caloric response in the operated ear. Given that the caloric test measures response from the lateral semicircular canal, whereas the surgery targets the posterior semicircular canal, the reduced vestibular function suggests the occurrence of unintended surgical trauma or postoperative labyrinthitis. Several authors of the case series acknowledged that singular nerve neurectomy is a technically challenging operation.

Table 3 summarizes the outcome of retrospective case series of posterior semicircular canal occlusion, showing resolution of BPPV in virtually all treated patients. All patients were completely cured of BPPV in the affected canal. Seven percent sustained various degrees of postoperative hearing loss greater than 10 dB pure tone average. The percentage of patients exhibiting reduced caloric response after surgery appears less with posterior canal occlusion (22%) than with singular nerve section, but remains a significant consideration. Overall, posterior canal occlusion appears to be a highly effective treatment option for intractable BPPV with some associated risks to hearing and vestibular function.

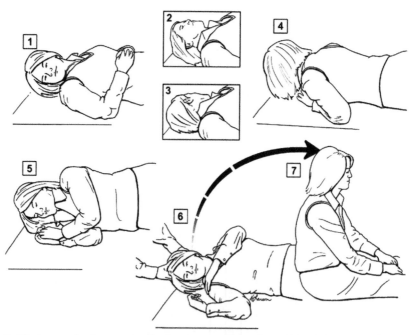

Fig. 5. The Lempert roll maneuver for treatment of lateral canal BPPV. The patient begins by lying supine with head turned 45° toward the affected side (1). The patient is then brought a series of step-wise 90° roll away from the affected side (2, 3, 4 and 5), holding each position for 10 to 30 seconds. From position 5, the patient returns to lying supine (6) in preparation for the rapid and simultaneous movement from the supine face up to the sitting position (7). (*Adapted from* Fife TD, Iverson DJ, Lempert T, et al. Practice parameter: therapies for benign paroxysmal positional vertigo (an evidence-based review): report of the Quality Standards Subcommittee of the American Academy of Neurology. Neurology 2008;70:2071; with permission.)

Repositioning Maneuvers for Lateral Canal BPPV

There are 3 particle repositioning methods for treatment of lateral canal BPPV:

1. Lempert roll[55] (**Fig. 5**)
2. Forced prolonged positioning[56]
3. Gufoni maneuver[57] (**Fig. 6**)

All 3 methods are designed to move the endolymphatic debris from the lateral semi-circular canal into the vestibule, where it does not cause vertigo.

The Lempert roll and its variations appear to be the most commonly used techniques based on prospective cohorts and retrospective case series.[29,30,55,58–63] Success rates ranged from 50% for the apogeotropic variant to 100% for the geotropic variant, although the endpoints differ widely among series, and there was no appropriate untreated or sham-treated control.

Forced prolonged positioning with the affected ear up and the unaffected ear down can be performed either alone or following the Lempert roll. In case series,[56,58,60,64,65] its success rates were 75% to 90%, but with the lack of control, the prolonged end

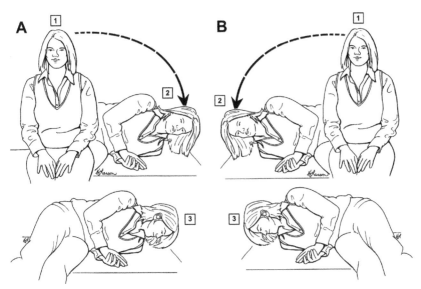

Fig. 6. The Gufoni maneuver for treatment of lateral canal BPPV. *(A)* For lateral canal BPPV with geotropic nystagmus, the patient is taken from the sitting position (step 1) to the straight side lying position on the unaffected side (left in this case) for 1 minute. Then the patient's head is quickly turned toward the ground 45° to 60° and held in position for 2 minutes. The patient then sits up again, with the head in the same position over the left shoulder. *(B)* For lateral canal BPPV with apogeotropic nystagmus, the patient is taken from the sitting position (step 1) to the straight side lying position on the affected side (right in this case) for 1 minute. Then the patient's head is quickly turned toward the ground 45° to 60° and held in position for 2 minutes. The patient then sits up again with the head in the same position over the right shoulder. *(Adapted from* Fife TD, Iverson DJ, Lempert T, et al. Practice parameter: therapies for benign paroxysmal positional vertigo (an evidence-based review): report of the Quality Standards Subcommittee of the American Academy of Neurology. Neurology 2008;70:2067–74 [supplemental figure 3B]; with permission.)

points can be difficult to distinguish from the relatively quick natural resolution of lateral canal BPPV.

The Gufoni maneuver is less well known, but it has garnered more support in recent literature.[57,66–68] A randomized controlled trial of 112 patients with geotropic variant of lateral canal BPPV compared Lempert roll plus forced prolonged position with Gufoni maneuver. The Gufoni maneuver was found to be statistically more successful than Lampert roll plus forced prolonged position after 1 treatment (86% vs 61%).[31]

BOTTOM LINE: WHAT DOES THE EVIDENCE SHOW?

BPPV is the most common diagnosis of vertigo in both primary care and subspecialty settings. A positive Dix-Hallpike maneuver is diagnostic for posterior canal BPPV. A positive supine roll test is diagnostic for lateral canal BPPV. Both Dix-Hallpike maneuver and supine roll test should be performed in the evaluation of vertigo or dizziness. Epley maneuver is the first-line treatment for posterior canal BPPV, with Semont maneuver an alternative treatment. Posterior semicircular canal occlusion is an effective treatment for recalcitrant posterior canal BPPV, with some risks to hearing and vestibular function. Lateral canal BPPV can be treated with Lempert roll, forced prolonged positioning, or Gufoni maneuver, although more controlled studies are needed to demonstrate efficacy of treatment, since lateral canal BPPV has a quick natural course of remission.

ACKNOWLEDGMENTS

The author would like to thank Louis Prahl for his assistance in the preparation of the manuscript.

REFERENCES

1. Blakley BW, Goebel J. The meaning of the word "vertigo". Otolaryngol Head Neck Surg 2001;125:147–50.
2. Drachman DA, Hart CW. An approach to the dizzy patient. Neurology 1972;22: 323–34.
3. Kroenke K, Price RK. Symptoms in the community. Prevalence, classification, and psychiatric comorbidity. Arch Intern Med 1993;153:2474–80.
4. Yardley L, Owen N, Nazareth I, et al. Prevalence and presentation of dizziness in a general practice community sample of working age people. Br J Gen Pract 1998;48:1131–5.
5. Hannaford PC, Simpson JA, Bisset AF, et al. The prevalence of ear, nose and throat problems in the community: results from a national cross-sectional postal survey in Scotland. Fam Pract 2005;22:227–33.
6. Mendel B, Bergenius J, Langius-Eklöf A. Dizziness: a common, troublesome symptom but often treatable. J Vestib Res 2010;20:391–8.
7. Neuhauser HK, von Brevern M, Radtke A, et al. Epidemiology of vestibular vertigo: a neurotologic survey of the general population. Neurology 2005;65: 898–904.
8. Sloane PD. Dizziness in primary care. Results from the National Ambulatory Medical Care Survey. J Fam Pract 1989;29:33–8.
9. Kerber KA, Meurer WJ, West BT, et al. Dizziness presentations in U.S. emergency departments, 1995–2004. Acad Emerg Med 2008;15:744–50.
10. Hanley K, O'Dowd T. Symptoms of vertigo in general practice: a prospective study of diagnosis. Br J Gen Pract 2002;52:809–12.

11. Kentala E, Rauch SD. A practical assessment algorithm for diagnosis of dizziness. Otolaryngol Head Neck Surg 2003;128:54–9.
12. Bhattacharyya N, Baugh RF, Orvidas L, et al. Clinical practice guideline: benign paroxysmal positional vertigo. Otolaryngol Head Neck Surg 2008;139:S47–81.
13. Welling DB, Parnes LS, O'Brien B, et al. Particulate matter in the posterior semi-circular canal. Laryngoscope 1997;107:90–4.
14. Herdman SJ, Tusa RJ. Complications of the canalith repositioning procedure. Arch Otolaryngol Head Neck Surg 1996;122:281–6.
15. Yimtae K, Srirompotong S, Srirompotong S, et al. A randomized trial of the canalith repositioning procedure. Laryngoscope 2003;113:828–32.
16. von Brevern M, Radtke A, Lezius F, et al. Epidemiology of benign paroxysmal positional vertigo: a population based study. J Neurol Neurosurg Psychiatr 2007;78:710–5.
17. Cakir BO, Ercan I, Cakir ZA, et al. What is the true incidence of horizontal semi-circular canal benign paroxysmal positional vertigo? Otolaryngol Head Neck Surg 2006;134:451–4.
18. Tomaz A, Ganança MM, Ganança CF, et al. Benign paroxysmal positional vertigo: concomitant involvement of different semicircular canals. Ann Otol Rhinol Laryngol 2009;118:113–7.
19. Dix MR, Hallpike CS. The pathology symptomatology and diagnosis of certain common disorders of the vestibular system. Proc R Soc Med 1952;45:341–54.
20. Hilton M, Pinder D. The Epley (canalith repositioning) manoeuvre for benign paroxysmal positional vertigo. Cochrane Database Syst Rev 2004;(2):CD003162.
21. Teixeira LJ, Machado JN. Maneuvers for the treatment of benign positional paroxysmal vertigo: a systematic review. Braz J Otorhinolaryngol 2006;72:130–9.
22. Halker RB, Barrs DM, Wellik KE, et al. Establishing a diagnosis of benign paroxysmal positional vertigo through the dix-hallpike and side-lying maneuvers: a critically appraised topic. Neurologist 2008;14:201–4.
23. Norré ME. Diagnostic problems in patients with benign paroxysmal positional vertigo. Laryngoscope 1994;104:1385–8.
24. Li JC, Li CJ, Epley J, et al. Cost-effective management of benign positional vertigo using canalith repositioning. Otolaryngol Head Neck Surg 2000;122:334–9.
25. Fife TD, Iverson DJ, Lempert T, et al. Practice parameter: therapies for benign paroxysmal positional vertigo (an evidence-based review): report of the Quality Standards Subcommittee of the American Academy of Neurology. Neurology 2008;70:2067–74.
26. McClure JA. Horizontal canal BPV. J Otolaryngol 1985;14:30–5.
27. Pagnini P, Nuti D, Vannucchi P. Benign paroxysmal vertigo of the horizontal canal. ORL J Otorhinolaryngol Relat Spec 1989;51:161–70.
28. Baloh RW, Jacobson K, Honrubia V. Horizontal semicircular canal variant of benign positional vertigo. Neurology 1993;43:2542–9.
29. Nuti D, Agus G, Barbieri MT, et al. The management of horizontal-canal paroxysmal positional vertigo. Acta Otolaryngol 1998;118:455–60.
30. White JA, Coale KD, Catalano PJ, et al. Diagnosis and management of lateral semicircular canal benign paroxysmal positional vertigo. Otolaryngol Head Neck Surg 2005;133:278–84.
31. Casani AP, Nacci A, Dallan I, et al. Horizontal semicircular canal benign paroxysmal positional vertigo: effectiveness of two different methods of treatment. Audiol Neurootol 2011;16:175–84.
32. Nakayama M, Epley JM. BPPV and variants: improved treatment results with automated, nystagmus-based repositioning. Otolaryngol Head Neck Surg 2005;133:107–12.

33. Cohen HS. Side-lying as an alternative to the Dix-Hallpike test of the posterior canal. Otol Neurotol 2004;25:130–4.
34. Imai T, Ito M, Takeda N, et al. Natural course of the remission of vertigo in patients with benign paroxysmal positional vertigo. Neurology 2005;64:920–1.
35. Imai T, Takeda N, Ito M, et al. Natural course of positional vertigo in patients with apogeotropic variant of horizontal canal benign paroxysmal positional vertigo. Auris Nasus Larynx 2011;38:2–5.
36. Oghalai JS, Manolidis S, Barth JL, et al. Unrecognized benign paroxysmal positional vertigo in elderly patients. Otolaryngol Head Neck Surg 2000;122:630–4.
37. Epley JM. The canalith repositioning procedure: for treatment of benign paroxysmal positional vertigo. Otolaryngol Head Neck Surg 1992;107:399–404.
38. Semont A, Freyss G, Vitte E. Curing the BPPV with a liberatory maneuver. Adv Otorhinolaryngol 1988;42:290–3.
39. Lynn S, Pool A, Rose D, et al. Randomized trial of the canalith repositioning procedure. Otolaryngol Head Neck Surg 1995;113:712–20.
40. Froehling DA, Bowen JM, Mohr DN, et al. The canalith repositioning procedure for the treatment of benign paroxysmal positional vertigo: a randomized controlled trial. Mayo Clin Proc 2000;75:695–700.
41. von Brevern M, Seelig T, Radtke A, et al. Short-term efficacy of Epley's manoeuvre: a double-blind randomised trial. J Neurol Neurosurg Psychiatr 2006;77:980–2.
42. Munoz JE, Miklea JT, Howard M, et al. Canalith repositioning maneuver for benign paroxysmal positional vertigo: randomized controlled trial in family practice. Can Fam Physician 2007;53:1048–53.
43. López-Escámez J, González-Sánchez M, Salinero J. Meta-analysis of the treatment of benign paroxysmal positional vertigo by Epley and Semont maneuvers. Acta Otorrinolaringol Esp 1999;50:366–70 [in Spanish].
44. Woodworth BA, Gillespie MB, Lambert PR. The canalith repositioning procedure for benign positional vertigo: a meta-analysis. Laryngoscope 2004;114:1143–6.
45. Prim-Espada MP, De Diego-Sastre JI, Pérez-Fernández E. Meta-analysis on the efficacy of Epley's manoeuvre in benign paroxysmal positional vertigo. Neurologia 2010;25:295–9 [in Spanish].
46. Helminski JO, Zee DS, Janssen I, et al. Effectiveness of particle repositioning maneuvers in the treatment of benign paroxysmal positional vertigo: a systematic review. Phys Ther 2010;90:663–78.
47. Devaiah AK, Andreoli S. Postmaneuver restrictions in benign paroxysmal positional vertigo: an individual patient data meta-analysis. Otolaryngol Head Neck Surg 2010;142:155–9.
48. Mandalà M, Santoro GP, Asprella Libonati G, et al. Double-blind randomized trial on short-term efficacy of the Semont maneuver for the treatment of posterior canal benign paroxysmal positional vertigo. J Neurol 2012;259(5):882–5.
49. Cohen HS, Kimball KT. Effectiveness of treatments for benign paroxysmal positional vertigo of the posterior canal. Otol Neurotol 2005;26:1034–40.
50. Salvinelli F, Casale M, Trivelli M, et al. Benign paroxysmal positional vertigo: a comparative prospective study on the efficacy of Semont's maneuver and no treatment strategy. Clin Ter 2003;154:7–11.
51. Soto Varela A, Bartual Magro J, Santos Pérez S, et al. Benign paroxysmal vertigo: a comparative prospective study of the efficacy of Brandt and Daroff exercises, Semont and Epley maneuver. Rev Laryngol Otol Rhinol (Bord) 2001;122:179–83.
52. Epley JM. Singular neurectomy: hypotympanotomy approach. Otolaryngol Head Neck Surg 1980;88:304–9.

53. Silverstein H, White DW. Wide surgical exposure for singular neurectomy in the treatment of benign positional vertigo. Laryngoscope 1990;100:701–6.

54. Parnes LS, McClure JA. Posterior semicircular canal occlusion in the normal hearing ear. Otolaryngol Head Neck Surg 1991;104:52–7.

55. Lempert T, Tiel-Wilck K. A positional maneuver for treatment of horizontal-canal benign positional vertigo. Laryngoscope 1996;106:476–8.

56. Vannucchi P, Giannoni B, Pagnini P. Treatment of horizontal semicircular canal benign paroxysmal positional vertigo. J Vestib Res 1997;7:1–6.

57. Gufoni M, Mastrosimone L, Di Nasso F. Repositioning maneuver in benign paroxysmal vertigo of horizontal semicircular canal. Acta Otorhinolaryngol Ital 1998;18: 363–7 [in Italian].

58. Appiani GC, Gagliardi M, Magliulo G. Physical treatment of horizontal canal benign positional vertigo. Eur Arch Otorhinolaryngol 1997;254:326–8.

59. Fife TD. Recognition and management of horizontal canal benign positional vertigo. Am J Otol 1998;19:345–51.

60. Casani AP, Vannucci G, Fattori B, et al. The treatment of horizontal canal positional vertigo: our experience in 66 cases. Laryngoscope 2002;112:172–8.

61. Tirelli G, Russolo M. 360-Degree canalith repositioning procedure for the horizontal canal. Otolaryngol Head Neck Surg 2004;131:740–6.

62. Prokopakis EP, Chimona T, Tsagournisakis M, et al. Benign paroxysmal positional vertigo: 10-year experience in treating 592 patients with canalith repositioning procedure. Laryngoscope 2005;115:1667–71.

63. Escher A, Ruffieux C, Maire R. Efficacy of the barbecue manoeuvre in benign paroxysmal vertigo of the horizontal canal. Eur Arch Otorhinolaryngol 2007;264: 1239–41.

64. Chiou WY, Lee HL, Tsai SC, et al. A single therapy for all subtypes of horizontal canal positional vertigo. Laryngoscope 2005;115:1432–5.

65. Boleas-Aguirre MS, Pérez N, Batuecas-Caletrío A. Bedside therapeutic experiences with horizontal canal benign paroxysmal positional vertigo (cupulolithiasis). Acta Otolaryngol 2009;129:1217–21.

66. Asprella Libonati G. Diagnostic and treatment strategy of lateral semicircular canal canalolithiasis. Acta Otorhinolaryngol Ital 2005;25:277–83.

67. Appiani GC, Catania G, Gagliardi M, et al. Repositioning maneuver for the treatment of the apogeotropic variant of horizontal canal benign paroxysmal positional vertigo. Otol Neurotol 2005;26:257–60.

68. Riggio F, Francesco R, Dispenza F, et al. Management of benign paroxysmal positional vertigo of lateral semicircular canal by Gufoni's manoeuvre. Am J Otol 2009;30:106–11.

69. Meyerhoff WL. Surgical section of the posterior ampullary nerve. Laryngoscope 1985;95:933–5.

70. Fernandes CM. Singular neurectomy in South African practice. S Afr J Surg 1993; 31:79–80.

71. Gacek RR, Gacek MR. Results of singular neurectomy in the posterior ampullary recess. ORL J Otorhinolaryngol Relat Spec 2002;64:397–402.

72. Pournaras I, Kos I, Guyot JP. Benign paroxysmal positional vertigo: a series of eight singular neurectomies. Acta Otolaryngol 2008;128:5–8.

73. Pace-Balzan A, Rutka JA. Non-ampullary plugging of the posterior semicircular canal for benign paroxysmal positional vertigo. J Laryngol Otol 1991;105:901–6.

74. Hawthorne M, el-Naggar M. Fenestration and occlusion of posterior semicircular canal for patients with intractable benign paroxysmal positional vertigo. J Laryngol Otol 1994;108:935–9.

75. Zappia JJ. Posterior semicircular canal occlusion for benign paroxysmal positional vertigo. Am J Otol 1996;17:749–54.
76. Pulec JL. Ablation of posterior semicircular canal for benign paroxysmal positional vertigo. Ear Nose Throat J 1997;76:17–22, 24.
77. Walsh RM, Bath AP, Cullen JR, et al. Long-term results of posterior semicircular canal occlusion for intractable benign paroxysmal positional vertigo. Clin Otolaryngol Allied Sci 1999;24:316–23.
78. Agrawal SK, Parnes LS. Human experience with canal plugging. Ann N Y Acad Sci 2001;942:300–5.
79. Shaia WT, Zappia JJ, Bojrab DI, et al. Success of posterior semicircular canal occlusion and application of the dizziness handicap inventory. Otolaryngol Head Neck Surg 2006;134:424–30.
80. Kisilevsky V, Bailie NA, Dutt SN, et al. Lessons learned from the surgical management of benign paroxysmal positional vertigo: the University Health Network experience with posterior semicircular canal occlusion surgery (1988–2006). J Otolaryngol Head Neck Surg 2009;38:212–21.

Evidence-Based Practice
Management of Adult Sensorineural Hearing Loss

Justin K. Chau, MD[a],*, John J.W. Cho, MD[b], Dieter K. Fritz, MD[a]

KEYWORDS

- Evidence-based medicine • Hearing loss, sensorineural
- Hearing loss, noise-induced • Hearing loss, sudden • Hearing loss, unilateral
- Magnetic resonance imaging • Glucocorticoids • Antiviral agents

KEY POINTS

The following points list the level of evidence based on the criteria of the Oxford Center for Evidence-Based Medicine. Additional critical points are provided and points here are expanded at the conclusion of this article.

- The best current evidence for oral corticosteroid treatment of sudden sensorineural hearing loss (SSNHL) is contradictory in outcome and does not permit a definitive treatment recommendation (level 1a).
- Treatment of SSNHL may be equally efficacious up to and potentially later than 10 days after the loss of hearing (level 1b).
- Transtympanic corticosteroids may be useful as either primary therapy or salvage therapy in patients with medical comorbidities who are at risk of serious adverse effects from oral corticosteroid administration (level 1b).
- There is insufficient evidence to recommend antiviral therapy as primary or steroid adjunctive therapy in patients with SSNHL (level 1a).
- There is limited evidence to suggest that primary hyperbaric oxygen therapy improves hearing in patients with idiopathic SSNHL and no evidence of a functionally significant improvement (level 1a).

OVERVIEW

Sensorineural hearing loss (SNHL) is a complex disease influenced by interactions between multiple internal and external causative factors. Genetics and age-related hearing changes may predetermine a patient's hearing throughout their lifetime, and

Faculty disclosure/conflict of interest: The authors have no funding, financial relationships, or conflicts of interest to disclose.
[a] Section of Otolaryngology, Department of Surgery, University of Calgary, 1403 29th Street NW, Calgary, Alberta T2N 2T9, Canada; [b] Paparella Ear Head & Neck Institute, Suite 200, 701 25th Ave South, Minneapolis, MN 55454, Minnesota
* Corresponding author.
E-mail address: justin.chau@gmail.com

any potential hearing changes over time may be accelerated by numerous external factors. This relationship becomes particularly complex if the patient's genetic makeup predisposes that individual to a hearing vulnerability from external influences such as chronic exposure to traumatic levels of noise or from the use of ototoxic pharmaceuticals.

The complexity of the diagnostic evaluation and potential treatment options for SNHL has increased because of multiple considerations. There is a downward trend in the presenting age and an increasing severity of hearing loss in patients from first-world (industrialized) nations.[1] Patterns of hearing loss have changed in relation to noise exposure because of various occupational hazards such as heavy industrial noise and firearms use in military and police occupations. Clinicians involved in the management of critically ill and complex medical patients are aware of the impact that pharmaceutical therapy for multisystem disease may have on hearing. Patients who have immigrated from developing countries may present with hearing loss caused by exposure to rare pathogens such as Lassa fever[2] or with a chronic otitis media complicated by a lack of primary care or access to an otolaryngologist in their country of origin. Thus, it is prudent for any practicing otolaryngologist to be aware of these and other factors that may influence their diagnostic and management approaches for patients presenting with SNHL.

The medical literature contains thousands of research papers on SNHL, the overall aim of which is to improve our ability as clinicians to diagnose and treat patients with hearing loss. The challenge lies in sifting through this wealth of data and applying them to our everyday practices, because the principles of evidence-based medicine have become integrated into our daily clinical interaction with patients. The goal of this article is to present the current best evidence available regarding the diagnostic process and treatments available for the management of hearing loss as it applies to the more controversial aspects of adult SNHL. The levels of evidence proposed by the Oxford Center for Evidence-Based Medicine are used throughout this article.[3]

Causes of Sensorineural Hearing Loss

Presbycusis is the most common cause of SNHL in industrialized nations. In 2003 to 2004, the prevalence of hearing loss in the adult US population aged 20 to 69 years was 16.1% (29 million Americans), and 31% of those had a high-frequency hearing loss. The prevalence of hearing loss was higher among the following set of individuals[4]:

- Men
- White
- Older age
- Less educated
- History of diabetes mellitus
- History of hypertension
- Greater than a 20 pack-year history of smoking

It can be expected that the prevalence and impact of hearing loss on society will increase as the elderly proportion of the population in many industrialized nations continues to grow.

Noise

The detrimental effect of noise on the inner ear is one of the most common causes of permanent hearing loss. Approximately 30 million American workers are exposed to hazardous work-related noise. Occupational and recreational exposure to firearms is also a significant cause of permanent noise-induced hearing loss. Permanent damage from firearms use in police officers was identified in a long-term study, even with the regular use of dual hearing protection.[5] Despite the increasing prevalence of hearing loss in the general population because of noise, this resultant hearing loss is preventable through engineering controls or with the use of regular and habitual hearing protection.[6]

Heredity and environment
Hereditary and developmental factors play a key role in influencing the development of SNHL. Multiple reviews have been published summarizing the complex role of genetics and hearing loss.[7,8] Dozens of genetic loci have been identified as the causes of numerous syndromic and nonsyndromic hearing loss with variable inheritance patterns (autosomal-dominant, autosomal-recessive, X-linked, mitochondrial). Genetic loci have been also identified that increase the potential for permanent SNHL caused by noise trauma or ototoxic medications such as aminoglycoside antibiotics.[9] Hearing losses caused by developmental disorders of the inner ear have also been linked to:

- Spontaneous or inherited genetic abnormalities, such as complete (Michel) aplasia
- Cochlear anomalies such as a Mondini malformation, labyrinthine anomalies, and ductal anomalies (enlarged vestibular aqueduct)

Infection
SNHL is a known complication of otologic or central nervous system infections such as acute labyrinthitis, meningitis, or as a sequela of chronic suppurative otitis media. Pediatric SNHL has been linked to multiple congenital infections such as toxoplasmosis and syphilis.[10,11] Labyrinthitis ossificans and permanent SNHL is a known sequela of bacterial meningitis.

Vascular
Vascular interruption of labyrinthine blood flow is another common suspected cause of SNHL, typically seen in an acute fashion after a cerebrovascular accident, acute interruption of posterior cerebral circulation,[12] or as the result of a coagulopathy or other hematologic anomaly. Several studies have examined the relationship between sudden SNHL (SSNHL) and cardiovascular and thrombophilic risk factors.[13,14]

Ototoxicity
Ototoxicity is a well-established complication of drug administration. The hearing loss can be reversible or permanent and can be accompanied by other otologic symptoms such as tinnitus and vertigo. Cisplatin chemotherapeutic agents, aminoglycoside antibiotics, and loop diuretics are frequently cited as the most common medications that can damage the inner ear. Critically ill patients are at particular risk of ototoxicity as a result of renal and hepatic compromise and the use of multiple ototoxic agents. Ototoxicity can also occur from the instillation of ototopical drops in the presence of a ventilation tube or tympanic membrane perforation.[15]

Trauma
Trauma to the ear and temporal bone are uncommon causes of SNHL. Fractures involving the otic capsule may result in permanent SNHL, vertigo, and facial nerve injury. Inner ear barotrauma from scuba diving or sudden and violent pressure changes to the external and middle ear causing damage to the oval or round windows may result in perilymph fistulization and subsequent hearing loss, tinnitus, and vertigo.

Autoimmune ear disease

Autoimmune inner ear disease (AIED) was first described in the medical literature in 1979,[16] and involvement of the inner ear in autoimmune disease has since become well established. Autoantibodies that target inner ear–specific antigens have been identified,[17] and numerous studies have confirmed the association between SNHL and systemic autoimmune diseases such as Cogan syndrome, rheumatoid arthritis, systemic lupus erythematosus, and Wegener granulomatosis.[18]

Neoplastic disease

Neoplastic disease of the cerebellopontine angle (CPA) can present with a progressive or sudden onset of hearing loss and other otologic symptoms; vestibular schwannoma is the most common diagnosis.[19] Early identification of CPA tumors poses a challenging diagnostic dilemma for otolaryngologists, and is discussed further in this article. Metastatic disease involving the temporal bone may also present in a similar clinical fashion to a CPA tumor.[20]

Endolymphatic hydrops and central nervous system disease

Although many other causes of SNHL exist, only 2 other causes are noted here. Endolymphatic hydrops is a primary otologic cause of SNHL, the cause of which remains in dispute. The classic presentation of Ménière syndrome (tinnitus, aural fullness, hearing loss, and peripheral vertigo) can often present as SSNHL or fluctuating SNHL affecting 1 or both ears. The diagnostic process can be challenging and prolonged before the diagnosis is made, usually after other more acute or life-threatening causes have been ruled out. Central nervous system disease such as cerebrovascular accidents or multiple sclerosis can also cause varying degrees of SNHL, which can be rapidly progressive, sudden, asymmetric, or bilateral.

Sudden Sensorineural Hearing Loss

SSNHL remains a diagnostic and therapeutic dilemma. Many aspects of this clinical entity are disputed in the medical literature, such as the definition of the syndrome, cause and clinical investigations, therapeutic interventions, and spontaneous rate of recovery. SSNHL is considered an otologic emergency primarily for expeditious treatment with corticosteroids as soon as possible after the onset of hearing loss. However, both the use of corticosteroids for sudden hearing loss and its status as an otologic emergency are under dispute.[21]

SSNHL is characterized by a rapid deterioration in hearing over seconds to days, with no universally accepted clinical definition. The most common definition in the literature is as defined by the National Institute on Deafness and Other Communications Disorder: an SNHL of 30 dB or more across at least 3 contiguous frequencies occurring within 72 hours.[22] Regional global variations in SSNHL definition exist, and numerous other criteria have been used for defining SSNHL in the literature. The incidence of SSNHL has been estimated by Byl[23] to range between 5 and 20 cases per 100,000 persons per year, but some consider this estimate to be lower than the actual number of cases because it is suspected that many cases of SSNHL resolve spontaneously before presentation to a hospital or physician. Most cases of SSNHL are unilateral, with bilateral involvement uncommon and simultaneous bilateral involvement rare. Factors that may influence the prognosis for hearing recovery include the age of the patient, severity and type of hearing loss, time between hearing loss onset and treatment, and presence of vertigo.

The cause of SSNHL was reviewed by the senior author.[24] The identifiable suspected causes included infectious disease in 12.8%, primary otologic disease in 4.7%, temporal bone and inner ear trauma in 4.2%, vascular or hematologic causes in 2.8%, neoplastic disease in 2.3%, and other causes in 2.2% of patients. Seventy-one percent of patients reviewed suffered from an idiopathic SSNHL, and it is these idiopathic cases that drive continuing research regarding sudden hearing loss.

Asymmetric/Unilateral Sensorineural Hearing Loss

The goal of evaluation for an asymmetric SNHL (ASNHL) is to rule out a retrocochlear cause such as vestibular schwannoma. Historically, clinicians relied on audiometric tests to identify patients with a retrocochlear pattern of disease and follow-up with a computed tomography (CT) scan. Advancements in technology have shifted our diagnostic reliance onto highly sensitive and specific diagnostic imaging tests such as magnetic resonance imaging (MRI), which can detect vestibular schwannomas at an early stage of presentation and potentially reduce the morbidity of any potential treatment. The high cost and limited availability of MRI in the past has influenced the development of cost-effective clinical diagnostic algorithms for asymmetric hearing loss evaluation. Refinements in MRI technology have allowed for more rapid acquisition of higher-resolution imaging at a reduced per-patient cost to the health care system. Despite these advancements, considerable debate continues regarding multiple factors such as the appropriate audiometric thresholds that should trigger radiographic evaluation of ASNHL as well as the continuing role of screening audiometric tests such as evoked auditory brainstem potentials to achieve a cost-effective evaluation.

Rapidly Progressive Sensorineural Hearing Loss

Rapidly declining or fluctuating SNHL presents in less than 1% of patients presenting with hearing loss and is often considered synonymous with the diagnosis of an AIED. McCabe's original article[16] reviewed 18 patients who presented with variable bilateral audiovestibular disease that improved with oral corticosteroids and intravenous cyclophosphamide. Autoimmune hearing loss is typically not as rapid as an SSNHL, but is significantly more pronounced than would be associated with presbycusis. It is typically bilateral, asymmetric, and rapidly progressive over weeks to months.[25]

Multiple ear diseases have been found to have a primary immunologic cause such as relapsing polychondritis, otosclerosis, Ménière disease, and sudden hearing loss. The ear can also be affected by systemic autoimmune diseases such as systematic lupus erythematosus, rheumatoid arthritis, Sjögren syndrome, Cogan syndrome, Wegener granulomatosis, and systemic sclerosis.[25]

EVIDENCE-BASED CLINICAL ASSESSMENT

A comprehensive history and physical examination are vital in the evaluation of a patient with hearing loss. The history should focus on the presence of other otologic symptoms such as tinnitus, vertigo, otalgia, aural fullness, and otorrhea, as well as a review of symptoms that assesses the status of the central nervous system. The patient's past medical history, family history, medication profile, and social history should be taken into consideration. Known causative causes for hearing loss should be reviewed and thoroughly evaluated if identified as potential risk factors on history and physical examination.

The diagnostic evaluation of a patient with SSNHL is a significant source of debate in the medical literature. Diagnostic regimens for SSNHL workup vary significantly amongst clinicians and there is no standardized battery of tests. Many centers have reported their results using diagnostic batteries for SSNHL with varying results.[26] Numerous research articles have been published examining various aspects of

SSNHL diagnosis, such as medical risk factor profiles, genetic predisposition toward prothrombotic and hypercoagulable states, autoimmune markers, the presence of infectious disease markers, and the usefulness of diagnostic imaging studies for diagnosing SSNHL.

Audiometric Testing

Standard pure tone audiometry (0.25 kHz–8 kHz) and speech discrimination testing are not only required to provide the criteria for any hearing loss diagnosis, but the characteristics of the initial audiogram provide a baseline for comparison and may also provide prognostic value. Serial audiometric evaluations are necessary to document recovery, monitor treatment response, screen for relapse, guide aural rehabilitation, and rule out hearing loss in the contralateral ear. If malingering is suspected, a Stenger test should be performed to rule out pseudohypoacusis.[27]

The definition of ASNHL is unclear in the literature. Many investigators have tried to validate a universal definition that can be clinically applied.[28–32] Commonly cited definitions include: 15 dB or greater (0.25–8 kHz),[32] 15 dB or greater at 2 or more frequencies or a 15% or greater difference in speech discrimination score,[28] or 20 dB or greater at 2 consecutive frequencies.[29] Saliba and colleagues[31] proposed a Rule 3000 after finding that an asymmetry of 15 dB or more at 3000 Hz had the highest odds-ratio association with a positive vestibular schwannoma finding on MRI in their retrospective study population. Gimsing[30] recently concluded that a patient with a 20-dB or greater asymmetry at 2 adjacent frequencies, unilateral tinnitus, or a 15-dB or greater asymmetry at 2 frequencies between 2 and 8 kHz on screening audiogram yielded the best compromise between sensitivity and specificity when attempting to rule out a vestibular schwannoma.

Auditory Brainstem Response

Auditory evoked potentials are commonly used for the detection of retrocochlear disease in asymmetric and sudden hearing loss. MRI has been shown to be a more sensitive diagnostic test for the detection of vestibular schwannoma than auditory brainstem response (ABR) (88% vs 99%), particularly for tumors measuring less than 1 cm in diameter (79%).[28] For cases in which MRI is not available or contraindicated, ABR may prove to be a suitable but less sensitive alternative test. Don and colleagues[33] showed improved sensitivity using stacked ABR (95%) in patients with vestibular schwannomas measuring less than 1 cm. The use of ABR for screening retrocochlear disease is also a less favorable diagnostic option from a practical standpoint, because sufficient residual hearing thresholds (<75 dbHL) must be present for an ABR response to be observed.

Vestibular Assessment

The presence of vertiginous symptoms with SSNHL is common and is generally believed to be a poor prognostic factor for hearing recovery. Objective vestibular assessment with electronystagmography (ENG) or vestibular evoked myogenic potentials (VEMP) testing is not a common part of an SSNHL test battery but may be useful in predicting the prognosis for hearing recovery. Korres and colleagues[34] identified a significantly higher number of abnormal ENG and VEMP results in patients with profound hearing loss, as well as a negative correlation between the severity of hearing loss and the likelihood of hearing recovery. These findings are similar to previously published findings in the literature.[35]

Magnetic Resonance Imaging

Radiologic evaluation of the CPA and internal acoustic meatus via MRI with gadolinium is indicated for the identification of potentially treatable causes of unilateral SSNHL and asymmetric hearing loss.[24,28] The sensitivity and specificity of MRI with gadolinium in the diagnosis of a vestibular schwannoma larger than 3 mm approaches nearly 100%.[28,36] Contrast-enhanced MRI can identify an abnormality in 10.7% to 57% of patients with SSNHL such as a CPA tumor, labyrinthine hemorrhage, cerebrovascular accident, or demyelinating process.[37–40] In patients with renal compromise, the risk of nephrogenic systemic fibrosis may contraindicate the use of gadolinium (relative glomerular filtration rate [GFR], 60 mL/min; absolute GFR <30 mL/min). In such cases, high-resolution MRI with constructive interference steady state sequence may be performed instead.[36,41]

Computed Tomography

Patients who are unable to receive an MRI scan (implanted ferromagnetic materials, claustrophobia) may undergo a CT scan with intravenous contrast of the head and temporal bones.[28] Such scans have reasonable sensitivity for lesions greater than 1.5 cm in diameter, although remain suboptimal in their diagnostic capabilities for retrocochlear lesions when compared with MRI.

Laboratory Tests

The evaluation of patients with SSNHL with laboratory tests is variable. Laboratory tests including complete blood count, electrolytes, basic metabolic panels, and erythrocyte sedimentation rate (ESR) are deemed reasonable but many clinicians may decide to forgo even these measures because of their low yield.[42] There is no evidence to support a shotgun approach to serologic testing for patients with SSNHL, because the positive yield of such testing remains unfavorably low.[43] However, when the history and physical examination suggest a possible cause, such information should be used to guide further specific serologic workup.

Serologic markers for metabolic disorders are commonly investigated in patients with SSNHL. Hypercholesterolemia has been identified in 35% to 40% of patients with idiopathic SSNHL, and hyperglycemia in 18% to 37% of patients.[26,43–45] Hypothyroidism is also common, with a prevalence of up to 15% in patients with SSNHL.[43,45,46] Most of these conditions have been identified on previous testing performed by the primary care physician before presentation to an otolaryngologist. Patients without a previously known diagnosis of these disorders may benefit from a screening evaluation when presenting with SSNHL.[43]

Hemostatic parameters such as thrombophilic genetic polymorphisms and coagulation studies have been investigated in patients with SSNHL. A higher rate of polymorphisms in factor V Leiden, prothrombin, methylenetetrahydrofolate reductase, and platelet GlyIIIa have been shown in patients with SSNHL,[13,47,48] but our clinical ability to identify these polymorphisms in the general population to stratify or minimize the risk of an SSNHL event before its occurrence is not feasible. Ballesteros and colleagues[47] showed that patients with SSNHL do not have a statistically significant difference in their coagulation profile compared with controls, suggesting that coagulation studies such as prothrombin time, activated partial thromboplastin time, and coagulation factors are of little diagnostic value in the clinical evaluation of SSNHL unless warranted by evidence of a systemic process by a comprehensive history and physical examination. Thus, the usefulness of routine evaluation of hemostatic parameters in SSNHL remains unlikely to provide significant clinical information that affects the incidence, therapy, or prognosis.

Infectious Diseases

Tests to identify possible infectious causes for SSNHL have been proposed in numerous diagnostic algorithms.[24] Numerous studies have attempted to associate a viral cause with SSNHL. Influenza B[49] and enterovirus[50] have been shown to have higher rates of seroconversion in patients with SSNHL in some studies. Other studies have failed to show an association between SSNHL and human herpes simplex virus,[50,51] varicella zoster,[50,51] cytomegalovirus,[51] influenza A1/A3,[49] parainfluenza viruses 1, 2, and 3,[49] enterovirus,[52] cytomegalovirus,[52] Epstein-Barr virus,[52] hepatitis C,[26] adenovirus,[49,53] rubella,[49,53] and respiratory syncytial virus.[49,53] There is currently little evidence to support the use of routine shotgun screening for a viral cause using polymerase chain reaction or preconvalescent and postconvalescent immunoglobulin titers in the workup of SSNHL. Convincing evidence of a causal relationship between a viral infection and SSNHL is lacking, and these investigations have not been shown to make a significant difference in guiding treatment or providing a benefit to patient outcomes.

Screening tests for nonviral infectious should be performed if a patient's history and physical examination are suggestive of an infectious cause. Hearing loss caused by Lyme disease rarely presents without other clinical symptoms, thus patients with history of exposure and positive clinical findings should be considered for serologic testing.[54] Confirmation of *Borrelia* infection can be performed by enzyme-linked immunosorbent assay (ELISA) testing or a serum immunoblot test, which is more specific than ELISA for anti-*Borrelia burgdorferi* antibodies.[41] If the possibility of congenital or latent syphilis is suspected, then screening should be performed with serum fluorescent treponemal antibody absorption or microhemagglutination-*Treponema pallidum* testing.[55]

Autoimmune Inner Ear Disease

Serologic markers for autoimmune disease are often ordered during the workup of sudden and rapidly progressive or fluctuating SNHL. Increase of the ESR is commonly seen in patients with SSNHL, although recent studies refute the prognostic usefulness of this marker.[43,56–58] Multiple studies have examined the relationship between SSNHL and various systemic autoimmune markers including antinuclear antibodies, rheumatoid factor, and anticardiolipin antibodies, all of which have been shown to be increased in patients with SSNHL.[43,58,59] Increased levels of antiphosphatidylserine antibodies[60] and antiendothelial cell autoantibodies[59] as well as a decrease in tumor necrosis factor α levels[58] and T-helper cell populations[61] have been shown in patients with SSNHL. All of these tests lack specificity for the diagnosis of an autoimmune-mediated SNHL, and the results are often clinically unhelpful because there is no identifiable positive association between the increase of a nonspecific inflammatory marker and a positive response to corticosteroid treatment of SSNHL in the medical literature.

Researchers have also investigated antibody responses to specific inner ear proteins. The 68-kDa antigen suspected to be heat shock protein 70 (hsp70) and its relationship with AIED has been researched extensively. Heat shock proteins are commonly expressed in multiple body tissues and in both healthy individuals and various disease states, thus limiting its diagnostic value in AIED.[58,62] Other potential inner ear antigens include cochlin,[63] β-tectorin,[63] choline transporterlike protein 2,[64] and myelin protein Po.[65] Routine testing for these antigens is not recommended, because the role of these inner ear antigens in AIED remains unclear.

EVIDENCE-BASED MANAGEMENT
Management of Sudden Sensorineural Hearing Loss

Oral corticosteroids
Although oral steroids are considered the gold standard in the treatment of SSNHL, their usefulness is a source of significant debate. Some consider that the first and best evidence for their use comes from a study by Wilson and colleagues,[66] which resulted in a statistically significantly greater rate of SSNHL recovery than oral placebo. Multiple placebo-controlled studies have since suggested value in the use of oral corticosteroids for the treatment of SSNHL,[66–68] but these studies have endured several criticisms, including being underpowered, nonrandomized, retrospective, and containing poorly defined clinical end points. A systematic review[69] and meta-analysis[70] by Conlin and Parnes concluded that a statistically significant treatment effect was no longer present when Wilson and colleagues' data[64] were pooled with data from a randomized, controlled trial by Cinamon and colleagues,[71] and a more recent Cochrane review found that these same 2 trials[66,71] were of low methodologic quality.[72] Thus, the current best evidence for oral corticosteroids obtained from randomized, controlled trials has been deemed to be contradictory in outcome and does not permit a definitive treatment recommendation.[72]

The timing of steroid therapy in SSNHL has been equally as contentious as the type of therapy itself. SSNHL has traditionally been considered an otologic emergency requiring prompt initiation of therapy for maximum efficacy and best chance of hearing recovery. A study by Huy and Sauvaget[21] found that a delay in initiating treatment from 24 hours to 1 week had no effect on the final degree of hearing loss. Other studies have also shown that the time between onset of SSNHL and initiation of corticosteroid therapy after hearing loss does not seem to affect hearing outcomes, with 1 study suggesting equal treatment efficacy 10 days or more after the onset of SSNHL.[73,74]

Transtympanic corticosteroids
Transtympanic corticosteroids (TTS) via injection into the middle ear have become increasingly popular. TTS have several theoretic advantages over oral corticosteroids, including the potential benefit of reduced systemic steroid exposure and the associated adverse effects. Animal studies have shown higher perilymph drug concentrations from TTS relative to either intravenous or oral steroid administration.[73,75] Three main protocols have been reported for TTS in the treatment of SSNHL: initial or primary therapy, adjunctive therapy with either oral or intravenous steroids, or salvage therapy after failure of systemic corticosteroid therapy. No consensus has been reached with respect to optimal steroid selection, because studies have been heterogeneous, with common usage of dexamethasone, prednisone, or methylprednisolone. Several studies have shown the potential benefits of using TTS as a salvage therapy.[76,77] Until recently, the use of TTS in primary therapy was uncommon. An inferiority trial by Rauch and colleagues[78] comparing TTS with oral treatment as primary therapy concluded that TTS were not inferior to oral steroids among patients with idiopathic SSNHL 2 months after treatment.

A review by Vlastarakos and colleagues[79] assessed the efficacy of TTS in the treatment of SSNHL with respect to each of the steroid delivery methods mentioned earlier. The study concluded that TTS seem to be effective as primary (grade A) or salvage treatment (grade B) in SSNHL but was unable to draw a definite conclusion regarding combination therapy because of heterogeneity among study results. It also concluded that primary TTS was the most effective modality in terms of complete hearing recovery, with a 34.4% cure rate, and that most complications of TTS were minor, temporary, and conservatively managed. This conclusion was further strengthened by a systematic review by Spear and Schwartz,[80] which found that TTS was equivalent to high-dose oral steroids, and with respect to salvage therapy offered the potential for additional hearing recovery. Both studies cautioned readers regarding the degree of significance of the objective hearing improvement and the percentage of patients who may subjectively experience benefit.

Antiviral therapy

Antivirals such as acyclovir and ganciclovir have been commonly used as a treatment adjunct with systemic corticosteroids for SSNHL therapy. A meta-analysis by Conlin and Parnes[70] determined that no significant treatment benefit was derived from treatment with oral corticosteroids and an antiviral over oral corticosteroids alone, and antivirals did not seem to improve recovery time or provide a hearing benefit. A more recent review has confirmed that there is insufficient evidence to recommend antiviral therapy in addition to corticosteroids in patients with SSNHL.[81] Despite the absence of scientific evidence supporting the efficacy of antiviral therapy, antivirals remain a common treatment adjunct across North America, likely because of the minimal risk and cost associated with treatment.

Rheopheresis

Rheopheresis has been used as a therapeutic option for SSNHL in Europe. The goal of therapy is to reduce acute microcirculatory impairment via plasmapheresis, which is used to eliminate a defined spectrum of high-molecular-weight plasma proteins, with a resultant reduction of plasma and whole blood viscosity. A recent German review reported on 2 main large randomized controlled trials[82,83] that showed equivalent efficacy to standard therapy with systemic corticosteroids and hemodilution.[84] These findings have been recognized by the German SSNHL guidelines, which propose similar treatments as part of a multimodality approach. Neither of these studies was without limitations, and further research is needed to further evaluate their encouraging findings.

Hyperbaric oxygen

Hyperbaric oxygen (HBO) therapy for the treatment of SSNHL has been studied as either a primary therapy or as an adjunctive therapy to systemic corticosteroids with mixed results. HBO was used as the primary therapy for SSNHL in 1 published study, in which it was found to provide an improved hearing outcome when compared with vasodilator therapy.[85] As an adjunctive therapy, a retrospective review by Alimoglu and colleagues[86] found that combined corticosteroid/HBO therapy for SSNHL had a higher rate of therapy response and complete recovery compared with primary HBO, oral, or intratympanic steroid therapies. Conversely, Cekin and colleagues[87] compared primary and adjunctive HBO and found no statistical benefit. A Cochrane review in 2007[88] found limited evidence that HBO therapy improves hearing in patients with idiopathic SSNHL and no evidence of a functionally significant improvement.

Management of Rapidly Progressive Sensorineural Hearing Loss

Studies have shown that corticosteroids are the only validated treatment option for AIED with significant but variable hearing gains.[89,90] Although a standard regimen of therapy does not exist, treatment with 1 mg/kg/d for 4 weeks followed by a slow taper over several weeks to a maintenance dose of 10 to 20 mg/d or the lowest dose that maintains hearing has been recommended.[25] Alexander and colleagues[91] conducted a study assessing corticosteroid safety in response to concerns regarding adverse affects from long-term corticosteroid use and found that with appropriate patient selection, monitoring, and patient education, high-dose corticosteroids were a safe and effective long-term treatment of AIED.

The audiovestibular symptoms of AIED typically follow a waxing and waning course, which can lead to an inability to wean off corticosteroids, or the symptoms can become refractory to steroid treatment. Corticosteroid-sparing treatments have been studied at length, with methotrexate showing initial promise in a retrospective study by Sismanis and colleagues,[92] but this trial was criticized for being retrospective and uncontrolled. A single randomized, controlled trial reported that methotrexate was no more effective than placebo in maintaining hearing improvement in patients with AIED despite an initial response to high-dose corticosteroids.[89]

Treatment with cyclophosphamide as adjunctive or salvage therapy has been described for patients who are either unresponsive to corticosteroid/methotrexate therapy or cannot be weaned from corticosteroid therapy.[16,93] Although cyclophosphamide remains a therapeutic alternative for refractory or chronic symptoms, patients may refuse therapy because of its potential toxicities such as myelosuppression, infertility, and increased risk of malignancy and elect for treatments such as cochlear implantation once their symptoms progress from severe to profound.

Other cytotoxic and proinflammatory antagonists such as etanercept and infliximab have been studied in the treatment of AIED. Most of these studies have been small and have shown the agents to be no better than placebo.[94,95] The studies were limited primarily by small sample size and may have been underpowered to detect a significant clinical difference. Therefore, larger trials are necessary to assess for potential benefit in the treatment of AIED.

Management of Asymmetric Sensorineural Hearing Loss

Despite having serviceable hearing from their remaining good ear, adult patients with profound ASNHL can suffer from significant hearing handicaps, including difficulties with speech perception in the presence of noise, localization of unseen sounds, and increased listening effort. Traditional treatment has been limited to the use of air-conduction contralateral routing of sound (CROS) hearing aids to reduce the head shadowing effect of monaural hearing as well as to improve speech perception. Limitations of CROS aids such as social stigma related to poor cosmesis and discomfort from occlusion of the better ear canal have led to increased interest in the potential benefits of bone-anchored hearing aids (BAHA).

A meta-analysis in 2006 comparing the usefulness of BAHA and CROS hearing aids found no significant improvement in auditory localization with either aid, but BAHA provided an advantage with both speech discrimination in noise and subjective auditory abilities.[96] A more recent contemporary review found that patients preferred BAHA over CROS hearing aids and that BAHA may offer enhancements in speech perception in noise over CROS aids.[97] Both of these studies recognized that the current best evidence regarding BAHA surgery for ASNHL suffers from several limitations, including a paucity of prospective randomized, controlled trials, and thus the investigators have advised clinicians to proceed with caution and await larger randomized trials.[96,97]

BOTTOM LINE: WHAT DOES THE EVIDENCE TELL US?

Significant gains have been made in our understanding of the genetics of hearing loss and how the interactions with our environment and other factors influence the auditory system. These advances have yet to translate into diagnostic tests and therapies that can effectively predict, prevent, or reverse sudden changes in hearing or delay the effects of age and noise on hearing. Advancements in the resolution and strength of diagnostic imaging techniques such as MRI have improved our ability to diagnose temporal bone, inner ear, or central nervous system causes of SNHL. Research continues toward the identification of laboratory tests that can diagnose the cause of an SSNHL with increased sensitivity and specificity, whether it is caused by an infectious disease or hematologic or coagulopathic disorder or is inflammatory/autoimmune in origin. Corticosteroids are a validated treatment of hearing loss caused by autoimmune and inflammatory disease, and also remain the primary treatment of idiopathic SSNHL despite the controversies regarding the effective timing, dosing, and true efficacy of corticosteroids for these patients.

CRITICAL POINTS WITH EVIDENCE

- Standard pure-tone audiometry and speech discrimination testing are essential for diagnosing patients with hearing loss. The Stenger test can be used to rule out pseudohypoacusis (level 1b).
- No clear definition of ASNHL exists in the literature (level 4).
- ABR is inferior to MRI in ruling out retrocochlear disease but can be considered if MRI is not available or is contraindicated (level 2b).
- MRI with gadolinium has a high sensitivity and specificity in diagnosing potentially treatable causes of ASNHL or unilateral hearing SNHL (level 2b). CT with intravenous contrast may be used to rule out large retrocochlear lesions (>1.5 cm) when MRI is contraindicated.
- Common metabolic disturbances associated with hearing loss such as hypercholesterolemia and hypothyroidism should be ruled out in previously unscreened patients (level 3b).
- The use of hemostatic parameters or coagulation studies is of little diagnostic value in the clinical evaluation of SSNHL unless warranted by evidence of a systemic process during a comprehensive history and physical examination (level 3b).
- There is a lack of evidence to support the use of routine screening for a viral cause in the workup of SSNHL (level 3b).
- Screening tests for nonviral infectious causes such as Lyme disease and syphilis should be performed in patients with a suggestive clinical history and physical examination (level 4).
- The use of systemic autoimmune markers in evaluating SSNHL, rapidly progressive SNHL, or fluctuating SNHL lack specificity and do not provide prognostic information (level 2b).
- Routine testing for hsp70 and inner ear antigens is not recommended because their role in the diagnosis and management of autoimmune ear disease is unclear (level 2b).
- The best current evidence for oral corticosteroid treatment of SSNHL is contradictory in outcome and does not permit a definitive treatment recommendation (level 1a).[69,70,72]
- SSNHL may not be an otologic emergency (level 2b).[21] Treatment may be equally efficacious up to and potentially later than 10 days after the loss of hearing (level 1b).[73,74,77]
- TTS may be useful as either primary therapy or salvage therapy in patients with medical comorbidities who are at risk of serious adverse effects from oral corticosteroid administration (level 1b).[78,79]

- There is insufficient evidence to recommend antiviral therapy as primary or steroid adjunctive therapy in patients with SSNHL (level 1a).[70,81]
- Rheolytic therapy may provide benefit for the treatment of SSNHL. Further research is needed to further evaluate these encouraging findings (level 1a).[84]
- There is limited evidence to suggest that primary HBO therapy improves hearing in patients with idiopathic SSNHL and no evidence of a functionally significant improvement (level 1a).[88]
- Corticosteroids are the only validated treatment option for AIED (level 2b).[89,90] There is limited evidence to recommend corticosteroid-sparing therapy, including cytotoxic (methotrexate) (level 1a) and proinflammatory antagonists (etanercept/infliximab) (level 4) in the treatment of AIED as a primary therapy.[16,89,93–95]
- BAHA surgery may be preferred by patients over CROS hearing aids for ASNHL and may provide improvement in speech discrimination in noisy environments (level 3a).[96,97]

REFERENCES

1. Shargorodsky J, Curhan S, Curhan G, et al. Change in prevalence of hearing loss in US adolescents. JAMA 2010;304:772–8.
2. Cummins D, McCorkick JB, Bennett D, et al. Acute sensorineural deafness in Lassa fever. JAMA 1990;264:2094–6.
3. OCEBM Levels of Evidence Working Group. The Oxford 2011 Levels of Evidence. Oxford Centre for Evidence-Based Medicine. 2011. Available at: http://www.cebm.net/index.aspx?o=1025. Accessed November 3, 2011.
4. Agrawal Y, Platz E, Niparko J. Prevalence of hearing loss and differences by demographic characteristics among US adults. Arch Intern Med 2008;168:1522–30.
5. NIOSH. Centers for disease Control and Prevention – National Institute for Occupational Safety and Health. Available at: http://www.cdc.gov/niosh/topics/noise. Accessed November 3, 2011.
6. Wu C, Young Y. Ten-year longitudinal study of the effect of impulse noise exposure from gunshot on inner ear function. Int J Audiol 2009;48:655–60.
7. Dror A, Avraham K. Hearing loss: mechanisms revealed by genetics and cell biology. Annu Rev Genet 2009;43:411–37.
8. Hone S, Smith R. Genetics of hearing impairment. Semin Neonatol 2001;6:531–41.
9. Bindu LH, Reddy PP. Genetics of aminoglycoside-induced and prelingual non-syndromic mitochondrial hearing impairment: a review. Int J Audiol 2008;47:702–7.
10. Brown ED, Chau J, Atashband S, et al. A systematic review of neonatal toxoplasmosis exposure and sensorineural hearing loss. Int J Pediatr Otorhinolaryngol 2009;73:787–92.
11. Chau J, Atashband S, Chang E, et al. A systematic review of pediatric sensorineural hearing loss in congenital syphilis. Int J Pediatr Otorhinolaryngol 2009;73:787–92.
12. Son EJ, Bang JH, Kang JG. Anterior inferior cerebellar artery infarction presenting with sudden hearing loss and vertigo. Laryngoscope 2007;117:556–8.
13. Capaccio P, Ottaviani F, Cuccarini V, et al. Genetic and acquired prothrombotic risk factors and sudden hearing loss. Laryngoscope 2007;117:547–51.
14. Marcucci R, Alessandrello Liotta A, Cellai A, et al. Cardiovascular and thrombophilic risk factors for idiopathic sudden sensorineural hearing loss. J Thromb Haemost 2005;3:929–34.

15. Haynes D, Rutka J, Hawke M, et al. Ototoxicity of ototopical drops–an update. Otolaryngol Clin North Am 2007;40:669–83.
16. McCabe BF. Autoimmune sensorineural hearing loss. Ann Otol Rhinol Laryngol 1979;88:585–9.
17. Bonaguri C, Orsoni J, Zavota L, et al. Anti-68 kDa antibodies in autoimmune sensorineural hearing loss. Autoimmunity 2007;40:73–8.
18. Mathews J, Kumar BN. Autoimmune sensorineural hearing loss [review]. Clin Otolaryngol 2003;28:479–88.
19. Swartz JD. Lesions of the cerebellopontine angle and internal auditory canal: diagnosis and differential diagnosis. Semin Ultrasound CT MR 2004;25:332–52.
20. Cureoglu S, Tulunay O, Ferlito A, et al. Otologic manifestations of metastatic tumors to the temporal bone. Acta Otolaryngol 2004;124:1117–23.
21. Huy PT, Sauvaget E. Idiopathic sudden sensorineural hearing loss is not an otologic emergency. Otol Neurotol 2005;26:896–902.
22. NIDCD. National Institute on Deafness and Other Communication Disorders. Available at http://www.nidcd.nih.gov/health/hearing/Pages/sudden.aspx. Accessed November 3, 2011.
23. Byl FM. Sudden hearing loss: eight years' experience and suggested prognostic table. Laryngoscope 1984;94:647–61.
24. Chau J, Lin JR, Atashband S, et al. Systematic review of the evidence for the etiology of adult sudden sensorineural hearing loss. Laryngoscope 2010;120: 1011–21.
25. Bovo R, Aimoni C, Martini A. Immune-mediated inner ear disease. Acta Otolaryngol 2006;126:1012–21.
26. Cadoni G, Scipione S, Ippolito S, et al. Sudden sensorineural hearing loss: our experience in diagnosis, treatment and outcome. J Otolaryngol 2005;34: 395–400.
27. Durmaz A, Karahatay S, Satar B, et al. Efficiency of Stenger test in confirming profound, unilateral pseudohypacusis. J Laryngol Otol 2009;123(8):840–4.
28. Cueva R. Auditory brainstem response versus magnetic resonance imaging for the evaluation of asymmetric sensorineural hearing loss. Laryngoscope 2004; 114:1686–92.
29. Dawes PJ, Jeannon JP. Audit of regional screening guidelines for vestibular schwannoma. J Laryngol Otol 1998;112(9):860–4.
30. Gimsing S. Vestibular schwannoma: when to look at it? J Laryngol Otol 2010;124: 258–64.
31. Saliba I, Bergeron M, Martineau G, et al. Rule 3,000: a more reliable precursor to perceive vestibular schwannoma on MRI in screened asymmetric sensorineural hearing loss. Eur Arch Otorhinolaryngol 2011;268:207–12.
32. Sheppard IJ, Milford CA, Anslow P. MRI in the detection of acoustic neuromas–a suggested protocol for screening. Clin Otolaryngol 1996;21:301–4.
33. Don M, Kwong B, Tanaka C, et al. The stacked ABR: a sensitive and specific screening tool for detecting small acoustic tumors. Audiol Neurootol 2005; 10(5):274–90.
34. Korres S, Stamatiou GA, Gkoritsa E, et al. Prognosis of patients with idiopathic sudden hearing loss: role of vestibular assessment. J Laryngol Otol 2011;125: 251–7.
35. Wilson WR, Laird N, Kavesh DA. Electronystagmographic findings in idiopathic sudden hearing loss. Am J Otol 1982;3:279–85.
36. Fortnum H, O'Neil C, Taylor R, et al. The role of magnetic resonance imaging in the identification of suspected acoustic neuroma: a systematic review of clinical

and cost effectiveness and natural history. Health Technol Assess 2009;13(18): 1–154.

37. Aarnisalo AA, Suoranta H, Ylikoski J. Magnetic resonance imaging findings in the auditory pathway of patients with sudden deafness. Otol Neurotol 2004;25(3):245–9.

38. Cadoni G, Cianfoni A, Agostino S, et al. Magnetic resonance imaging findings in sudden sensorineural hearing loss. J Otolaryngol 2006;35(5):310–6.

39. Chaimoff M, Nageris BI, Sulkes J, et al. Sudden hearing loss as a presenting symptom of acoustic neuroma. Am J Otol 1999;20(3):157–60.

40. Sugiura M, Nakashima T, Naganawa S, et al. Sudden sensorineural hearing loss associated with inner ear anomaly. Otol Neurotol 2005;26(2):241–6.

41. Kuhn M, Heman-Ackah SE, Shaikh JA, et al. Sudden sensorineural hearing loss: a review of diagnosis, treatment, and prognosis. Trends Amplif 2011; 15(3):91–105.

42. O'Malley MR, Haynes DS. Sudden hearing loss. Otolaryngol Clin North Am 2008; 41(3):633–49.

43. Heman-Ackah SE, Jabbour N, Huang TC. Asymmetric sudden sensorineural hearing loss: is all this testing necessary. J Otolaryngol Head Neck Surg 2010; 39(5):486–90.

44. Aimoni C, Bianchini C, Borin M, et al. Diabetes, cardiovascular risk factors and idiopathic sudden sensorineural hearing loss: a case-control study. Audiol Neurootol 2010;15(2):111–5.

45. Oiticica J, Bittar RS. Metabolic disorders prevalence in sudden deafness. Clinics (Sao Paulo) 2010;65(11):1149–553.

46. Narozny W, Kuczkowski J, Mikaszewski B. Thyroid dysfunction–underestimated but important prognostic factor in sudden sensorineural hearing loss. Otolaryngol Head Neck Surg 2006;135(6):995–6.

47. Ballesteros F, Alobid I, Tassies D, et al. Is there an overlap between sudden neurosensorial hearing loss and cardiovascular risk factors? Audiol Neurootol 2009; 14(3):139–45.

48. Capaccio P, Cuccarini V, Ottaviani F, et al. Prothrombotic gene mutations in patients with sudden sensorineural hearing loss and cardiovascular thrombotic disease. Ann Otol Rhinol Laryngol 2009;118(3):205–10.

49. Wilson WR, Veltri RW, Laird N, et al. Viral and epidemiologic studies of idiopathic sudden hearing loss. Otolaryngol Head Neck Surg 1983;91(6):653–8.

50. Mentel R, Kaftan H, Wegner U, et al. Are enterovirus infections a co-factor in sudden hearing loss? J Med Virol 2004;72(4):625–9.

51. Mishra B, Panda N, Singh MP, et al. Viral infections in sudden hearing loss. Do we have enough evidence. Kathmandu Univ Med J (KUMJ) 2005;3(3): 230–3.

52. Gross M, Wolf DG, Elidan J, et al. Enterovirus, cytomegalovirus, and Epstein-Barr virus infection screening in idiopathic sudden sensorineural hearing loss. Audiol Neurootol 2007;12(3):179–82.

53. Jaffe BF. Clinical studies in sudden deafness. Adv Otorhinolaryngol 1973;20:221–8.

54. Gagnebin J, Maire R. Infection screening in sudden and progressive idiopathic sensorineural hearing loss: a retrospective study of 182 cases. Otol Neurotol 2002;23(2):160–2.

55. Yimtae K, Srirompotong S, Lertsukprasert K. Otosyphilis: a review of 85 cases. Otolaryngol Head Neck Surg 2007;136(1):67–71.

56. Chang NC, Ho KY, Kuo WR. Audiometric patterns and prognosis in sudden sensorineural hearing loss in southern Taiwan. Otolaryngol Head Neck Surg 2005;133(6):916–22.

57. Mattox DE, Simmons FB. Natural history of sudden sensorineural hearing loss. Ann Otol Rhinol Laryngol 1977;86:463–80.
58. Suslu N, Yilmaz T, Gursel B. Utility of anti-HSP 70, TNF-α, ESR, antinuclear antibody, and antiphospholipid antibodies in the diagnosis and treatment of sudden sensorineural hearing loss. Laryngoscope 2009;119(2):341–6.
59. Cadoni G, Fetoni AR, Agostino S, et al. Autoimmunity in sudden sensorineural hearing loss: possible role of anti-endothelial cell autoantibodies. Acta Otolaryngol Suppl 2002;548:30–3.
60. Bachor E, Kremmer S, Kreuzfelder E, et al. Antiphospholipid antibodies in patients with sensorineural hearing loss. Eur Arch Otorhinolaryngol 2005; 262(8):622–6.
61. Garcia Berrocal JR, Ramirez-Camacho R, Vargas JA, et al. Does the serological testing really play a role in the diagnosis of immune-mediated inner ear disease? Acta Otolaryngol 2002;122:243–8.
62. Soliman AM. Autoantibodies in inner ear disease. Acta Otolaryngol 1997;117(4): 501–4.
63. Tebo AE, Szankasi P, Hillman TA, et al. Antibody reactivity to heat shock protein 70 and inner ear-specific proteins in patients with idiopathic sensorineural hearing loss. Clin Exp Immunol 2006;146:427–32.
64. Nair TS, Kozma KE, Hoefling NL, et al. Identification and characterization of choline transporter-like protein 2, an inner ear glycoprotein of 68 and 72 KDa that is the target of antibody-induced hearing loss. Neuroscience 2004;24:1172–9.
65. Cao MY, Dupriez VJ, Rider MH, et al. Myelin protein Po as a potential autoantigen in autoimmune inner ear disease. FASEB J 1996;10:1635–40.
66. Wilson WR, Byl FM, Laird N. The efficacy of steroids in the treatment of idiopathic sudden hearing loss. A double-blind clinical study. Arch Otolaryngol 1980; 106(12):772–6.
67. Chen CY, Halpin C, Rauch SD. Oral steroid treatment of sudden sensorineural hearing loss: a ten year retrospective analysis. Otol Neurotol 2003;24: 728–33.
68. Slattery WH, Fisher LM, Iqbal Z, et al. Oral steroid regimens for idiopathic sudden sensorineural hearing loss. Otolaryngol Head Neck Surg 2005;132:5–10.
69. Conlin AE, Parnes LS. Treatment of sudden sensorineural hearing loss: I. A systematic review. Arch Otolaryngol Head Neck Surg 2007;133(6):573–81.
70. Conlin AE, Parnes LS. Treatment of sudden sensorineural hearing loss: II. A meta-analysis. Arch Otolaryngol Head Neck Surg 2007;133(6):582–6.
71. Cinamon U, Bendet E, Kronenberg J. Steroids, carbogen, or placebo for sudden hearing loss: a prospective double-blind study. Eur Arch Otorhinolaryngol 2001; 258(9):477–80.
72. Wei BPC, Mubiru S, O'Leary S. Steroids for idiopathic sudden sensorineural hearing loss. Cochrane Database of Syst Rev 2009;(4):CD003998. DOI: 10.1002/14651858.
73. Parnes LS, Sun AH, Freeman DJ. Corticosteroid pharmacokinetics in the inner ear fluids: an animal study followed by clinical application. Laryngoscope 1999;109(7 Pt 2):1–117.
74. Dispenza F, Amodio E, De Stefano A, et al. Treatment of sudden sensorineural hearing loss with transtympanic injection of steroids as single therapy: a randomized clinical study. Eur Arch Otorhinolaryngol 2011;268:1273–8.
75. Chandrasekhar SS, Rubinstein RY, Kwartler JA, et al. Dexamethasone pharmacokinetics in the inner ear: comparison of route of administration and use of facilitating agents. Otolaryngol Head Neck Surg 2000;122(4):521–8.

76. Haynes DS, O'Malley M, Cohen S, et al. Intratympanic dexamethasone for sudden sensorineural hearing loss after failure of systemic therapy. Laryngoscope 2007;117:3–15.
77. Ho GM, Lin HG, Shu MT. Effectiveness of intratympanic dexamethasone injection in sudden deafness patients as salvage treatment. Laryngoscope 2004;114: 1184–9.
78. Rauch SD, Halpin CF, Antonelli PJ, et al. Oral vs intratympanic corticosteroid therapy for idiopathic sudden sensorineural hearing loss: a randomized trial. JAMA 2011;305(20):2071–9.
79. Vlastarakos PV, Papacharalampous G, Maragoudakis P, et al. Are intratympanically administered steroids effective in patients with sudden deafness? Implications for current clinical practice. Eur Arch Otorhinolaryngol 2012; 269(2):363–80.
80. Spear SA, Schwartz SR. Intratympanic steroids for sudden sensorineural hearing loss: a systematic review. Otolaryngol Head Neck Surg 2011;145(4):534–43.
81. Shaikh JA, Roehm PC. Does addition of antiviral medication to high-dose corticosteroid therapy improve hearing recovery following idiopathic sudden sensorineural hearing loss? Laryngoscope 2011;121(11):2280–1.
82. Suckfull M. Fibrinogen and LDL apheresis in treatment of sudden hearing loss: a randomised multicentre trial. Lancet 2002;360:1811–7.
83. Mosges R, Koberlein J, Heibges A, et al. Rheopheresis for idiopathic sudden hearing loss: results from a large prospective, multicenter, randomized, controlled trial. Eur Arch Otorhinolaryngol 2009;266:943–53.
84. Klingel R, Heibges A, Uygun-Kiehne S, et al. Rheopheresis for sudden sensorineural hearing loss. Atheroscler Suppl 2009;10:102–6.
85. Fattori B, Berrettini S, Casani A, et al. Sudden hypoacusis treated with hyperbaric oxygen therapy: a controlled study. Ear Nose Throat J 2001;80(9):655–60.
86. Alimoglu Y, Inci E, Edizer DT, et al. Efficacy comparison of oral steroid, intratympanic steroid, hyperbaric oxygen and oral steroid + hyperbaric oxygen treatments in idiopathic sudden sensorineural hearing loss cases. Eur Arch Otorhinolaryngol 2011;268:1735–41.
87. Cekin E, Cincik H, Ulubil SA, et al. Effectiveness of hyperbaric oxygen therapy in management of sudden hearing loss. J Laryngol Otol 2009;123:609–12.
88. Bennett MH, Kertesz T, Yeung P. Hyperbaric oxygen for idiopathic sudden sensorineural hearing loss and tinnitus. Cochrane Database Syst Rev 2007;(1): CD004739.
89. Harris JP, Weisman MH, Derebery JM, et al. Treatment of corticosteroid-responsive autoimmune inner ear disease with methotrexate: a randomized controlled trial. JAMA 2003;290:1875–83.
90. Niparko JK, Wang NY, Rauch SD, et al. Serial audiometry in a clinical trial of AIED treatment. Otol Neurotol 2005;26:908–17.
91. Alexander TH, Weisman MH, Derebery JM, et al. Safety of high-dose corticosteroids for the treatment of autoimmune inner ear disease. Otol Neurotol 2009;30: 443–8.
92. Sismanis A, Wise CM, Johnson GD. Methotrexate management of immune-mediated cochleovestibular disorders. Otolaryngol Head Neck Surg 1997;116: 146–52.
93. McCabe BF. Autoimmune inner ear disease. Am J Otol 1989;10(3):196–7.
94. Cohen S, Shoup A, Weisman MH, et al. Etanercept treatment for autoimmune inner ear disease: results of a pilot placebo-controlled study. Otol Neurotol 2005;26:903–7.

95. Liu YC, Rubin R, Sataloff RT. Treatment-refractory autoimmune sensorineural hearing loss: response to infliximab. Ear Nose Throat J 2011;90(1):23–8.
96. Baguley DM, Bird J, Humphriss RL, et al. The evidence base for the application of contralateral bone anchored hearing aids in acquired unilateral sensorineural hearing loss in adults. Clin Otolaryngol 2005;31(1):6–14.
97. Bishop CE, Eby TL. The current status of audiologic rehabilitation for profound unilateral sensorineural hearing loss. Laryngoscope 2010;120(3):552–6.

Cochlear Implants
Clinical and Societal Outcomes

Yevgeniy R. Semenov, MA, Rodrigo Martinez-Monedero, MD,
John K. Niparko, MD*

KEYWORDS

- Cochlear implantation outcomes • Speech perception • Language development
- Cost utility • Quality of life • Education

KEY POINTS

- The primary goal of cochlear implantation in children is to facilitate comprehension and expression through the use of spoken language.
- Early educational intervention is associated with improvements in language development after cochlear implantation.
- Recent analyses show that in adults, the age at implantation carries minimal or even statistically insignificant predictive power on postimplantation outcomes. The duration of deafness and preoperative speech-perception scores have the highest predictive power on postimplantation outcomes across the adult population.
- Age-related degeneration of the spiral ganglion and progressive central auditory dysfunction raise potential concerns about the efficacy of cochlear prostheses in the elderly, but comparable gains in speech understanding have been reported for both elderly and younger groups of implant recipients.

INTRODUCTION

Over the past 30 years, hearing care clinicians have increasingly relied on cochlear implants to restore auditory sensitivity in selected patients with advanced sensorineural hearing loss (SNHL). This article examines the impact of intervention with cochlear implantation in children and adults. The authors report a range of clinic-based results and patient-based outcomes reflected in the reported literature on cochlear implants. The authors describe the basic assessment of the physiologic

No relevant disclosures.
All figures are derived from articles authored by John K. Niparko, who is the corresponding author for this article.
Department of Otolaryngology-Head and Neck Surgery, Johns Hopkins Hospital, Johns Hopkins University School of Medicine, 601 N. Caroline Street, Baltimore, MD 21287-0910, USA
* Corresponding author.
E-mail address: jnipark@jhmi.edu

Otolaryngol Clin N Am 45 (2012) 959–981
http://dx.doi.org/10.1016/j.otc.2012.06.003
0030-6665/12/$ – see front matter © 2012 Elsevier Inc. All rights reserved.

response to auditory nerve stimulation; measures of receptive and productive benefit; and surveys of life effects as reflected measures of quality of life, educational attainment, and economic impact.

AUDITORY OUTCOMES

Auditory performance is measured at preimplant and postimplant intervals, allowing the assessment of candidacy criteria and longitudinal tracking of the patients' progress. Measurement variables associated with auditory testing should be standardized as much as possible. Clinicians can choose between closed-set tests (eg, forced choice of 1 answer from a list of 4) and open-set tests (auditory alone without context) of words and/or sentences. Closed-set tests and sentence tests typically produce substantially higher correct percentages than do open-set tests and tests of single words. This difference reflects the amount of contextual information available when word and sentence material are presented. Voice presentation can also affect speech-perception scores,[1] with live presentations typically producing higher rates of correct responses than taped presentations.

Trends toward higher rates of open-set speech recognition with newer implant technology and longer implant experience have prompted calls for more stringent assessments of receptive capability. Increasing the difficulty of a speech-perception test has the effect of limiting the ceiling effect that results from testing with simple, everyday phrases. For the purpose of generating more meaningful comparative data, increasing the test difficulty tends to normalize distributions across populations, thereby enabling more powerful statistical analyses of differences between groups.

TESTS OF IMPLANT PERFORMANCE

The Minimum Speech Test Battery (MSTB) for adult cochlear implant users is a standardized set of comprehensive tests of preoperative and postoperative speech recognition.[2] To minimize the effects of learning and memorization, the word and sentence tests have different lists for at least 6 testing trials. The average and range of performance of cochlear implant users are critical to defining audiologic performance boundaries for implant candidacy, monitor postimplantation results, and facilitate in comparisons across implant designs and coding strategies.

The major components of the MSTB are the Hearing in Noise Test (HINT) and the Consonant/Nucleus/Consonant (CNC) test. The HINT[3] provides a measure of speech-reception thresholds for sentences in quiet and in noise. For high levels of recognition in quiet, the background noise is filtered to match the long-term average spectrum of the sentences. In the MSTB, the HINT sentence lists are presented at 70 dB in quiet and at a +10 dB signal-to-noise ratio (ie, noise at 60 dB). Smaller signal-to-noise ratios (eg, +5 dB or 0 dB) may also be used to avoid ceiling effects. Normal-hearing listeners can comprehend sentences effectively with signal-to-noise ratios down to −3 dB, whereas implant recipients typically show degraded speech recognition when signal-to-noise ratios are lowered beyond +10 dB.

The CNC test consists of monosyllabic words with equal phonemic distribution, with each list of words having approximately the same phonemic distribution as the English language.[4] CNC lists enable performance testing that is likely to represent daily experience with speech stimuli. These tests measure the percentage of words correctly recognized. Revised CNC lists[5] were developed to eliminate relatively uncommon words and proper nouns. More recent observations have stressed the importance of speech test materials that reduce contextual cues in the interest of assessing auditory performance (bottom-up processing) rather than cognitive (top-down processing) components of speech recognition.[6]

Improved speech perception is the primary goal of cochlear implantation. Initial clinical series judged implant efficacy mostly on environmental sound perception and performance on closed-set tests, whereas greater emphasis is now placed on measures of open-set speech comprehension. Speech-perception results from early clinical trials have served to guide the evolution of cochlear implantation.

Clinical observations in patients with current processors indicate that for patients with implant experience beyond 6 months, the mean score on open-set word testing approximates 30% to 60%, with a range of 0% to 100%.[7-10] Results achieved with the most recently developed speech-processing strategies reveal mean scores more than 75% on words-in-sentence testing, although once again with a wide range of 0% to 100%. Although patients perform substantially poorer on single-word testing, these mean scores continue to improve as the speech-processing strategy evolves.[11] After implantation, speech recognition by telephone[12] and music appreciation are often observed. Again, these benefits seem to be best achieved through more recently developed processing strategies.

The high prevalence of SNHL among the elderly has prompted evaluations of the benefit of cochlear implantation in this age group.[10,13-16] For recipients of the cochlear implant after the age of 65 years, open-set speech-recognition scores are not as high as those reported in younger cohorts, potentially representing an effect of longer duration of deafness as opposed to age per se. Nonetheless, implant usage is high among elderly recipients, with nonuse observed in few patients.

PREDICTORS OF BENEFIT IN ADULTS

The evaluation of the benefit of cochlear implantation in adults has largely focused on measuring gains in speech perception. Assessments of speech recognition in implanted adults offer the opportunity to develop models of benefit prediction. As investigators identify the salient predictive factors, patients' choices regarding candidacy, device and processing strategy, and the degree of postoperative auditory rehabilitation necessary can be better informed. Various statistical methods have been used to assess speech comprehension using cochlear implants. Multivariate analysis, a statistical technique that determines the contribution of individual factors to variations in performance, is the most commonly used methodology.[7,8,17-19] The following factors have been evaluated:

- Patient variables: age of onset, age of implantation, deafness duration, cause, preoperative hearing, survival and location of spiral ganglion cells, patency of the scala tympani, cognitive skills, personality, visual attention, motivation, engagement, communication mode, and auditory memory.
- Device variables: processor, implant, electrode geometry, electrode number, duration and pattern of implant use, and the strategy used by the speech processing unit.

Although the factors identified as most determinative have varied with different study populations, the most recent analyses[8,17-19] showed that age at implantation carries minimal or even statistically insignificant predictive power on postimplantation outcomes. Rather, it was the duration of deafness and preoperative speech perception scores that had the highest predictive power on postimplantation outcomes across the adult population.

The resulting models of postimplantation outcomes follow a similar mathematical structure with a patient's postoperative word score starting at a constant value k, which is either increased by the addition of a term dependent on the pre–cochlear-implant sentence score or decreased by the subtraction of a term dependent on the duration of deafness.

Predicted percentage of words in everyday sentences = k − (Dur Yrs df) + (% words pre-CI)

where *CI* is cochlear implant, *Dur Yrs df* is duration of deafness in years from onset and *% words pre-CI* is consonant-nucleus-consonant (CNC) monosyllabic word score before implantation.

In addition to the previously mentioned factors, the choice of which ear to implant has been a frequently discussed issue. Several studies, particularly the Iowa model, have emphasized the utility of implanting the better-hearing ear. At Johns Hopkins Hospital, the authors have advocated the implantation of the poorer-hearing ear. Although greater data are needed, the authors' studies thus far reveal no significant difference in implant performance based on whether the better- or worse-hearing ear is implanted. **Fig. 1** shows a regression plot of the predicted postoperative word scores for each patient as modeled by the Johns Hopkins (implant poorer ear) and Iowa formulas (better ear).[17] There are virtually identical scores predicted from each patient's duration of deafness and preoperative sentence recognition scores. These data suggest that results obtained through cochlear implantation of the poorer-hearing ear are

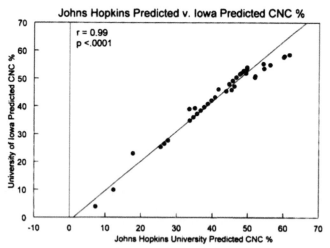

Fig. 1. Regression plot of the predicted postoperative word scores for each patient as modeled by the Johns Hopkins (implant poorer ear) and Iowa formulas (better ear). There are virtually identical scores predicted from each patient's duration of deafness and preoperative sentence-recognition scores. These data suggest that results obtained through cochlear implantation of the poorer-hearing ear are statistically equivalent to results obtained through implantation of the better-hearing ear. The similarity of results obtained through both methods suggests that implantation may have a beneficial effect on central auditory pathway development regardless of sidedness. (*Adapted from* Friedland DR, Venick HS, Niparko JK. Choice of ear for cochlear implantation: the effect of history and residual hearing on predicted postoperative performance. Otol Neurotol 2003;24(4):582–9; with permission.)

statistically equivalent to results obtained through implantation of the better-hearing ear. The similarity of results obtained through both methods suggests that implantation may have a beneficial effect on central auditory pathway development regardless of the choice of ear to be implanted, a finding which was later confirmed by Francis and colleagues[20] (2005).

Another variable that influences speech perception is technological sophistication of the implanted device. Improvements in speech perception have been associated with generational improvements in signal processing strategies, speech processors, and electrode arrays,[21,22] but may reflect clinical trends in patient selection as well as technological advances.

IMPLANT PERFORMANCE IN CHILDREN

The era of pediatric cochlear implantation began with House-3M single-channel implants (a collaboration between House Ear Institute and Minnesota Mining and Manufacturing Company) in 1980. Investigational trials with multiple-channel cochlear implants began with adolescents (aged 10 through 17 years) in 1985 and with children (aged 2 through 9 years) in 1986. Implantation of infants and toddlers younger than 2 years of age began in 1995.[23] Although clinical experience with cochlear implantation is considerably shorter in children than in adults, a large body of evidence is now available (reviewed by[24,25]).

AUDITORY PERFORMANCE ASSESSMENTS FOR CHILDREN

Auditory performance in children is assessed with a battery of audiological tests that can address the wide range of perceptual skills exhibited by children with severe to profound sensorineural hearing loss. Although substantial auditory gains are apparent in implanted children, the range of quantifiable improvement varies widely between children and depends heavily on the duration of use of the device as well as preoperative variables. For this reason, testing should survey a range of levels of speech recognition, including simple awareness of sound, pattern perception (discrimination of time and stress differences of utterance), closed-set (multiple choice) speech recognition, and open-set (auditory only) recognition.

Methodological variables must be considered when attempting to objectively rate the effect of cochlear implants on the development of speech perception in children who are deaf. There are obvious difficulties inherent in objectively rating communication competence in very young children; older children may exhibit advantages by virtue of greater familiarity with a test's context, independent of perceptual skills.[1] Objective assessment also mandates a structured setting. Given its unfamiliarity, children may not be in an optimal frame of mind in cooperating with testing. Investigators must also account for discontinuity in the age-appropriate measures necessary for longitudinal assessment.[26] Kirk and colleagues[1] (1997) have examined the methodological challenges and developmental considerations inherent in pediatric implant assessment and categorized variables relating to

- The child's age and level of language and cognitive development (internal variables)
- The child's ability and willingness to respond as influenced by reinforcement and required memory task (external variables)
- The procedure of voice presentation, the test administered, and the available options from which to choose a response (methodological variables)

Tests of speech perceptions typically used for childhood assessment have been described in detail[1,27–29] and typically consist of closed-set tests that assess word identification among a limited set of options with auditory cues only, open-set tests (scored by percentage of individual words correctly repeated), and structured interviews of parents using criteria-based surveys to assess the response to sound in everyday situations and behaviors related to spoken communication.

SPEECH COMPREHENSION RESULTS IN CHILDREN WITH COCHLEAR IMPLANTS

Early assessments of pediatric hearing outcomes were performed by House and colleagues[30] (1983) and showed substantial improvement in auditory thresholds and closed-set speech recognition, albeit with limited open-set speech recognition using early technology (House-3M single-channel implant). In 1994, Miyamoto and colleagues[31] provided systematic, well-controlled assessments of childhood cohorts and consistently demonstrated performance advantages of multichannel over single-channel implants. Other early studies by Fryauf-Bertschy and colleagues[32] (1992), Waltzman and colleagues[33] (1994), Miyamoto and colleagues[34] (1993), and Gantz and colleagues[35] (1994) observed that implanted children gain substantial speech-perception capabilities for 5 years after implantation. Furthermore, the fact that many of the implanted children tracked in these studies were congenitally or prelingually deaf indicates that implantation can provide auditory access during critical developmental stages to form the early correlates of spoken language. More recent auditory outcomes publications reflect advances in implant technology and information processing, yielding ever-improving means in speech recognition results.

Over the past 15 years, a wealth of reports has documented further gains in speech recognition in young children who are deaf using multichannel cochlear implants.[26,27,36,37] Miyamoto and colleagues[34] (1993) noted that in 29 children with 1 to 4 years of experience with a cochlear implant, roughly half achieved open-set speech recognition. Subsequent assessments using greater duration of postimplantation follow-up suggest that this percentage has increased through the rest of the 1990s and 2000s, with open-set speech-recognition scores averaging as high as 80%.[37–39]

Variability in speech-perception performance across patients is widely recognized.[7,26,40,41] Factors implicated in speech recognition variability include

- Amount of residual hearing[42,43]
- Age of implantation[40,44,45]
- Mode of communication[33,46]
- Family support[47]
- Length of deafness[43,48]

Miyamoto and colleagues[31] (1994) found that the duration of deafness, communication mode, age at onset of deafness, and the processor used accounted for roughly 35% of the variance in closed-set testing, with the length of implant use accounting for the largest percentage of variance in measures of speech perception. O'Donoghue and colleagues[40] (2000) found that age at implantation and mode of communication had a significant effect on speech-perception development in young children after implantation.

Zwolan and colleagues[44] (2004) and Manrique and colleagues[45] (2004) reported improved speech perception in children implanted at younger than 2 years of age compared with children implanted at an older age. Multicenter data reported by Osberger (2002)[49] indicate that implantation performance of children implanted at younger than 2 years of age is significantly better than that of children implanted between 2 and 3 years of age. However, Osberger also identified an important confounding variable that exists in the children who receive a cochlear implant at a younger age: they are more likely to use an oral mode of communication. This finding, by itself, may be a predictor of higher implant performance, which is an observation borne out in early studies of a national childhood cohort assembled by Geers and colleagues[46] (2000).

Osberger (2002) also found that children with more residual hearing were undergoing implantation relative to earlier cohorts. Gantz and colleagues[50] (2000) compiled data from across centers that indicate children with some degree of preoperative open-set speech recognition obtain substantially higher levels of speech comprehension. Taken together, these studies suggest the strongest potential for benefit exists with implantation at a young age, when intervention is provided early and, in the case of a progressive loss, before auditory input is lost completely.

Cheng and colleagues[24] (1999) performed a meta-analysis of relevant literature on speech recognition in children with cochlear implants. Of 1916 reports on cochlear implants published since 1966, 44 provided sufficient patient data to compare speech recognition results between published (n = 1904 children) and unpublished (n = 261) trials. Meta-analysis was complicated by the diversity of tests required to address the full spectrum of speech reception in implanted children. An expanded format of the Speech Perception Categories[51] was designed to integrate results across studies. The main conclusions of this meta-analysis were that earlier implantation is consistently associated with a greater trajectory of gain in speech-recognition performance with an absence of a plateau in speech-recognition benefits over time. More than 75% of the children with cochlear implants reported in peer-reviewed publications have achieved substantial open-set speech recognition after 3 years of implant use.

In an effort to provide the first reference for evaluating postimplant speech recognition in children with cochlear implants, Wang and colleagues[26] (2008) mapped the speech-recognition trajectory of implanted children from baseline up to the 24-month post–cochlear-implant evaluation (**Fig. 2**). The growth in speech-recognition development over the first 24 months after the implantation was spread widely among children with cochlear implants. A substantial number of children implanted at younger ages demonstrated growth patterns very similar in range or well into the trajectories of the normal-hearing children. A few children implanted at older ages showed slower trajectories of development after implantation. In contrast, the trajectories of speech-recognition development among normal-hearing children showed much less variability, forming a much tighter band of normal development.

LANGUAGE DEVELOPMENT IN CHILDREN

The above-mentioned studies have helped to characterize gains in speech recognition. However, the primary goal of implantation in children is to facilitate comprehension and expression through the use of spoken language.

By improving auditory access, cochlear implants augment sound and phrase structure. Although difficult to characterize, benefits in receptive language skills and language production after implantation are the crucial measure by which effectiveness of implants in young children should be assessed. One approach is to compare language performance on standardized tests.

The Reynell Developmental Language Scale evaluates both receptive and expressive skills independently.[52] These scales have been normalized by performance levels of hearing children over an age range of 1 to 8 years and have been used extensively in populations of children who are deaf. Children who are deaf without cochlear implants

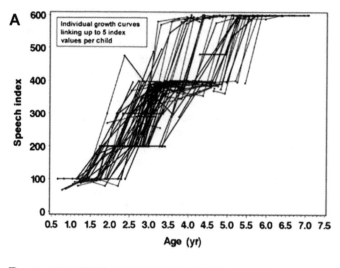

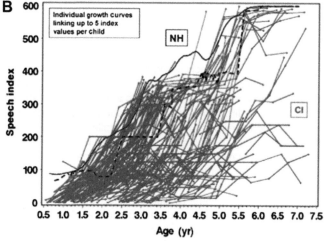

Fig. 2. Growth trajectories between baseline and 24-month follow-up visit using Speech recognition in quiet (SRI-Q) index for (A) 97 normal-hearing (NH) children in *black solid lines* and (B) 188 children with cochlear implants (CI) in *red solid lines*. The *black solid curve* (B) indicates the nonparametric mean trajectory of SRI-Q index by age for all 97 NH children. The *black dashed line* indicates the estimated lower boundary of SRI-Q score, by age, achieved by the NH children. (*Adapted from* Wang NY, Eisenberg LS, Johnson KC, et al. Tracking development of speech recognition: longitudinal data from hierarchical assessments in the Childhood Development after Cochlear Implantation Study. Otol Neurotol 2008;29(2):240–5; with permission.)

achieved language competence at half the rate of their normal-hearing peers, whereas implanted patients exhibited language-learning rates that matched, on average, those of their normal-hearing peers[52,53] (Niparko and colleagues,[54] 2010). In a study of 188 children deafened before 3 years of age assessed language development following cochlear implantation. The average age of implantation in this cohort was approximately 27 months. They found that cochlear implantation is consistently associated with a significant improvement in comprehension and expression of spoken language over the first 3 years of implant use. The development of spoken language was positively associated with younger age at implantation and greater residual hearing before implantation. The rate of improvement in performance on spoken-language measures was less steep in children undergoing cochlear implantation at later ages, with clinical gaps that persist with longitudinal follow-up (**Fig. 3**). The implication of this study is that cochlear implantation not only improves spoken-language expression and comprehension of children who are severely to profoundly deaf but does so early at a significantly increased rate in infants and toddlers.

In addition to younger ages at implantation, Moog and colleagues[55] (2010) found that early educational intervention is also associated with improvements in language development after cochlear implantation. The effect of this benefit was increased when implantation took place at younger ages. Moreover, a recent study by Geers and colleagues[56] (2009) showed that more than half of implanted children who used early educational intervention exhibited age-appropriate vocabulary scores by kindergarten.

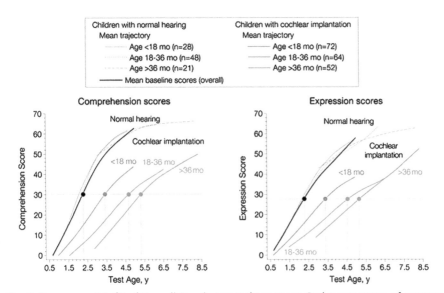

Fig. 3. Nonparametric fit of Reynell Developmental Language Scales raw scores of comprehension and expression stratified by age at baseline and test age. The effect of cochlear implantation in children on language development. The horizontal dotted line projects the chronologic age at which the mean scores of normal-hearing children at baseline (30.1 for comprehension and 27.6 for expression) were obtained by subgroups of children undergoing cochlear implantation at different ages. Vertical drop lines indicate ages at which this score was obtained for each group of children. On the comprehension scale, the ages were 2.3 years for normal-hearing children and among children undergoing cochlear implantation, 3.4 years for children younger than 18 months at implant, 4.7 years for those aged 18 to 36 months at implant, and 5.3 years for those older than 36 months at implant. On the expression scale, the ages were 2.3 years for hearing children and among children undergoing cochlear implantation, 3.4 years for children younger than 18 months at implant, 4.5 years for those aged 18 to 36 months at implant, and 5.2 years for those older than 36 months at implant. (*Adapted from* Niparko JK, Tobey EA, Thal DJ, et al. Spoken language development in children following cochlear implantation. JAMA 2010;303(15): 1498–506; with permission.)

From a communication perspective, Robbins and colleagues[52] (1997) noted that implantation improved language-learning rates for children in both oral- and total-communication settings based on the Reynell Developmental Language Scale. Geers and colleagues[46] (2000), also assessing language skills in implanted children enrolled in oral and total communication (TC) settings, found that the groups did not differ in language level, although the oral group demonstrated significantly better intelligibility in their speech production. Additionally, performance on language measures can be influenced by the child's mode of communication such that results may not directly reflect the influences of auditory perception or prosthetic intervention.[57,58] Clinical findings, however, support the hypothesis that some children who are deaf are able to use the acoustic-phonetic cues provided by the implant in ways that may reduce the language gap between normal-hearing and deaf children.

Central nervous system processing is a primary determinant of the level of verbal language ultimately attained after cochlear implantation. Pisoni and colleagues[59] (1995) assessed performance in 2 groups of pediatric cochlear implant users:

1. *Stars* were children whose Phonetically Balanced Kindergarten (PBK) test scores placed them in the top 20%.
2. The second group, children with scores in the bottom 20%, composed the control group.

Children with superior implant performance were consistently better on measures of speech perception (ie, vowel and consonant recognition), spoken-word recognition, comprehension, language development, and speech intelligibility than the control children. However, the two groups did not differ in their vocabulary knowledge, nonverbal intelligence, visual-motor integration, or visual attention. It was concluded that a star performance on measures of spoken-language processing and speech intelligibility was not caused by global differences in overall performance but to differences specifically in the task of processing auditory information provided by the cochlear implant. A strength-of-correlation analyses revealed a highly significant association between spoken-word recognition, language development, and speech intelligibility for the stars group but not for the control group. A star performance seemed to result from an increased ability to process language and to develop phonological and lexical representations for words.

Pisoni and colleagues[60] (2000) further posit that the exceptional performance of the stars seems to be caused by their superior abilities to perceive, encode, and retrieve information about spoken words from lexical memory. They described the capacity for processing tasks that require the manipulation and transformation of the phonological representations of spoken words as "working memory."

OUTCOMES AFTER COCHLEAR IMPLANTATION
Educational Placement and Support of Implanted Children

Children with hearing impairments are at substantial risk for educational under-achievement.[61,62] Educational achievement by children with hearing impairments can be enhanced by verbal communication, and traditional methods of speech instruction are more successful with children who have enough residual hearing to benefit from early devices of hearing rehabilitation.[63] Improved speech perception and production provided by cochlear implants offer the possibility of increased access to oral-based education and enhanced educational independence.

Koch and colleagues[64] (1997) and Francis and colleagues[65] (1999) tracked the educational progress of implanted children by using an educational resource matrix to map educational and rehabilitative resource use. The matrix was developed from observations that changes in classroom settings (eg, into a mainstream classroom) are often compensated by an initial increase in interpreter and speech-language therapy. A follow-up of 35 school-aged children with implants indicated that, relative to age-matched hearing-aid users with equivalent baseline hearing, implanted students are mainstreamed at a substantially higher rate, although this effect is not immediate and requires rehabilitative support to be achieved. Within 5 years after implantation, the rate of full-time assignment to a mainstream classroom increases from 12% to 75% (**Fig. 4**).

This greater rate of mainstream education in the implanted population has, in turn, led to increased benefits for implanted children. In one of the most comprehensive studies of the effects of educational placement on outcomes from cochlear implantation, Geers and colleagues[66] (2008) has followed a group of 85 patients from the elementary grades to high school. A battery of tests was used to assess student performance in speech perception, language, and reading. Speech-perception scores improved significantly with long-term cochlear implant use. Mean language scores improved at a faster-than-normal rate, but reading scores did not keep pace with normal development. Not surprisingly, oral communication at school (an educational

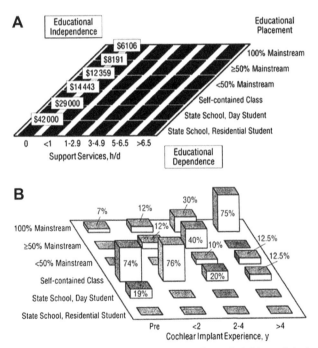

Fig. 4. Matrix of educational resources usage by implanted children. (*A*) The Educational Resource Matrix plot classroom placement (*ordinate*) versus rehabilitative (speech-language and interpretive) support (*abscissa*). (*B*) Relationship between educational placement and duration of implant experience. Patterns of change in use of educational resources in a cohort of children within 6 years of implantation. Note the higher levels of mainstreaming and reduced use of support services with prolonged use of the cochlear implant. (*Adapted from* Francis HW, Koch ME, Wyatt JR, et al. Trends in educational placement and cost-benefit considerations in children with cochlear implants. Arch Otolaryngol Head Neck Surg 1999;125(5):499–505; with permission.)

mode used in mainstream classes) contributed significantly to the improvement in the previously mentioned categories. However, the study observed that implant recipients achieving high scores on the previously mentioned tests in elementary school also continued performing better than the rest of the study population in high school, suggesting the presence of additional factors, such as nonverbal intelligence, influencing postimplantation outcomes.

Quality of Life and Cost-Effectiveness

Prior studies of the cost utility of cochlear implants have assessed quality of life and health status to determine the utility gained from cochlear implants.[67–70] Utility is a concept that reflects the true value of a good or service. Cost-utility methods determine the ratio of monetary expenditure to change in utility as defined by a change in quality of life over a given period. The assessment of cost utility is based on the following:

$$\text{Cost-utility} = \text{costs (in \$)}/\Delta(\text{quality-adjusted life-years})$$
$$= \text{costs (in \$)}/\Delta(\text{life-years} \times \text{health utility})$$

The term life-years is the mean anticipated number of years of implant experience based on a life-expectancy analysis of the participating cohort. The change in health utility reflects the difference between preimplant and postimplant scores on survey instruments that have been designed and validated to reflect quality of life. In the early 2000s, health interventions with a cost-utility ratio less than \$25 000 were generally considered to represent an acceptable value for the money expended (ie, they are cost-effective).[71–73] More recent studies in the United Kingdom have used a £30 000 (\$46 000) societal willingness-to-pay cutoff in the determination of cost-effective interventions in health care.[74]

STUDIES IN ADULTS AND THE ELDERLY

Costs per quality-adjusted life-year (QALY) for the cochlear implant in adult users were determined using cost data that account for the preoperative, postoperative, and operative phases of cochlear implantation.[67,68,70,75,76] Benefits were determined by the functional status and quality of life. The precise cost-utility results varied between studies mostly because of methodological differences in the determination of benefit, level of benefit obtained, and differences in costs associated with the intervention. Nonetheless, these appraisals consistently indicated that the multichannel cochlear implant in adult populations is associated with cost-utility ratios in the range of \$14 000 to \$16 000 per QALY for unilateral implantation in the United States, indicating a highly favorable position in terms of cost-effectiveness (**Table 1**). Moreover, recent studies have focused on evaluating the cost-effectiveness of bilateral cochlear implantation. Although not as cost-effective as the first implant, Bichey and colleagues[76] (2008) showed that bilateral cochlear implantation carried an incremental cost-utility ratio of \$38 198 per QALY in US adults and still ranks among the most cost-effective interventions in health care.

Hearing impairment is one of the most common clinical conditions affecting elderly people in the United States.[77] Hearing loss is so profound in 10% of the aged hearing-impaired population that little or no benefit is gained with conventional amplification.[78] Assessing the effectiveness of cochlear implants in the elderly requires consideration of both audiological and psychosocial factors. The social isolation associated with acquired hearing loss in the elderly[79] is accompanied by a significant decline in quality of life and an increase in emotional handicaps.[80] The rehabilitation of hearing loss is,

Table 1
Cost-utility ratio of the cochlear implant in adults and children

| | | | | Cost-Utility Ratio ($)/QALY | |
| | | | | Unilateral vs | Bilateral vs |
Study	Instrument	Country	Population	No CI	Unilateral CI
Summerfield et al,[74] 2010	TTO	United Kingdom	Children	34 824	37 100
	VAS			23 026	30 973
Bond et al,[70] 2009	HUI	United Kingdom	Children	25 519	70 470
	HUI		Adults	33 132	86 425
Bichey et al,[76] 2008	HUI	United States	Children	10 221	39 115
	HUI		Adults	11 092	38 189
Summerfield et al,[75] 2002	HUI	United Kingdom	Adults	45 215	118 387
Cheng et al,[69] 2000	TTO	United States	Children	9029	—
	VAS			7500	
	HUI			5197	
Palmer et al,[96] 1999	HUI	United States	Adults	14 670	—
Wyatt et al,[68] 1996	HUI	United States	Adults	15 928	—

Variability on cost-utility metrics is largely attributable to different methodologies of direct cost calculation across countries. A threshold of $25 000/QALY or lower is considered an acceptable cost-utility ratio for a given health intervention in the United States and Canada. A £30 000 ($46 000) willingness-to-pay threshold has been recently proposed as a cutoff threshold in the United Kingdom.

Abbreviations: CI, cochlear implant; HUI, Health Utilities Index; TTO, time trade-off; VAS, visual analog scale.

therefore, an important goal in this vulnerable population, providing both functional and psychological contributions to quality of life.

Age-related degeneration of the spiral ganglion[81,82] and progressive central auditory dysfunction[83,84] raise potential concerns about the efficacy of cochlear prostheses in the elderly. Comparable gains in speech understanding have been reported for both elderly and younger groups of implant recipients,[85] but the implications of these functional gains on the quality of life of older adults have not been well characterized. The determination of both auditory efficacy and quality of life is critical to any cost-benefit analysis in the elderly and may help guide clinical resource allocation, particularly in light of the high costs associated with cochlear implantation as a non–life-saving intervention.

Reports of quality-of-life gains in elderly patients with cochlear implants have been favorable[86–88] but are based on questionnaires that are difficult to correlate with function and cost utility. Francis and colleagues[14] (2002) evaluated 47 patients with multichannel cochlear implants, aged 50 to 80 years, who completed the Ontario Health Utilities Index Mark 3 (HUI 3) survey as well as a quality-of-life survey. This study assessed preimplantation and postimplantation (6 months and 1 year after implantation) responses to questions related to device use and quality of life. There was a significant mean gain in health utility of 0.24 (SD 0.33) associated with cochlear implantation ($P<.0001$) (**Fig. 5**). Improvements in hearing and emotional health attributes were primarily responsible for this increase in health-related quality-of-life measure. There was a significant increase in speech-perception scores at 6 months after surgery ($P<.0001$ for both the Central Institute for the Deaf (CID) everyday sentence and monosyllabic word tests) and a strong correlation between the magnitude of health-utility gains and postoperative enhancement of speech perception ($r = 0.45$, $P<.05$).

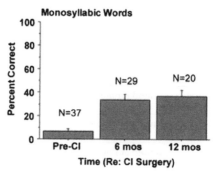

Fig. 5. Impact of cochlear implants (CI) on the functional health status of older adults. Mean monosyllabic word scores obtained in older adult patients with postlingual hearing impairment just before CI surgery and at 6 and 12 months afterward (error bar = 1 SE). Monosyllabic word scores, which are generally considered one of the most difficult tests of speech perception, clearly increase during the first year after CI. (*Adapted from* Francis HW, Chee N, Yeagle J, et al. Impact of cochlear implants on the functional health status of older adults. Laryngoscope 2002;112(8 Pt 1):1482–8; with permission.)

Speech-perception gain was also correlated with improvements in emotional status and the hours of daily implant use. The investigators concluded that cochlear implantation has a statistically significant and cost-effective impact on the quality of life of older patients who are deaf.

STUDIES IN CHILDREN

Published cost-utility analyses of the cochlear implant in children have been limited by using either health utilities obtained from adult patients[70,72,74–76,89] or hypothetically estimated utilities of a child who is deaf.[90–93] These studies yielded cost-utility ratios that spread out over a wide range ($3141 to $25 450 per QALY). Utility assessments derived from adult-patient surveys may not capture the impact of issues unique to childhood deafness.[24] To address this issue more rigorously, Cheng and colleagues[69] (2000) surveyed parents of 78 children (average age 7.4 years, with 1.9 years of cochlear implant use) who received multichannel implants at the Johns Hopkins Hospital to determine direct and total cost to society per QALY. Parents of children who were profoundly deaf (n = 48) awaiting cochlear implantation served as a comparison group to assess the validity of recall. Parents rated their child's health state now, immediately before, and 1 year before the cochlear implant using the time trade-off (TTO), visual analog scale (VAS), and HUI 3. Mean VAS scores increased 0.27 on a scale of 0 to 1 (from 0.59–0.86), TTO scores increased 0.22 (from 0.75–0.97), and HUI scores increased 0.39 (from 0.25–0.64) (**Fig. 6**). Discounted direct medical costs were $60 228, yielding cost-utility ratios of $9029 per QALY using the TTO, $7500 per QALY using the VAS, and $5197 per QALY using the HUI 3. Including indirect costs, such as reduced educational expenses, the cochlear implant yielded a calculated net savings of $53 198 per child. Based on assessments of this cohort based in a single center, childhood cochlear implantation produces a positive impact on quality of life at reasonable direct costs and results in societal savings.

The educational resource matrix used by Koch and colleagues[64] (1997) and Francis and colleagues[65] (1999) also offers a basis for assessing overall cost-benefit ratios. Although initial educational costs for implanted students remained static or increased

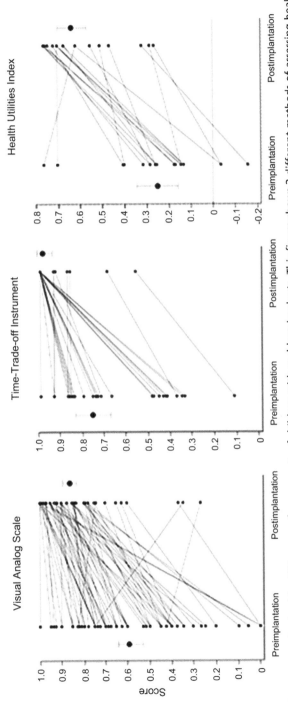

Fig. 6. Retrospective health utility scores from parents of children with cochlear implants. This figure shows 3 different methods of assessing health-utility scores. The mean change in utility (postintervention − preintervention scores) was 0.27 for the VAS, 0.22 for the TTO instrument, and 0.39 for the HUI 3. The error bars on the side of each graph show mean scores with 95% confidence intervals. (*Adapted from* Cheng AK, Rubin HR, Powe NR, et al. Cost-utility analysis of the cochlear implant in children. JAMA 2000;284(7):850–6; with permission.)

over the first 3 years, an ultimate achievement of educational independence for most implanted children produced net savings that ranged from $30 000 to $100 000 per child, including the costs associated with initial cochlear implantation and postoperative rehabilitation. Language- and education-related outcomes in children with cochlear implants have been supplemented with parental perspectives of quality-of-life effects to yield cost-utility ratings.[69,89] Even with conservative assumptions, both studies supported the view that cochlear implantation is, relative to other medical and surgical interventions, highly cost-effective in young children who are profoundly hearing impaired.

Recent trends in cost-effectiveness have aimed at analyzing the comparative effectiveness of pediatric cochlear implantation by the age at procedure. These studies have shown that younger ages at implantation are associated not only with more favorable auditory outcomes but also with lower direct and indirect costs.[45,94,95]

SUMMARY

Cochlear implants offer an option in the auditory rehabilitation of congenital, as well as acquired, profound SNHL for candidates across the age spectrum. Although a cochlear implant facilitates sensitive hearing reliably, actual listening capabilities are less easily characterized. Speech-recognition results are variable, and there is increasing awareness that epiphenomena surrounding implantation and the postimplant experience affect performance. Thus, expected results depend heavily on the environment in which cochlear implants are used as well as case selection. Children with early onset deafness lack a base of auditory memory with which to pair implant-mediated percepts and they may harbor other disabilities that may prevent instinctive language learning. Such conditions can produce a wide range of individual variability, particularly when intervention with a cochlear implant is delayed. Adults with cochlear implants exhibit a similarly wide range of results usually owing in large part to factors outside of the device per se. These facts mandate comprehensive pre-implant assessment. Screening for other handicapping conditions, particularly those that will impair the acquisition of receptive and productive communication skills, will help determine candidacy and direct rehabilitative strategies. By enabling simultaneous input of multiple perspectives, a multidisciplinary team is the most effective approach to assessing a candidate's needs and desires and the potential for an implant to meet them.

In the 1980s, candidacy requirements for a cochlear implant required total or near-total sensorineural hearing losses as characterized by a pure-tone average of 100 dB or greater, amplified thresholds that failed to reach 60 dB, and an absence of open-set speech recognition despite the use of powerful, best-fit hearing aids. Because clinical experience has indicated that the mean speech-reception scores of implant recipients generally exceed the aided results of individuals with lesser impairments, the audiologic criteria have been progressively relaxed over the past 30 years to include those with a range of pure-tone averages, focusing instead on functional benefits provided by amplification. In children, initial reports suggest that implantation before the age of 3 years provides distinct advantages over later implantation in cases of early onset deafness. Whether earlier implantation may yield greater benefits will require longitudinal follow-up of the development of the ever-younger infants undergoing implantation.

Additionally, postimplantation rehabilitation can be important for some adult implant recipients but seems critical for children to optimize the usefulness of an implant. It is often assumed that effective interactive skills and language comprehension directly result from the sensitivity with which sound is perceived through a cochlear implant.

However, hearing is not a sufficient condition for these higher skills, and there is a compelling rationale for a high priority to be placed on auditory rehabilitation to enhance fundamental skills in verbal communication.

REFERENCES

1. Kirk K. Assessing speech perception in children. In: Mendel L, Danhauer J, editors. Audiologic evaluation and management and speech perception assessment. San Diego (CA): Singular; 1997. p. 101–32.
2. Nilsson M, McCaw V, Soli S. Minimum speech test battery for adult cochlear implant users. User's manual. Los Angeles (CA): House Ear Institute; 1997.
3. Nilsson M, Soli SD, Sullivan JA. Development of the hearing in noise test for the measurement of speech reception thresholds in quiet and in noise. J Acoust Soc Am 1994;95(2):1085–99. Available at: http://www.ncbi.nlm.nih.gov/pubmed/ 8132902. Accessed November 18, 2011.
4. Lehiste I. Linguistic considerations in the study of speech intelligibility. J Acoust Soc Am 1959;31(3):280. Available at: http://link.aip.org/link/?JASMAN/31/280/1. Accessed January 23, 2012.
5. Peterson GE, Lehiste I. Revised CNC lists for auditory tests. J Speech Hear Disord 1962;27:62–70. Available at: http://www.ncbi.nlm.nih.gov/pubmed/14485785. Accessed January 23, 2012.
6. Gifford RH, Shallop JK, Peterson AM. Speech recognition materials and ceiling effects: considerations for cochlear implant programs. Audiol Neurootol 2008; 13(3):193–205. Available at: http://www.ncbi.nlm.nih.gov/pubmed/18212519. Accessed January 23, 2012.
7. Waltzman SB, Fisher SG, Niparko JK, et al. Predictors of postoperative performance with cochlear implants. Ann Otol Rhinol Laryngol Suppl 1995;165:15–8. Available at: http://www.ncbi.nlm.nih.gov/pubmed/7717629. Accessed January 24, 2012.
8. Rubinstein JT, Parkinson WS, Tyler RS, et al. Residual speech recognition and cochlear implant performance: effects of implantation criteria. Am J Otol 1999; 20(4):445–52. Available at: http://www.ncbi.nlm.nih.gov/pubmed/10431885. Accessed January 24, 2012.
9. Hamzavi J, Baumgartner WD, Pok SM, et al. Variables affecting speech perception in postlingually deaf adults following cochlear implantation. Acta Otolaryngol 2003;123(4):493–8. Available at: http://informahealthcare.com/doi/abs/10.1080/ 0036554021000028120. Accessed January 5, 2012.
10. Budenz CL, Cosetti MK, Coelho DH, et al. The effects of cochlear implantation on speech perception in older adults. J Am Geriatr Soc 2011;59(3):446–53. Available at: http://www.ncbi.nlm.nih.gov/pubmed/21361884. Accessed January 5, 2012.
11. Skinner MW, Fourakis MS, Holden TA, et al. Identification of speech by cochlear implant recipients with the multipeak (MPEAK) and spectral peak (SPEAK) speech coding strategies II. Consonants. Ear Hear 1999;20(6):443–60. Available at: http://www.ncbi.nlm.nih.gov/pubmed/10613383. Accessed January 24, 2012.
12. Cohen NL. Cochlear implant soft surgery: fact or fantasy? Otolaryngol Head Neck Surg 1997;117(3 Pt 1):214–6. Available at: http://www.ncbi.nlm.nih.gov/pubmed/ 9334767. Accessed January 23, 2012.
13. Shin YJ, Fraysse B, Deguine O, et al. Benefits of cochlear implantation in elderly patients. Otolaryngol Head Neck Surg 2000;122(4):602–6. Available at: http://oto. sagepub.com/content/122/4/602.full. Accessed January 24, 2012.

14. Francis HW, Chee N, Yeagle J, et al. Impact of cochlear implants on the functional health status of older adults. Laryngoscope 2002;112(8 Pt 1):1482–8. Available at: http://www.ncbi.nlm.nih.gov/pubmed/12172266. Accessed January 23, 2012.

15. Veronique Chatelin EK. Cochlear implant outcomes in the elderly. Cochlear Implants Int 2003;4(Suppl 1):55–6. Available at: http://www.ncbi.nlm.nih.gov/pubmed/18792178. Accessed January 23, 2012.

16. Haensel J, Ilgner J, Chen YS, et al. Speech perception in elderly patients following cochlear implantation. Acta Otolaryngol 2005;125(12):1272–6. Available at: http://www.ncbi.nlm.nih.gov/pubmed/16303673. Accessed January 5, 2012.

17. Friedland DR, Venick HS, Niparko JK. Choice of ear for cochlear implantation: the effect of history and residual hearing on predicted postoperative performance. Otol Neurotol 2003;24(4):582–9. Available at: http://www.ncbi.nlm.nih.gov/pubmed/12851549. Accessed January 24, 2012.

18. Leung J, Wang NY, Yeagle JD, et al. Predictive models for cochlear implantation in elderly candidates. Arch Otolaryngol Head Neck Surg 2005;131(12):1049–54. Available at: http://archotol.ama-assn.org/cgi/content/abstract/131/12/1049. Accessed January 23, 2012.

19. Roditi RE, Poissant SF, Bero EM, et al. A predictive model of cochlear implant performance in postlingually deafened adults. Otol Neurotol 2009;30(4):449–54. Available at: http://www.ncbi.nlm.nih.gov/pubmed/19415041. Accessed January 24, 2012.

20. Francis HW, Yeagle JD, Bowditch S, et al. Cochlear implant outcome is not influenced by the choice of ear. Ear Hear 2005;26(Suppl 4):7S–16S. Available at: http://www.ncbi.nlm.nih.gov/pubmed/16082263. Accessed January 5, 2012.

21. Wilson B. Cochlear implant technology. In: Niparko J, Kirk K, Mellon N, et al, editors. Cochlear implants: principles and practices. Philadelphia: Lippincott, Williams & Wilkins; 2000. p. 109–27.

22. Krueger B, Joseph G, Rost U, et al. Performance groups in adult cochlear implant users: speech perception results from 1984 until today. Otol Neurotol 2008;29(4):509–12. Available at: http://www.ncbi.nlm.nih.gov/pubmed/18520586. Accessed January 23, 2012.

23. NIH Consensus development statement: cochlear implants in adults and children. JAMA 1995;274:1955–61.

24. Cheng AK, Niparko JK. Cost-utility of the cochlear implant in adults: a meta-analysis. Arch Otolaryngol Head Neck Surg 1999;125(11):1214–8. Available at: http://www.ncbi.nlm.nih.gov/pubmed/10555692. Accessed January 5, 2012.

25. Yoon PJ. Pediatric cochlear implantation. Curr Opin Pediatr 2011;23(3):346–50. Available at: http://www.ncbi.nlm.nih.gov/pubmed/21572386. Accessed January 6, 2012.

26. Wang NY, Eisenberg LS, Johnson KC, et al. Tracking development of speech recognition: longitudinal data from hierarchical assessments in the Childhood Development after Cochlear Implantation Study. Otol Neurotol 2008;29(2):240–5. Available at: http://www.pubmedcentral.nih.gov/articlerender.fcgi?artid=2733235&tool=pmcentrez&rendertype=abstract. Accessed January 24, 2012.

27. Osberger MJ, Kalberer A, Zimmerman-Phillips S, et al. Speech perception results in children using the Clarion Multi-Strategy Cochlear Implant. Ann Otol Rhinol Laryngol Suppl 2000;185:75–7. Available at: http://www.ncbi.nlm.nih.gov/pubmed/11141014. Accessed January 23, 2012.

28. Kirk K. Challenges in the clinical investigation of cochlear implant outcomes. In: Niparko J, Kirk K, Mellon N, et al, editors. Cochlear implants: principles & practices. Philadelphia: Lippincott, Williams & Wilkins; 2000. p. 225–58.

29. Eisenberg LS, Johnson KC, Martinez AS, et al. Comprehensive evaluation of a child with an auditory brainstem implant. Otol Neurotol 2008;29(2):251–7. Available at: http://www.researchgate.net/publication/5821242_Comprehensive_evaluation_of_a_child_with_an_auditory_brainstem_implant. Accessed January 23, 2012.
30. House WF, Berliner KI, Eisenberg LS. Experiences with the cochlear implant in preschool children. Ann Otol Rhinol Laryngol 1983;92(6 Pt 1):587–92. Available at: http://www.ncbi.nlm.nih.gov/pubmed/6689257. Accessed January 23, 2012.
31. Miyamoto RT, Osberger MJ, Todd SL, et al. Variables affecting implant performance in children. Laryngoscope 1994;104(9):1120–4. Available at: http://www.ncbi.nlm.nih.gov/pubmed/8072359. Accessed January 23, 2012.
32. Fryauf-Bertschy H, Tyler RS, Kelsay DM, et al. Performance over time of congenitally deaf and postlingually deafened children using a multichannel cochlear implant. J Speech Hear Res 1992;35(4):913–20. Available at: http://www.mendeley.com/research/performance-time-congenitally-deaf-postlingually-deafened-children-using-multichannel-cochlear-implant/. Accessed January 23, 2012.
33. Waltzman SB, Cohen NL, Gomolin RH, et al. Long-term results of early cochlear implantation in congenitally and prelingually deafened children. Am J Otol 1994;15(Suppl 2):9–13. Available at: http://www.ncbi.nlm.nih.gov/pubmed/8572107. Accessed January 24, 2012.
34. Miyamoto RT, Osberger MJ, Robbins AM, et al. Prelingually deafened children's performance with the nucleus multichannel cochlear implant. Am J Otol 1993;14(5):437–45. Available at: http://www.ncbi.nlm.nih.gov/pubmed/8122704. Accessed January 23, 2012.
35. Gantz BJ, Tyler RS, Woodworth GG, et al. Results of multichannel cochlear implants in congenital and acquired prelingual deafness in children: five-year follow-up. Am J Otol 1994;15(Suppl 2):1–7. Available at: http://www.ncbi.nlm.nih.gov/pubmed/8572105. Accessed January 23, 2012.
36. Eisenberg LS, Johnson KC, Martinez AS, et al. Speech recognition at 1-year follow-up in the childhood development after cochlear implantation study: methods and preliminary findings. Audiol Neurotol 2006;11(4):259–68. Available at: http://www.mendeley.com/research/speech-recognition-1year-followup-childhood-development-after-cochlear-implantation-study-methods-preliminary-findings/. Accessed January 23, 2012.
37. Davidson LS, Geers AE, Blamey PJ, et al. Factors contributing to speech perception scores in long-term pediatric cochlear implant users. Ear Hear 2011;32(Suppl 1):19S–26S. Available at: http://www.pubmedcentral.nih.gov/articlerender.fcgi?artid=3187573&tool=pmcentrez&rendertype=abstract. Accessed January 24, 2012.
38. Beadle EA, McKinley DJ, Nikolopoulos TP, et al. Long-term functional outcomes and academic-occupational status in implanted children after 10 to 14 years of cochlear implant use. Otol Neurotol 2005;26(6):1152–60. Available at: http://www.ncbi.nlm.nih.gov/pubmed/16272934. Accessed January 24, 2012.
39. Uziel AS, Sillon M, Vieu A, et al. Ten-year follow-up of a consecutive series of children with multichannel cochlear implants. Otol Neurotol 2007;28(5):615–28. Available at: http://www.ncbi.nlm.nih.gov/pubmed/17667770. Accessed January 24, 2012.
40. O'Donoghue GM, Nikolopoulos TP, Archbold SM. Determinants of speech perception in children after cochlear implantation. Lancet 2000;356(9228):466–8. Available at: http://www.thelancet.com/journals/a/article/PIIS0140-6736(00http://www.thelancet.com/journals/a/article/PIIS0140-6736(00)02555-1/fulltext. Accessed January 23, 2012.

41. O'Neill C, O'Donoghue GM, Archbold SM, et al. Variations in gains in auditory performance from pediatric cochlear implantation. Otol Neurotol 2002;23(1): 44–8. Available at: http://www.ncbi.nlm.nih.gov/pubmed/11773845. Accessed January 23, 2012.

42. Zwolan TA, Zimmerman-Phillips S, Ashbaugh CJ, et al. Cochlear implantation of children with minimal open-set speech recognition skills. Ear Hear 1997;18(3): 240–51. Available at: http://www.ncbi.nlm.nih.gov/pubmed/9201459. Accessed January 24, 2012.

43. Meyer TA, Svirsky MA, Kirk KI, et al. Improvements in speech perception by children with profound prelingual hearing loss: effects of device, communication mode, and chronological age. J Speech Lang Hear Res 1998;41(4):846–58. Available at: http://www.ncbi.nlm.nih.gov/pubmed/9712131. Accessed January 23, 2012.

44. Zwolan TA, Ashbaugh CM, Alarfaj A, et al. Pediatric cochlear implant patient performance as a function of age at implantation. Otol Neurotol 2004;25(2): 112–20. Available at: http://www.ncbi.nlm.nih.gov/pubmed/15021769. Accessed January 24, 2012.

45. Manrique M, Cervera-Paz FJ, Huarte A, et al. Advantages of cochlear implantation in prelingual deaf children before 2 years of age when compared with later implantation. Laryngoscope 2004;114(8):1462–9. Available at: http://www.ncbi.nlm.nih.gov/pubmed/15280727. Accessed January 23, 2012.

46. Geers AE, Nicholas J, Tye-Murray N, et al. Effects of communication mode on skills of long-term cochlear implant users. Ann Otol Rhinol Laryngol Suppl 2000;185:89–92. Available at: http://www.ncbi.nlm.nih.gov/pubmed/11141021. Accessed January 23, 2012.

47. Fryauf-Bertschy H, Tyler RS, Kelsay DM, et al. Cochlear implant use by prelingually deafened children: the influences of age at implant and length of device use. J Speech Lang Hear Res 1997;40(1):183–99. Available at: http://jslhr.asha.org/cgi/content/abstract/40/1/183. Accessed January 23, 2012.

48. Vieu A, Mondain M, Blanchard K, et al. Influence of communication mode on speech intelligibility and syntactic structure of sentences in profoundly hearing impaired French children implanted between 5 and 9 years of age. Int J Pediatr Otorhinolaryngol 1998;44(1):15–22. Available at: http://www.ncbi.nlm.nih.gov/pubmed/9720675. Accessed January 24, 2012.

49. Osberger MJ, Zimmerman-Phillips S, Koch DB. Cochlear implant candidacy and performance trends in children. Ann Otol Rhinol Laryngol Suppl 2002;189:62–5. Available at: http://www.ncbi.nlm.nih.gov/pubmed/12018351. Accessed January 23, 2012.

50. Gantz BJ, Rubinstein JT, Tyler RS, et al. Long-term results of cochlear implants in children with residual hearing. Ann Otol Rhinol Laryngol Suppl 2000;185:33–6. Available at: http://www.ncbi.nlm.nih.gov/pubmed/11140995. Accessed January 23, 2012.

51. Geers AE, Moog JS. Predicting spoken language acquisition of profoundly hearing-impaired children. J Speech Hear Disord 1987;52(1):84–94. Available at: http://jshd.asha.org/cgi/content/abstract/52/1/84. Accessed January 23, 2012.

52. Robbins AM, Svirsky M, Kirk KI. Children with implants can speak, but can they communicate? Otolaryngol Head Neck Surg 1997;117(3 Pt 1):155–60. Available at: http://www.ncbi.nlm.nih.gov/pubmed/9334759. Accessed January 24, 2012.

53. Svirsky MA, Robbins AM, Kirk KI, et al. Language development in profoundly deaf children with cochlear implants. Psychol Sci 2000;11(2):153–8. Available at: http://www.ncbi.nlm.nih.gov/pubmed/11273423. Accessed January 24, 2012.

54. Niparko JK, Tobey EA, Thal DJ, et al. Spoken language development in children following cochlear implantation. JAMA 2010;303(15):1498–506. Available at: http://www.pubmedcentral.nih.gov/articlerender.fcgi?artid=3073449&tool=pm centrez&rendertype=abstract. Accessed January 23, 2012.
55. Moog JS, Geers AE. Early educational placement and later language outcomes for children with cochlear implants. Otol Neurotol 2010;31(8):1315–9. Available at: http://www.ncbi.nlm.nih.gov/pubmed/20729785. Accessed January 23, 2012.
56. Geers AE, Moog JS, Biedenstein J, et al. Spoken language scores of children using cochlear implants compared to hearing age-mates at school entry. J Deaf Stud Deaf Educ 2009;14(3):371–85. Available at: http://jdsde.oxford journals.org/cgi/content/abstract/14/3/371. Accessed June 20, 2011.
57. Levitt H, McGarr N, Geffner D. Development of language and communication skills in hearing-impaired children, vol. 26. Rockville (MD): ASHA Monogr; 1987. p. 1–158.
58. Moeller MP, Osberger MJ, Eccarius M. Language and learning skills of hearing-impaired students. Receptive language skills. ASHA Monogr 1986;23:41–53. Available at: http://www.ncbi.nlm.nih.gov/pubmed/3730031. Accessed January 23, 2012.
59. Kirk KI, Pisoni DB, Osberger MJ. Lexical effects on spoken word recognition by pediatric cochlear implant users. Ear Hear 1995;16(5):470–81. Available at: http://www.mendeley.com/research/lexical-effects-spoken-word-recognition-pediatric-cochlear-implant-users/. Accessed January 23, 2012.
60. Pisoni DB, Geers AE. Working memory in deaf children with cochlear implants: correlations between digit span and measures of spoken language processing. Ann Otol Rhinol Laryngol Suppl 2000;185:92–3. Available at: http://www.ncbi.nlm.nih.gov/pubmed/11141023. Accessed January 23, 2012.
61. Trybus RJ, Karchmer MA. School achievement scores of hearing impaired children: national data on achievement status and growth patterns. Am Ann Deaf 1977;122(2):62–9. Available at: http://www.ncbi.nlm.nih.gov/pubmed/868721. Accessed January 24, 2012.
62. Holt JA. Stanford achievement test, 8th edition: reading comprehension subgroup results. Am Ann Deaf 1996;138:172–5.
63. Geers AE, Moog JS. Evaluating the benefits of cochlear implants in an education setting. Am J Otol 1991;12(Suppl):116–25. Available at: http://www.ncbi.nlm.nih.gov/pubmed/2069172. Accessed January 23, 2012.
64. Koch ME, Wyatt JR, Francis HW, et al. A model of educational resource use by children with cochlear implants. Otolaryngol Head Neck Surg 1997;117(3 Pt 1): 174–9. Available at: http://www.ncbi.nlm.nih.gov/pubmed/9334762. Accessed January 23, 2012.
65. Francis HW, Koch ME, Wyatt JR, et al. Trends in educational placement and cost-benefit considerations in children with cochlear implants. Arch Otolaryngol Head Neck Surg 1999;125(5):499–505. Available at: http://www.ncbi.nlm.nih.gov/pubmed/10326806. Accessed January 25, 2012.
66. Geers A, Tobey E, Moog J, et al. Long-term outcomes of cochlear implantation in the preschool years: from elementary grades to high school. Int J Audiol 2008;47(Suppl 2):S21–30. Available at: http://www.ncbi.nlm.nih.gov/pubmed/19012109. Accessed July 13, 2011.
67. Summerfield A. Cochlear implantation in the UK 1990-1994: report by the MRC Institute of Hearing Research on the Evaluation of the National Cochlear Implant Programme: executive summary and synopsis. London: H.M.S.O; 1995.

Available at: http://www.worldcat.org/title/cochlear-implantation-in-the-uk-1990-1994-report-by-the-mrc-institute-of-hearing-research-on-the-evaluation-of-the-national-cochlear-implant-programme-executive-summary-and-synopsis/oclc/33897591. Accessed January 24, 2012.

68. Wyatt JR, Niparko JK, Rothman M, et al. Cost utility of the multichannel cochlear implants in 258 profoundly deaf individuals. Laryngoscope 1996;106(7):816–21. Available at: http://www.ncbi.nlm.nih.gov/pubmed/8667975. Accessed January 24, 2012.

69. Cheng AK, Rubin HR, Powe NR, et al. Cost-utility analysis of the cochlear implant in children. JAMA 2000;284(7):850–6. Available at: http://www.ncbi.nlm.nih.gov/pubmed/10938174. Accessed July 5, 2011.

70. Bond M, Mealing S, Anderson R, et al. The effectiveness and cost-effectiveness of cochlear implants for severe to profound deafness in children and adults: a systematic review and economic model. Health Technol Assess 2009;13(44):1–330. Available at: http://www.ncbi.nlm.nih.gov/pubmed/19799825. Accessed July 22, 2011.

71. Gold MR, Siegel JE, Russell LB, et al. Cost-effectiveness in health and medicine. New York: Oxford University Press; 1996.

72. Summerfield AQ, Marshall DH, Archbold S. Cost-effectiveness considerations in pediatric cochlear implantation. Am J Otol 1997;18(Suppl 6):S166–8. Available at: http://www.ncbi.nlm.nih.gov/pubmed/9391647. Accessed January 24, 2012.

73. Azimi NA, Welch HG. The effectiveness of cost-effectiveness analysis in containing costs. J Gen Intern Med 1998;13(10):664–9. Available at: http://www.pubmedcentral.nih.gov/articlerender.fcgi?artid=1500894&tool=pmcentrez&rendertype=abstract. Accessed January 24, 2012.

74. Summerfield AQ, Lovett RE, Bellenger H, et al. Estimates of the cost-effectiveness of pediatric bilateral cochlear implantation. Ear Hear 2010;31(5):611–24. Available at: http://www.ncbi.nlm.nih.gov/pubmed/20473177. Accessed January 24, 2012.

75. Summerfield AQ, Marshall DH, Barton GR, et al. A cost-utility scenario analysis of bilateral cochlear implantation. Arch Otolaryngol Head Neck Surg 2002;128(11):1255–62. Available at: http://www.ncbi.nlm.nih.gov/pubmed/12431166. Accessed July 5, 2011.

76. Bichey BG, Miyamoto RT. Outcomes in bilateral cochlear implantation. Otolaryngol Head Neck Surg 2008;138(5):655–61. Available at: http://www.ncbi.nlm.nih.gov/pubmed/18439474. Accessed October 10, 2011.

77. Campbell VA, Crews JE, Moriarty DG, et al. Surveillance for sensory impairment, activity limitation, and health-related quality of life among older adults - United States, 1993-1997. MMWR CDC Surveill Summ 1999;48:131–56.

78. Havlik R. Aging in the eighties, impaired senses for sound and light in persons age 65 years and over preliminary data from the supplement on aging to the public health. National Center for Health Statistics 1986. Accessed January 23, 2012.

79. Weinstein BE, Ventry IM. Hearing impairment and social isolation in the elderly. J Speech Hear Res 1982;25(4):593–9. Available at: http://jslhr.asha.org/cgi/content/abstract/25/4/593. Accessed January 24, 2012.

80. Mulrow CD, Aguilar C, Endicott JE, et al. Association between hearing impairment and the quality of life of elderly individuals. J Am Geriatr Soc 1990;38(1):45–50. Available at: http://www.ncbi.nlm.nih.gov/pubmed/2295767. Accessed January 23, 2012.

81. Otte J, Schunknecht HF, Kerr AG. Ganglion cell populations in normal and pathological human cochleae. Implications for cochlear implantation. Laryngoscope 1978;88(8 Pt 1):1231–46. Available at: http://www.ncbi.nlm.nih.gov/pubmed/672357. Accessed January 23, 2012.

82. Ng M, Niparko JK, Nager GT. Inner ear pathology in severe to profound sensori-neural hearing loss. In: Niparko JK, Kirk KI, Mellon NK, et al, editors. Cochlear implants: principles and practices. Philadelphia: Lippincott, Williams and Wilkins; 2000. p. 57–100.

83. Welsh LW, Welsh JJ, Healy MP. Central presbycusis. Laryngoscope 1985;95(2): 128–36. Available at: http://www.ncbi.nlm.nih.gov/pubmed/3968946. Accessed January 24, 2012.

84. Stach BA, Spretnjak ML, Jerger J. The prevalence of central presbyacusis in a clinical population. J Am Acad Audiol 1990;1(2):109–15. Available at: http://www.ncbi.nlm.nih.gov/pubmed/2132585. Accessed January 24, 2012.

85. Kelsall DC, Shallop JK, Burnelli T. Cochlear implantation in the elderly. Am J Otol 1995;16(5):609–15. Available at. http://www.ncbi.nlm.nih.gov/pubmed/8588665. Accessed January 23, 2012.

86. Horn KL, McMahon NB, McMahon DC, et al. Functional use of the Nucleus 22-channel cochlear implant in the elderly. Laryngoscope 1991;101(3):284–8. Available at: http://www.ncbi.nlm.nih.gov/pubmed/2000016. Accessed January 23, 2012.

87. Facer GW, Peterson AM, Brey RH. Cochlear implantation in the senior citizen age group using the Nucleus 22-channel device. Ann Otol Rhinol Laryngol Suppl 1995;166:187–90. Available at: http://www.mendeley.com/research/cochlear-implantation-senior-citizen-age-group-using-nucleus-22channel-device/. Accessed January 23, 2012.

88. Orabi AA, Mawman D, Al-Zoubi F, et al. Cochlear implant outcomes and quality of life in the elderly: Manchester experience over 13 years. Clin Otolaryngol 2006; 31(2):116–22. Available at: http://www.ncbi.nlm.nih.gov/pubmed/16620330. Accessed January 23, 2012.

89. O'Neill C. Cost-utility analysis of pediatric cochlear implantation. Laryngoscope 2000;110(7):1239. Available at: http://www.ncbi.nlm.nih.gov/pubmed/10646733. Accessed December 15, 2011.

90. Lea A. Cochlear implants. Health technology series, No. 6. Canberra (Australia): Australian Institute of Health; 1991.

91. Lea AR, Hailey DM. The cochlear implant. A technology for the profoundly deaf. Med Prog Technol 1995;21(1):47–52. Available at: http://www.ncbi.nlm.nih.gov/pubmed/7791692. Accessed January 23, 2012.

92. Hutton J, Politi C, Seeger T. Cost-effectiveness of cochlear implantation of children. A preliminary model for the UK. Adv Otorhinolaryngol 1995;50:201–6. Available at: http://www.ncbi.nlm.nih.gov/pubmed/7610962. Accessed January 24, 2012.

93. Carter R, Hailey D. Economic evaluation of the cochlear implant. Int J Technol Assess Health Care 1999;15(3):520–30. Available at: http://www.ncbi.nlm.nih.gov/pubmed/10874379. Accessed January 24, 2012.

94. Govaerts PJ, De Beukelaer C, Daemers K, et al. Outcome of cochlear implantation at different ages from 0 to 6 years. Otol Neurotol 2002;23(6):885–90. Available at: http://www.ncbi.nlm.nih.gov/pubmed/12438851.

95. Colletti L, Mandalà M, Shannon RV, et al. Estimated net saving to society from cochlear implantation in infants: a preliminary analysis. Laryngoscope 2011; 121(11):2455–60. Available at: http://www.ncbi.nlm.nih.gov/pubmed/22020896. Accessed December 15, 2011.

96. Palmer CS, Niparko JK, Wyatt J, Rothman M, de Lissovoy G. A Prospective Study of the Cost-Utility of the Multichannel Cochlear Implant. Arch Otolaryngol Head Neck Surg 1999;125(11):1221–8.

Evidence-Based Practice
Reflux in Sinusitis

Michael Lupa, MD, John M. DelGaudio, MD*

KEYWORDS

- Sinusitis • Reflux • Evidence base • Aerodigestive • Vagus nerve • Gastric acid

KEY POINTS

- There is a strong body of evidence showing a high prevalence of pharyngeal reflux events in patients with surgically refractory chronic rhinosinusitis (CRS).
- In medically refractory CRS, most studies show a high prevalence of pharyngeal reflux events.
- The studies looking directly at the value of treatment of reflux in patients with CRS show some benefit, although more powerful randomized studies are required for a more definitive conclusion.
- There is significant evidence for a link between postnasal drip symptomatology and the presence of pharyngeal reflux, with good evidence for empiric treatment of postnasal drip with proton-pump inhibitors.

OVERVIEW

Chronic rhinosinusitis (CRS) remains one of the most common health care problems in the United States.[1-3] The pathophysiology of the disease process is complex but involves inflammatory changes in the nasal and sinus mucosa, resulting in edema and obstruction. These changes in turn cause mucus stasis with subsequent infection.[4] The initiating insult causing these changes can be due to a variety of sources including viral infection, environmental pollutants, and immune-mediated processes such as environmental allergy or allergic fungal sinusitis. In addition, laryngopharyngeal reflux (LPR) has recently been implicated as a potential contributor to the pathophysiology of CRS. This concept is consistent with the widespread role extraesophageal reflux has been found to play in the pathophysiology of diseases throughout both the upper and lower aerodigestive tract.[1]

Department of Otolaryngology, Emory University Hospital Midtown, 550 Peachtree Street, 11th floor, Atlanta, GA 30308, USA
* Corresponding author.
E-mail address: jdelgau@emory.edu

Otolaryngol Clin N Am 45 (2012) 983–992
http://dx.doi.org/10.1016/j.otc.2012.06.004
0030-6665/12/$ – see front matter © 2012 Elsevier Inc. All rights reserved.

The exact mechanism by which LPR contributes to the pathophysiology of CRS is unclear. There are currently 3 main theories:

1. The first theory proposes direct exposure of the nasopharynx and nose to gastric acid. The acidic refluxate causes mucosal inflammation and impaired mucociliary clearance.[5]
2. The second proposed mechanism is through a vagus nerve–mediated reflex, which has been described to exist in the lower airway.[6] Evidence to support this concept is reported by Wong and colleagues,[7] who showed a tendency for an increase in nasal mucus production, nasal symptom scores, and to a lesser extent nasal inspiratory peak flow in subjects who had direct administration of both nasal saline and HCl-containing fluid at the level of the gastroesophageal junction.
3. The third mechanism involves a direct role of *Helicobacter pylori*. Koc and colleagues[8] found *H pylori* to be present in polyp tissue but not normal mucosa taken during surgery for concha bullosa, although the numbers were small. In another study, Morinaka and colleagues[9] found that 3 of 19 specimens from patients undergoing surgery for CRS contained *H pylori* by polymerase chain reaction. This study did not contain a nondiseased tissue comparison.

Whether one of these processes mediates the effects seen in CRS, alone or in combination, is still unclear, and further research is required.

EVIDENCE-BASED CLINICAL MANAGEMENT

Evidence for the role of LPR in the etiology of CRS comes mainly from research using multisensor pH-probe studies looking for the presence of acid in the esophagus, hypopharynx, and nasopharynx in patients with CRS. It is further derived from studies looking at the correlation of LPR and other associated sinonasal diseases such as postnasal drip (PND) and vasomotor rhinitis (VR), and from evidence concerning pediatric sinonasal disease.

Evidence from Pediatric Studies

Evidence for a relationship between gastroesophageal reflux (GER) and pediatric sinonasal disease comes from a variety of sources and study designs (**Table 1**). Carr and colleagues,[10] in a retrospective study of children younger than 2 years, reported a history of reflux in 42% of children undergoing adenoidectomy compared with 7% of children undergoing tympanostomy tube placement alone. The study was hampered by multiple inclusion criteria for the diagnosis of GER and few patients receiving pH studies for diagnosis. El-Serag and colleagues[11] retrospectively looked at a large cohort of children with and without a diagnosis of GER disease (GERD), and found a higher prevalence of sinusitis in the GERD group (4.2% vs 1.4%). The study was weakened by the lack of any standardized criteria for establishing a diagnosis of GERD (group inclusion was based on presence of reflux ICD-9 code) and the heterogeneous nature of the 2 groups (the GERD group was older).

Phipps and colleagues[12] looked at a cohort of patients with CRS refractory to medical therapy. The goal was to determine the prevalence of GERD in these patients with CRS using dual-sensor pH monitoring. In this cohort 63% of patients were diagnosed with GERD. Of those patients with GERD, 32% were found to have nasopharyngeal reflux (NPR). In patients who were diagnosed with GERD, reflux treatment was instituted, achieving a 79% improvement in sinusitis symptoms based on parental opinion. The investigators concluded that this cohort had a higher prevalence of GERD than would be expected for their population, and secondly that treatment improved

Table 1
Pediatric studies linking reflux to sinonasal disease

Authors,[Ref.] Year	Type	Size	Measurement	Result	EBM Level
Carr et al,[10] 2001	Case-control	194	Presence of GERD by gastric scintiscan, pH probe, or reflux on barium swallow	42% GERD in adenoidectomy group vs 7% in the PE tube group	2b
El-Serag et al,[11] 2001	Case-control	9900	Presence of sinusitis and other upper airway diseases in patients with or without a diagnosis of GERD	4.2% sinusitis in GERD group vs 1.4% sinusitis in the non-GERD group	3b
Phipps et al,[12] 2000	Prospective cohort	30	Percentage of CRS patients with GERD	63% of CRS patients had GERD by dual-channel pH monitor	4
Contencin et al,[13] 1991	Prospective case-control	31	Presence of nasopharyngeal reflux in patients with sinonasal disease vs control	Significantly more time spent with pH below threshold in the sinonasal disease group, $P<.00005$	2b
Megale et al,[14] 2006	Retrospective case series	45	Percentage of patients with GERD and sinonasal complaints who respond to antireflux therapy	83.87% improvement in chronic nasal obstruction, and 85.7% in nasal secretions	4
Bothwell et al,[15] 1999	Retrospective cohort	28	Avoidance of surgery if treated for GERD	83% of patients in study successfully avoided surgery	4

Abbreviations: CRS, chronic rhinosinusitis; EBM, evidence-based medicine; GERD, gastroesophageal reflux disease; PE, pressure equalization.

patients' sinusitis symptoms. Their study is hampered by the lack of a control group. Contencin and Narcy[13] evaluated 31 children for the presence of NPR by performing 24-hour nasopharyngeal pH studies. The study group consisted of 13 children with recurrent or chronic rhinitis or rhinopharyngitis. The control group of 18 children was free of any nasopharyngeal disease. The study group was found to have significantly more time in the nasopharynx with a pH below the threshold (pH less than 6). Because a single-channel pH monitor was used in this study, it was impossible to determine whether some of the reflux events were nasopharyngeal reflux of gastric contents or artifact.

Other pediatric studies looked directly at the results of treating reflux in the presence of sinonasal disease. Megale and colleagues[14] retrospectively looked at a cohort of children diagnosed with GERD by single-probe pH monitor and history. This study evaluated patients' response to treatment with antireflux interventions including prokinetic agents, proton-pump inhibitor (PPI) therapy, and reflux surgeries. Therapy for GERD significantly improved the symptoms of chronic nasal obstruction and nasal secretion by 83.87% and 85.7%, respectively. Unfortunately, about half the number of the treated patients with these complaints also received antihistamine therapy at the same time as the antireflux medication, therefore confounding the result. This confounder, in addition to the lack of a control group in the study design, greatly weakens the strength of the results. Bothwell and colleagues[15] looked retrospectively at a cohort of pediatric patients who had met the criteria to undergo functional endoscopic sinus surgery (ESS) for CRS. It was found that in patients treated with a variety of different antireflux therapies, sinus surgery could be avoided in 89% of patients.

Evidence from Studies Looking at Associated Sinonasal Disorders

Studies looking at the relationship between reflux and other inflammatory sinonasal disorders also allude to the role of reflux in creating, or contributing to, an environment conducive to the presence of sinusitis (**Table 2**). Loehrl and colleagues[16] sought to look at the relationship between extraesophageal reflux (EER) and VR, which was defined by the symptom of nasal congestion for at least 3 months without any signs of current infection, pregnancy, nasal polyps, or allergy. The study included 3 groups: patients with VR without EER, patients with VR with EER (by history and physical examination), and normal controls without VR. The amount of reflux was documented by 4 sensor pH probes in all groups. The amount of autonomic dysfunction present in each group was also measured using the composite autonomic scoring scale (CASS). The group with VR with EER by history and physical examination had a higher CASS score than both the VR-free control group and the VR-alone group. The investigators further confirmed the presence of EER via a 4-sensor pH study, finding that the VR-with-EER group had nasopharyngeal reflux events present in 9 of 10 patients. This study shows that EER can change the environment in the sinonasal cavity, in this case by altering the body's autonomic response.

Other investigators have looked at the relationship between the patient complaint of PND and reflux. Wise and colleagues[17] looked at the relationship between PND, defined as an increased awareness of the movement of the pharyngeal mucus blanket, and LPR in a cohort of 68 patients. These patients were first asked to complete both the validated SNOT-20 questionnaire and the modified Reflux Symptoms Index questionnaire, and then underwent 24-hour pH testing with a triple-sensor pH probe. The pH probe had sensors at the nasopharynx, hypopharynx (1 cm above the upper esophageal sphincter), and distal esophagus. The investigators found that in patients with nasopharyngeal reflux events with a pH less than 5, there were significantly more PND symptoms reported on the SNOT-20 and the modified

Table 2
Studies linking reflux to related sinonasal disorders

Authors,[Ref.] Year	Type	Size	Measurement	Result	EBM Level
Loehrl et al,[16] 2002	Case-control	30	Prevalence of autonomic dysfunction in VR patients with or without EER and normal controls	Significantly increased autonomic dysfunction in VR patients with EER compared with those without EER	2b
Wise et al,[17] 2006	Cohort	68	Association between PND symptoms and the presence of NPR and LPR by 3-channel pH probe	Significantly more PND symptoms in patients with NPR and LPR	4
Vaezi et al,[18] 2010	Randomized controlled trial	75	Improvement in PND symptoms following treatment with lansoprazole	Significantly greater percentage improvement in the treatment arm vs control	1b

Abbreviations: EER, extraesophageal reflux; LPR, laryngopharyngeal reflux; NPR, nasopharyngeal reflux; PND, postnasal drip; VR, vasomotor rhinitis.

Reflux Symptom Index survey, compared with patients without reflux in this area. Patients with LPR also had more PND symptoms on the SNOT-20 survey when compared with patients without LPR.

Vaezi and colleagues[18] asked the question of whether directly treating reflux would improve patients' PND symptoms. To answer this question they performed a double-blinded study on 75 patients with complaints of PND without any signs of chronic sinusitis or allergy, randomizing them to either twice-daily lansoprazole or placebo. Patients completed validated sinus disease questionnaires (SNOT-20 and RSOM-31) and the Quality Of Life in Reflux And Dyspepsia questionnaires (QOLRAD) and underwent ambulatory pH and impedance monitoring before the institution of therapy. This pretreatment pH monitoring was performed in only 65% of participants but in equal amounts for each of the study groups. The primary outcome measure was a visual analog scale describing the percentage resolution of the PND sensation. Patients were then followed up after 8 and 16 weeks of therapy. Patients given lanso-prazole therapy had a 3.12-fold greater (at 8 weeks of therapy) and 3.5-fold greater (at 16 weeks of therapy) chance of improving compared with controls. At 16 weeks the median improvement in the treatment arm was 50% compared with 5% in the placebo arm. In addition, there was a statistically significant improvement in the SNOT-20 and QOLRAD outcomes for the treatment arm. Of note, no link was reported between the presence of reflux on pH study and the response to treatment. The technique used, however, only assessed the presence of reflux into the esophagus and not into the nasopharynx. The investigators state that the study results do support a role for reflux in causing PND symptoms in this group of patients, but comment that alternative causes for the benefit seen may come from possible intrinsic anti-inflammatory properties of the PPI drugs and a putative decrease in nonacid reflux created by PPI drugs.[18]

Evidence from Adults with CRS

Several studies have looked directly at the relationship between reflux and CRS (**Table 3**). Ulualp and colleagues[19] evaluated a diverse group of patients with upper airway and sinonasal complaints, and found a statistically higher incidence of hypo-pharyngeal acid reflux events in patients with both persistent CRS after sinus surgery and posterior laryngitis (4 of 6 patients, 67%) compared with healthy controls (7 of 34, 21%) or with patients with CRS without posterior laryngitis (4 of 12, 33%). There was no difference between the distal and proximal esophageal reflux parameters between these groups. The investigators concluded that LPR may play a role in a subset of patients with CRS, and posterior laryngitis may be the common thread among reflux-induced aerodigestive tract disorders. The small number of sinusitis patients is a drawback of this study. Ulualp's group[20] also looked directly at a cohort of 11 patients with medically refractory CRS, and found a higher prevalence of pharyngeal acid reflux compared with a group of 11 healthy controls (7 of 11, 64% vs 2 of 11, 18%). A study by Jecker and colleagues[21] evaluated 20 patients with CRS who had previously failed surgical therapy, and compared them with a group of normal controls. In these patients dual-sensor pH readings were obtained 6 weeks after the patients' revision sinus surgery. The CRS patients had a higher number of reflux events and percentage of time with pH spent below 4 in comparison with the control group. These results, interestingly, were not found in the hypopharynx. The investigators concluded that there was a link between GERD and CRS but not between EER and CRS. This study was hampered by its small size and heterogeneous groups.

Ozmen and colleagues[22] conducted a prospective case-control study with 33 patients recruited for ESS because of CRS unresponsive to medical therapy, and

Table 3
Adult studies linking CRS to reflux

Authors,[Ref.] Year	Type	Size	Measurement	Result	EBM Level
Ulualp et al,[19] 1999	Case-control	18	Presence of proximal reflux by 3-channel pH probe in patients who failed sinus surgery	Higher percentage of reflux in CRS patients with laryngitis and CRS patients alone compared with controls	2b
Ulualp et al,[20] 1999	Case-control	22	Presence of proximal reflux by 3-channel pH probe in patients with medically refractory CRS	Higher percentage of reflux in CRS patients compared with controls	2b
Jecker et al,[21] 2005	Case-control	40	Presence of LPR or GERD by dual-channel pH probe	Significantly more GER events in the CRS patients than in controls, but not in hypopharynx	2b
Ozmen et al,[22] 2008	Case-control	52	Presence of LPR by dual-channel pH probe and presence of pepsin in middle meatus aspirate	More pharyngeal acid events in CRS group; 88% vs 55%, pepsin was found in most patients with reflux	2b
DelGaudio,[4] 2005	Case-control	68	Presence of NPR, reflux at UES or GERD by 3-channel pH probe	Significantly more reflux events in the NP, UES, and LES in the CRS group compared with successful treatment and controls	2b
Wong et al,[23] 2004	Cohort	37	Presence of acid reflux into the nasopharynx by 4-channel pH probe in CRS patients failing medical therapy	Found nasopharyngeal reflux in only 2 of 37 patients (5%); GER was found in 12 of 37 patients (32.4%)	4
DiBaise et al,[24] 2002	Cohort	11	Response to twice daily PPI therapy in patients with CRS	Modest symptom improvement	2b
Pincus et al,[25] 2006	Cohort	15	Response to daily PPI therapy in patients with medically and surgically refractory CRS	Modest symptom improvement	4

Abbreviations: GER, gastroesophageal reflux; LES, lower esophageal sphincter; NP, nasopharynx; PPI, proton-pump inhibitor; UES, upper esophageal sphincter.

compared them with a group of 20 patients without CRS who were to undergo sinus and nasal surgery for endonasal anatomic variations (concha bullosa or other endonasal deformities). Using a dual-channel pH probe, they found that there was a higher incidence of pharyngeal acid reflux events in patients with CRS (29 of 33, 88%) when compared with controls (11 of 20, 55%). This difference was found to be statistically significant. In addition, they looked at the relationship between the presence of pepsin in sinonasal tissue and the presence of LPR as determined by the pH studies. To determine the presence of pepsin in the sinonasal tissues, 3 mL of saline was administered into the middle meatus of each patient under endoscopic guidance. The collected fluid was then subjected to a pepsin assay. In all patients with pepsin present LPR was documented by pH study, with only 3 patients with LPR having a negative pepsin assay. Of note, 50% of the control patients were found to have pepsin in the middle meatus by the pepsin assay. The investigators suggest that pepsin may be a good indicator for the presence of LPR and may play an etiologic role in the relationship between LPR and CRS, given that pepsin activity can be present at pH levels greater than 4.[22]

DelGaudio[4] looked at a cohort of 38 patients with a history of CRS who had failed surgical therapy and had persistent CRS symptoms and endoscopic signs of inflammation, and compared them with a group of patients who had undergone ESS and were symptom-free for at least 1 year postoperatively, and with a control group with no history of CRS or sinus surgery. Using 3-channel pH probes, significantly more nasopharyngeal reflux (NPR) was found in the persistent CRS group than in the 2 control groups, at pH less than 4 (39% vs 7%) and pH less than 5 (76% vs 24%). The CRS patients also had statistically significantly more reflux above the upper esophageal sphincter as well as in the distal esophagus in comparison with the pooled control groups. In addition, the difference between the groups increased further when the CRS patients with frontal sinus disease alone were excluded from the analysis.

Wong and colleagues[23] evaluated patients with CRS refractory to medical treatment and were candidates for ESS. This study evaluated 40 patients and tested them using 4-channel pH probes, including a nasopharyngeal sensor. Little nasopharyngeal reflux was found to be present in this group of patients. In comparison with the study by DelGaudio, whose study group consisted of surgically refractory CRS patients, the study group in the Wong study consisted of medically refractory CRS patients only. This group would most closely correlate to the successful ESS control group in the DelGaudio study, which had much less nasopharyngeal reflux than the study group. In addition, the Wong study only evaluated for pH less than 4, and not pH less than 5, thereby likely missing a substantial number of nasopharyngeal reflux events.

EVIDENCE-BASED MEDICAL MANAGEMENT

Evidence for the value of GERD treatment in improving CRS comes from studies of associated disorders such as that performed by Vaezi and colleagues[18] for PND, and from pediatric studies such as those performed by Bothwell and colleagues[15] and Megale and colleagues[14] already discussed. There are also a limited number of studies looking at the efficacy of GERD treatment in adults with CRS. DiBaise and colleagues[24] performed a prospective study on 11 patients who had failed both medical and surgical therapy for CRS, comparing this cohort with a group of GERD patients without CRS. All subjects underwent 2-channel pH studies and obtained baseline symptom severity scores. A similar percentage of abnormal pH tests between the 2 groups (82% in the CRS group and 79% in the GERD group) was found. The CRS group was then begun on twice-daily omeprazole and was reassessed symptomatically at 4, 8, and 12 weeks of therapy. There was modest improvement in patients' CRS symptoms, as well as overall satisfaction, with treatment. Dramatic improvement in CRS symptoms in this study was infrequent. Though encouraging, this study does lack a control group and is hampered by small numbers.

In a study by Pincus and colleagues,[25] the prevalence of GERD in patients with medically and surgically refractory CRS was evaluated by pH study, followed by treatment with PPIs. The main outcome measure was symptoms severity as recorded by phone interview after 1 month of treatment. Twenty-five of the 30 patients who underwent pH-probe evaluation had reflux. Fourteen of 15 patients who completed the course of PPIs had improvement in their symptoms. These improved patients included 7 who experienced a complete or near complete resolution in their symptoms. Again this study was an uncontrolled cohort study, and further study looking at the value of treatment of GERD for CRS is necessary.

SUMMARY

There is moderate evidence linking reflux to CRS. The means whereby this relationship takes place is likely direct reflux of gastric contents into the nasopharynx and nasal cavity. There is evidence for the use of reflux therapy in the treatment of medically and surgically refractory CRS. The strongest evidence for the use of PPI comes not from the treatment of CRS but from the treatment of PND via the randomized controlled study performed by Vaezi and colleagues[18] (Evidence-Based Medicine [EBM] Grade 1b). Overall EBM is Grade B.

REFERENCES

1. Lindstrom DR, Wallace J, Loehrl TA, et al. Nissen fundoplication surgery for extra-esophageal manifestations of gastroesophageal reflux (EER). Laryngoscope 2002;112(10):1762–5.
2. Ylitalo R, Ramel S, Hammarlund B, et al. Prevalence of extraesophageal reflux in patients with symptoms of gastroesophageal reflux. Otolaryngol Head Neck Surg 2004;131(1):29–33.
3. Benninger MS, Ferguson BJ, Hadley JA, et al. Adult chronic rhinosinusitis: definitions, diagnosis, epidemiology, and pathophysiology. Otolaryngol Head Neck Surg 2003;129(Suppl 3):S1–32.
4. DelGaudio JM. Direct nasopharyngeal reflux of gastric acid is a contributing factor in refractory chronic rhinosinusitis. Laryngoscope 2005;115(6):946–57.
5. Delehaye E, Dore MP, Bozzo C, et al. Correlation between nasal mucociliary clearance time and gastroesophageal reflux disease: our experience on 50 patients. Auris Nasus Larynx 2009;36(2):157–61.
6. Lodi U, Harding SM, Coghlan HC, et al. Autonomic regulation in asthmatics with gastroesophageal reflux. Chest 1997;111(1):65–70.
7. Wong IW, Rees G, Greiff L, et al. Gastroesophageal reflux disease and chronic sinusitis: in search of an esophageal-nasal reflex. Am J Rhinol Allergy 2010; 24(4):255–9.
8. Koc C, Arikan OK, Atasoy P, et al. Prevalence of *Helicobacter pylori* in patients with nasal polyps: a preliminary report. Laryngoscope 2004;114(11):1941–4.
9. Morinaka S, Ichimiya M, Nakamura H. Detection of *Helicobacter pylori* in nasal and maxillary sinus specimens from patients with chronic sinusitis. Laryngoscope 2003;113(9):1557–63.
10. Carr MM, Poje CP, Ehrig D, et al. Incidence of reflux in young children undergoing adenoidectomy. Laryngoscope 2001;111(12):2170–2.

11. El-Serag HB, Gilger M, Kuebeler M, et al. Extraesophageal associations of gastroesophageal reflux disease in children without neurologic defects. Gastroenterology 2001;121(6):1294–9.
12. Phipps CD, Wood WE, Gibson WS, et al. Gastroesophageal reflux contributing to chronic sinus disease in children: a prospective analysis. Arch Otolaryngol Head Neck Surg 2000;126(7):831–6.
13. Contencin P, Narcy P. Nasopharyngeal pH monitoring in infants and children with chronic rhinopharyngitis. Int J Pediatr Otorhinolaryngol 1991;22(3):249–56.
14. Megale SR, Scanavini AB, Andrade EC, et al. Gastroesophageal reflux disease: its importance in ear, nose, and throat practice. Int J Pediatr Otorhinolaryngol 2006;70(1):81–8.
15. Bothwell MR, Parsons DS, Talbot A, et al. Outcome of reflux therapy on pediatric chronic sinusitis. Otolaryngol Head Neck Surg 1999;121(3):255–62.
16. Loehrl TA, Smith TL, Darling RJ, et al. Autonomic dysfunction, vasomotor rhinitis, and extraesophageal manifestations of gastroesophageal reflux. Otolaryngol Head Neck Surg 2002;126(4):382–7.
17. Wise SK, Wise JC, DelGaudio JM. Association of nasopharyngeal and laryngopharyngeal reflux with postnasal drip symptomatology in patients with and without rhinosinusitis. Am J Rhinol 2006;20(3):283–9.
18. Vaezi MF, Hagaman DD, Slaughter JC, et al. Proton pump inhibitor therapy improves symptoms in postnasal drainage. Gastroenterology 2010;139(6): 1887–1893.e1 [quiz: e11].
19. Ulualp SO, Toohill RJ, Shaker R. Pharyngeal acid reflux in patients with single and multiple otolaryngologic disorders. Otolaryngol Head Neck Surg 1999;121(6): 725–30.
20. Ulualp SO, Toohill RJ, Hoffmann R, et al. Possible relationship of gastroesophagopharyngeal acid reflux with pathogenesis of chronic sinusitis. Am J Rhinol 1999;13(3):197–202.
21. Jecker P, Orloff LA, Wohlfeil M, et al. Gastroesophageal reflux disease (GERD), extraesophageal reflux (EER) and recurrent chronic rhinosinusitis. Eur Arch Otorhinolaryngol 2006;263(7):664–7.
22. Ozmen S, Yucel OT, Sinici I, et al. Nasal pepsin assay and pH monitoring in chronic rhinosinusitis. Laryngoscope 2008;118(5):890–4.
23. Wong IW, Omari TI, Myers JC, et al. Nasopharyngeal pH monitoring in chronic sinusitis patients using a novel 4 channel probe. Laryngoscope 2004;114(9): 1582–5.
24. DiBaise JK, Olusola BF, Huerter JV, et al. Role of GERD in chronic resistant sinusitis: a prospective, open label, pilot trial. Am J Gastroenterol 2002;97(4):843–50.
25. Pincus RL, Kim HH, Silvers S, et al. A study of the link between gastric reflux and chronic sinusitis in adults. Ear Nose Throat J 2006;85(3):174–8.

Evidence-Based Practice
Balloon Catheter Dilation in Rhinology

Pete S. Batra, MD, FACS

KEYWORDS

- Chronic rhinosinusitis • Frontal sinusitis • Recurrent acute rhinosinusitis • Evidence
- Balloon dilation • Balloon catheter • Technology • Sinus ostia dilation

KEY POINTS

The following points list the level of evidence as based on Oxford Center for Evidence-Based Medicine. Additional critical points are provided and points here are expanded at the conclusion of this article.

- Numerous studies have evaluated the usefulness of balloon catheter technology for surgical management of adult CRS, with overarching existing data deemed to be level 4.
- One study reporting the use of BCD for frontal sinus disease provides level 2b evidence, suggesting possible usefulness of the technology for this indication.
- Level 4 evidence is available for the use of BCD in the office and intensive care unit setting, although both may represent potentially important applications of balloon devices.
- The overall recommendation is grade C for use of BCD for paranasal sinus inflammatory disease, but well-controlled randomized trials are needed.

BACKGROUND ON CHRONIC RHINOSINUSITIS

Chronic rhinosinusitis (CRS) represents a clinical disorder characterized by inflammation of the mucosa of the nose and paranasal sinuses of 12 weeks' duration.[1] A European Position Paper on Rhinosinusitis and Nasal Polyposis clinically defines CRS by 2 or more symptoms, 1 of which is nasal blockage/obstruction/congestion or nasal discharge with or without facial pain/pressure and/or reduction or loss of smell.[2] Symptomatology is supported by endoscopic evidence of mucopurulence, edema, or polyps, and/or computed tomography (CT), presence of mucosal thickening, or air-fluid levels in the sinuses. CRS is one of the most common chronic medical

Disclosures: Medtronic (research grant), American Rhinologic Society (research grant).
Department of Otolaryngology – Head and Neck Surgery, Comprehensive Skull Base Program, University of Texas Southwestern Medical Center, 5323 Harry Hines Boulevard, Dallas, TX 75390, USA
E-mail address: pete.batra@utsouthwestern.edu

Otolaryngol Clin N Am 45 (2012) 993–1004
http://dx.doi.org/10.1016/j.otc.2012.06.005
0030-6665/12/$ – see front matter © 2012 Elsevier Inc. All rights reserved.

conditions in the United States, afflicting approximately 31 million Americans.[3] The illness accounts for 18 million to 22 million office visits annually, resulting in an estimated $6 billion in direct and indirect health care expenditures.[4] CRS not only causes physical symptoms but also results in significant functional and emotional impairment, with quality of life scores similar to those of patients with other chronic debilitating illnesses, including congestive heart failure, angina, and back pain.[5] The pathophysiologic mechanisms resulting in CRS remain elusive. A variety of host and environmental factors have been implicated, including derangements in innate and adaptive immunity, ciliary dysfunction, inhalant allergies, infectious agents (viral, bacterial, and/or fungal), superantigens, biofilms, and osteitis.

Medical therapy remains the cornerstone in the overall management schema of patients with CRS. This therapy typically entails various oral and topical agents, such as antibiotics, steroids, antihistamines, leukotriene receptor antagonists, saline irrigations, and mucolytics.

Functional endoscopic sinus surgery (FESS) represents the main surgical strategy for management of medically recalcitrant CRS. FESS is a minimally invasive, mucosal-sparing surgical technique that is designed to achieve 1 or more of the following goals:

1. Open the sinuses to facilitate ventilation and drainage
2. Remove polyps and/or osteitic bone fragments to reduce the inflammatory load
3. Enlarge the sinus ostia to achieve optimal instillation of topical therapies
4. Obtain bacterial and fungal cultures and tissue for histopathology

FESS has been shown to be effective in improving symptoms and quality of life (QOL) in adult patients with CRS.[6] A recent multi-institutional prospective trial showed improvement in QOL in both medically and surgically treated patients with CRS; however, the FESS group experienced significantly more improvement in disease-specific QOL, reduction in need for systemic antibiotics and steroids, and decrease in missed work/school days.[7]

OVERVIEW OF BALLOON CATHETER TECHNOLOGIES
Balloon Sinuplasty TM

The use of balloon catheters for frontal sinus dilation was initially described by Lanza[8] in 1993. He used Fogarty balloon catheters under endoscopic guidance in post-FESS patients to achieve temporary ventilation and drainage of the frontal recess. In 2002, California-based engineers started the process of adapting cardiac catheters to perform paranasal sinus balloon dilation.[9] Balloon catheter technology cleared the US Food and Drug Administration (FDA) 510(k) pathway in April 2005, being launched as balloon sinuplasty (Acclarent, Inc., Menlo Park, CA).[10] In contrast with traditional balloons that are compliant and conform to regional anatomy, the new device is semi-rigid and noncompliant, with the ability to displace adjacent bone and tissue on inflation. The basic premise of balloon catheter dilation (BCD) is the Seldinger technique, with initial access being gained by endoscopic placement of a guide catheter. A flexible guide is introduced through the guide catheter and its position in the targeted sinus confirmed by fluoroscopy, transillumination, or image guidance. The balloon catheter is then advanced over the guidewire and gradually inflated to dilate the obstructed sinus ostium.[10]

The initial cadaver study on BCD was presented at the annual American Rhinologic Society meeting in 2005.[11] Technical feasibility and safety were evaluated by dilation of 31 sinus ostia (9 maxillary, 11 sphenoid, 11 frontal) in 6 cadaver heads. BCD successfully dilated all 31 sinuses and did not result in adjacent skull base or orbital injury in any cases. The investigators posited that balloon technology also seemed to impart less mucosal trauma than standard endoscopic instruments, although no comparative analysis was performed in the study. This work was followed by the first patient trial on BCD in 10 patients with persistent CRS after failed medical therapy.[12] A total of 18 sinuses were dilated, with 8 of 10 patients undergoing concurrent ethmoidectomy. All sinuses were successfully dilated without adverse events, though the investigators noted that the maxillary sinus was the most difficult to cannulate given the position of the natural ostium relative to the uncinate process. This study served as proof of concept in a limited number of patients without any follow-up period. The impact on the underlying disease process was unclear.

LacriCATH

The LacriCATH system (Quest Medical, Inc., Allen, TX) is an established balloon device used for dilation of the lacrimal outflow system for chronic epiphora.[13] Citardi and Kanowitz[14] performed endoscopic paranasal sinus dissection in 3 cadaver heads using conventional FESS instrumentation concurrently with the lacrimal balloon for BCD. Frontal recess dissection was successfully performed in all 6 sinuses with FESS instruments and BCD, and all 6 sphenoid sinuses were also successfully dilated. It was not feasible to reliably pass the balloon through the maxillary natural ostium, with only 3 of 6 being successfully dilated with this technique. This study provided proof of concept in a cadaver model, precluding extrapolation of the intervention in patients with CRS. The study highlighted the potential technical limitation of BCD of the maxillary sinus in patients with an intact uncinate process.

FinESS

FinESS (Functional Infundibular Endoscopic Sinus System [Entellus Medical, Inc., Maple Grove, MN]) obtained FDA clearance in April 2008 and was launched at the annual American Academy of Otolaryngology meeting later that year.[10] The transantral dilation system uses a flexible 0.5-mm endoscope and dual-channel cannula to localize the maxillary sinus ostia via the canine fossa approach. BCD of the maxillary ostium and ethmoid infundibulum is then performed under endoscopic visualization. The initial data on this device were reported in a multicenter study (Balloon Remodeling Antrostomy Therapy [BREATHE] I) assessing outcomes and safety in patients with CRS.[15] Fifty-five of 58 (94.8%) maxillary ostia were successfully treated, with 97% being performed under local anesthesia with or without minimal sedation. Mean Sinonasal Outcome Test (SNOT-20) scores had statistically improved at 6 months, with patency in 95.8% by CT imaging. Follow-up data showed sustained improvement in all 4 domains on SNOT-20 at 1 year.[16] These 2 studies provide a proof of clinical concept of this technology. The technology may be applicable to patients with limited disease focused at the maxillary infundibulum; however, broader application to the larger subset of CRS is not afforded by the data.

EVIDENCE-BASED CLINICAL ASSESSMENT

Given the paucity of controlled studies with a comparator group, the role of the various balloon catheter devices in the management of CRS and its subtypes remains to be elucidated. Thus, definitive recommendations on how to evaluate patients thought suitable for BCD are not possible. Nonetheless, the available database shows multitude of potential applications in patients with paranasal sinus inflammatory disease. Studies have reported on both adult and pediatric CRS refractory to maximal medical therapy.[17–24] Patients with limited sinus disease have also been evaluated.[15,16]

Several studies have explored the usefulness of BCD in frontal sinus disease.[25–31] Studies have also evaluated the use of BCD in the office and intensive care unit (ICU) settings.[32–34] The evidence base available for the various applications is evaluated later.

EVIDENCE-BASED SURGICAL TECHNIQUE
Adult Medically Refractory CRS

Multiple retrospective case series have reported on the usefulness of BCD on medically refractory adult CRS. The present analysis focuses on the salient studies to highlight the current state of the evidence.

CLEAR study

The initial large-scale investigation, dubbed the Clinical Evaluation to Confirm Safety and Efficacy of Sinuplasty in the Paranasal Sinuses (CLEAR) study, reported on 109 patients with nonpolypoid CRS unresponsive to medical management undergoing planned FESS.[17] Follow-up evaluations were performed at 1, 2, 12, and 24 weeks, with main outcome measures being ostial patency, SNOT-20 scores, and global rating of improvement. Overall, 52% of patients underwent concomitant ethmoidectomy, or so-called hybrid procedures. The mean Lund-Mackay scores for the balloon-only and hybrid groups were 6.1 and 10.4, respectively.

Most procedures were performed uneventfully without any cases of cerebrospinal fluid (CSF) leaks, orbital injury, or epistaxis requiring packing. BCD seemed to be technically feasible, although there were 12 device malfunctions. Endoscopic sinus ostial patency rates at 24 weeks were 91% for maxillary sinus, 82% at frontal sinus, and 60% for sphenoid sinus. A significant number of frontal (17%) and sphenoid (39%) sinuses were not evaluable because of inadequate postoperative endoscopic visualization. A statistically significant decrease in SNOT-20 scores was noted for both the balloon and hybrid groups: scores for the patients who had balloons decreased from 2.14 to 1.27, whereas the hybrid scores improved from 2.42 to 1.02.

One-year follow-up data were reported on 66 patients from the original cohort.[18] The remainder was excluded from the analysis because of attrition, loss to follow-up, and loss of study sites. Postoperative ostial patency by endoscopy and CT was 93.5% for maxillary sinus, 91.9% for frontal sinus, and 86.1% for sphenoid sinus. Mean SNOT-20 scores for balloon-only and hybrid subsets improved to 0.95 and 0.87, respectively. Additional 2-year follow-up data were published on 65 of the patients.[19] The SNOT-20 scores for the balloon-only and hybrid groups decreased to 1.09 and 0.66, respectively. The Lund-Mackay scores improved from 5.7 to 1.8 and from 12.1 to 3.3 for balloon-only and hybrid patients, respectively. Overall, 85% of patients reported symptom improvement, with 15% remaining the same and 0% worse.

Many important observations can be gleaned from the CLEAR series. It attests to the technical feasibility and safety of the balloon to achieve sinus ostia dilatation. Further, 1-year and 2-year follow-up studies showed the potential for reasonable ostial patency over this time period. However, many questions remain unanswered. The patient cohort for these studies was not clearly defined; moreover, a uniform management algorithm was not applied to tailor the medical and surgical therapy. Thus, it is unclear whether the data can be generalized to all patients with CRS.

The CLEAR study serves as a representative example of a single-arm, uncontrolled, observational study that has been historically accepted in rhinology to justify surgical interventions, including FESS. However, the lack of a comparison group limits meaningful interpretation of the results; it precludes any efficacy claims relative to FESS.

Comparison of the mean SNOT-20 scores for the balloon-only and hybrid groups offers some insights.[35] The balloon-only group improved from a baseline of 2.14 to 0.99 and 1.09 at 1 year and 2 years, respectively. In contrast, the hybrid group started at higher mean SNOT-20 score of 2.42, improving to 0.68 and 0.64 at 1 year and 2 years, respectively. This finding suggests that patients undergoing concurrent ethmoidectomy not only have higher baseline SNOT-20 scores but also derive greater benefit from surgery. Although the data were intended to be interpreted in this manner, they highlight the potential usefulness of direct comparative trials to better understand the role of BCD compared with FESS.

BCD outcomes: retrospective study from a multicenter registry
In the largest retrospective study to date, Levine and colleagues[20] reported outcomes of BCD on 1036 patients from a multicenter registry. BCD was used in 3276 sinuses, with a mean of 3.2 sinuses per patient. Sinonasal symptoms improved in 95.2%, were unchanged in 3.8%, and were worse in 1.0% of patients. Postoperative infections were significantly less frequent and less severe compared to before surgery. No major adverse events were attributable to balloons, although 2 CSF leaks were documented in patients undergoing concurrent ethmoidectomy. Six cases had minor bleeding requiring packing or cautery. Perhaps the most important observation that stems from the data is the safety profile of BCD. However, the study does make it possible to reliably assess the impact of BCD on CRS. The data are pooled across 27 sites with no standardization of medical treatment or indications for surgery. The starting burden of disease was not defined by endoscopy and/or CT. The use of subjective symptom improvement as the primary endpoint and lack of validated outcome measures prevents robust assessment of BCD on the underlying disease process.

BCD versus FESS: comparative retrospective analysis
Friedman and colleagues[21] performed a comparative retrospective analysis of prospectively collected data in 70 patients undergoing BCD versus FESS. Inclusion criteria included recurrent rhinosinusitis in patients with either a persistently abnormal CT after 4 weeks of continuous therapy or an abnormal CT during treatment, with posttreatment normalization and 3 or more recurrences per year. Exclusion criteria included Lund-McKay scores greater than 12, significant polyposis, osteoneogenesis, or systemic disease. Thirty-five patients in each treatment arm were assessed by SNOT-20 scores, global patient assessment, postoperative narcotic usage, and cost at a minimum of 3 months follow-up. The SNOT-20 scores improved from 2.8 to 0.78 for the balloon group and 2.7 to 1.29 from the FESS group, showing clinically and statistically significant improvement in both groups. Patient satisfaction was higher and narcotic usage was lower in the BCD group. The average cost of BCD ($12,657) was less than that of FESS ($14,471); the lower charges were attributed to shorter operative and recovery times and reduced need for general anesthesia with BCD.

The results may suggest the superiority of BCD compared with FESS in this comparative study. However, closer analysis of the data shows that the study represents a highly selectively patient sample that did not undergo matching or randomization. The patients decided on their surgical intervention, thus likely influencing the symptom and satisfaction scores. Furthermore, the study did not report on ostial patency for this patient group, acknowledging the inherent limitations in adequate endoscopic visualization in patients with an intact uncinate process. The short follow-up period in a chronic inflammatory process that often spans years is an additional drawback that precludes meaningful interpretation of the data. In addition, the operative charges are an estimation at best.

Pediatric Medically Refractory CRS

BCD for medically recalcitrant CRS

Ramadan[22] reported initial data on technical feasibility and safety of BCD in children.[22] Thirty children with medically recalcitrant CRS underwent BCD; concurrent adenoidectomy was performed in 13 patients (43%). The procedures were technical feasible in 51 of 56 sinuses (91%) with no complications attributable to BCD. The feasibility rate was 98% in normal sinuses, decreasing to 60% in hypoplastic sinuses. The average fluoroscopy time was 18 seconds per sinus; mean fluoroscopy exposure was 0.18 mGy. The preliminary data again attest to the safety of BCD. They suggest that, although technically feasible in children, the inherent limitations posed by the smaller, especially hypoplastic, sinuses result in a lower cannulation rate in children. The study provides proof of concept in pediatric patients with CRS. The short-term or long-term impact on the underlying disease process is unclear.

BCD and/or adenoidectomy for CRS

In a follow-up study, Ramadan and Terrell[24] presented experience on 49 pediatric patients with CRS undergoing BCD and/or adenoidectomy with postoperative follow-up of 1 year. The groups were matched except for age, with the adenoidectomy-alone group being statistically younger (4.8 years) than the balloon group (7.7 years). The comparative groups included adenoidectomy alone[19] or BCD[30]; 17 in the latter group also underwent adenoidectomy. Symptom improvement, defined as a decrease of 0.5 or more on Sinonasal-5 (SN-5) questionnaire, was seen in 24 (80%) and 10 (52.6%) in the balloon-alone and adenoidectomy-alone groups, respectively. These data suggest the potential usefulness of BCD in pediatric patients. However, similarly to the study by Friedman and colleagues,[21] the 2 groups represent highly selective samples without any attempt at randomization. Given that 17 of the 30 in the balloon group underwent concomitant adenoidectomy, the impact of BCD on the underlying disease process and SN-5 scores is unclear. The intervention of adenoidectomy in both groups confounds the ability to interpret the findings.

BCD in children with CRS: prospective, multicenter, nonrandomized study

A subsequent prospective, multicenter, nonrandomized study evaluated the efficacy of BCD in 32 children with CRS.[23] Concurrent adenoidectomy was performed in 15 patients. Twenty-four patients (75%) completed the 52 weeks follow-up. BCD was successful in 56 of 63 (89%) sinuses. Of the 7 failed sinuses, 3 were hypoplastic maxillary sinuses, 3 were sphenoid sinuses, and 1 was a frontal sinus. The SN-5 score improved from 4.9 at baseline to 2.95 at 52 weeks. Overall, improvement was significant in 50%, moderate in 29%, and mild in 8%. One had no improvement, whereas 2 worsened in the postoperative period. Although this study makes a compelling case for BCD in pediatric patients, the impact of BCD is difficult to discern, given that 15 (46.9%) had simultaneous adenoidectomy and 6 (18.9%) had concurrent ethmoidectomy. The potential beneficial effect of adenoidectomy in pediatric patients with CRS cannot be understated. The adenoid may serve as a reservoir of potentially pathogenic bacteria; the overall adenoid bacterial isolation rate has been noted to be as high as 79%, with isolate rate increasing with sinusitis grade.[36] A recent meta-analysis of adenoidectomy in medically refractory CRS showed improvement of sinusitis symptoms or outcomes in 69.3% of the patients.[37] Given its simplicity, effectiveness, and low-risk profile, adenoidectomy likely represents a first-line therapy for uncomplicated pediatric CRS. Direct comparative trials of adenoidectomy, BCD, and FESS are required to better understand the role of balloons in the management algorithm of pediatric CRS.

Limited Disease

Two studies using the FinESS system have explored the usefulness of BCD for limited disease focused in the maxillary sinus with or without involvement of the ethmoid infundibulum.[15,16] As mentioned earlier, the data has shown technical feasibility in 94.8%, with improvement in SNOT-20 scores at 6 months and 1 year. These data have provided proof of concept for the new device, suggesting potential usefulness in patients with limited disease. However, careful evaluation of the BREATHE I 6-month data shows that they mirror many of the deficiencies evident in the CLEAR study.[17] The patient population for the study group in not clearly defined. CT imaging, showing an air-fluid level or maxillary ostial or infundibular narrowing with greater than or equal to 2-mm maxillary mucosal thickening served as the inclusionary criteria; however, the degree of maxillary opacification or level of infundibular narrowing were not objectively characterized beyond the point of inclusion. The medical therapy was inconsistently applied across the patient group. Furthermore, given that 2 simultaneous interventions (transantral approach, maxillary ostia BCD) were used, the impact of each is difficult to discern from the study design. Nonetheless, the data suggest that this may be a potential option for limited disease, especially in the office setting, and deserves additional investigation.

Frontal Sinus Disease

BCD has been proposed as a potential minimally invasive alternative to endoscopic frontal sinusotomy (EFS) for frontal sinus disease. Several studies have evaluated the usefulness of balloons in this regard (**Table 1**).[25–32] Khalid and colleagues[26] performed frontal recess BCD in 8 cadaver heads to evaluate the patterns of fracture of bony lamellae and change in frontal recess dimensions using preintervention and postintervention endoscopy and CT. This, in turn, was compared with the degree of change seen with EFS. BCD resulted in statistically less change in mean coronal

Table 1
Evidence base of studies on BCD for frontal sinus disease

Author	Indication	N	Study Design	EBM Level	Outcome
Catalano and Payne,[25] 2009	Chronic frontal sinusitis ± polyps	20	Retrospective	4	Mixed
Khalid et al,[26] 2010	Anatomic dimensions in normal sinuses	8	Cadavers	5	Mixed
Heimgartner et al,[27] 2011	Chronic frontal sinusitis	64	Retrospective	4	Mixed
Hopkins et al,[28] 2009	Acute frontal sinusitis	1	Case report	5	Positive
Wycherly et al,[29] 2010	Revision frontal sinus surgery	13	Retrospective	4	Positive
Plaza et al,[30] 2011	CRS with polyposis	32	Prospective	3	Positive
Andrews et al,[31] 2010	Recurrent sinus barotrauma	1	Case report	5	Negative
Luong et al,[32] 2008	Postoperative frontal stenosis	6	Retrospective	4	Positive

Abbreviation: EBM, evidence-based medicine.

(0.9 mm vs 2.6 mm) and sagittal (1.0 mm vs 4.0 mm) dimensions compared with EFS. The most commonly fractured lamella after BCD was the anterior face of the ethmoid bulla (56%). The clinical significance of these 2 interventions on frontal sinus disease is not evident from the cadaveric data; from a technical perspective, it suggests that BCD results in smaller frontal sinus outflow tract dimensions and may not produce consistent fracture patterns of the bony lamellae of the frontal recess cells.

BCD for medically refractory chronic frontal sinusitis

Catalano and Payne[25] performed BCD in 20 patients with medically refractory chronic frontal sinusitis. A total of 29 frontal sinuses were accrued with either complete opacification or partial opacification with total Lund-McKay score of greater than or equal to 10. The disease was categorized grade I (<5 mm of mucosal thickening), II ($\geq$5 mm of mucosal thickening, partial opacification, air-fluid level), and III (total opacification) in 10, 5, and 14 frontal sinuses, respectively. Overall, improvement was noted in 14 of 29 (48.3%) frontal sinuses using CT as the primary outcome measure. Success rate by disease subtype for Samter triad, CRS with polyposis, and CRS without polyposis was 36.4%, 40%, and 61.5%, respectively. The investigators posited that "...50% of the frontal sinuses in this study group were spared aggressive endoscopic intervention and its associated morbidity...."[25] It could also be argued that the failure rate of BCD in patients with chronic frontal sinusitis approximates 50%, approaching 60% to 65% in patients with hyperplastic disease. It is possible that the reported failure rate was high given that many of the frontal mucosal changes seen on CT may be potentially irreversible in patients with severe polyp disease and, thus, not respond favorably to BCD. Furthermore, the study did not consider patient symptoms or endoscopic patency for outcome measures.

BCD for medically refractory chronic frontal sinusitis: retrospective evaluation

Heimgartner and colleagues[27] retrospectively evaluated the limitation of BCD in frontal sinus surgery to determine the technical failure rate and to assess the potential reasons for failed access to the frontal sinus. BCD was unsuccessful in 12 (12%) of 104 frontal sinuses. The CT anatomy of the failed cases revealed that complex frontal recess pneumatization pattern, such as agger nasi cell, frontoethmoidal cell, and/or frontal bullar cell, or the presence of significant osteoneogenesis, may result in BCD being challenging or impossible. This study underscores the potential limitation of BCD in difficult anatomic configurations; it also emphasizes the need for the surgeon to be able to perform EFS or other endoscopic frontal sinus procedures if BCD is unable to achieve the desired result.

BCD for medically refractory chronic frontal sinusitis: randomized clinical trial

Plaza and colleagues[30] performed the only randomized clinical trial of BCD and Draf I for frontal sinus disease to date. A total of 40 patients with CRS with polyposis were enrolled, with 32 successfully concluding the study. All patients had failed an 8-week course of antibiotics, oral steroids, and saline irrigations. Exclusion criteria included previous sinus surgery; advanced CRS, defined as Samter triad or symptomatic asthma; severe systemic disease (ie, diabetes); and smoking more than 20 cigarettes daily. All patients underwent hybrid procedures, which included a minimum of maxillary antrostomy and anterior ethmoidectomy, with posterior ethmoidectomy and sphenoidotomy being performed in select cases. Preoperative and 12-month postoperative measures were obtained, including visual analog scores (VAS), Rhinosinusitis Disability Index (RSDI), olfactory threshold, Lund-McKay scores, and frontal recess patency.

The VAS, RSDI, olfactory thresholds, and polyp scores were statistically improved in both groups. The frontal sinus Lund-McKay scores improved from 1.9 to 0.5 and 2.0 to

0.4 in the BCD and Draf I groups, respectively, with both being statistically significant. Resolution of frontal sinus disease was more common after BCD compared with Draf I or Draf IIa procedures (80.8% vs 75%), although neither was statistically significant. Frontal patency was statistically more common after BCD (73.1% vs 62.5%), whereas synechiae formation was more common in the BCD, although not statistically significant.

This is the first prospective comparative analysis of BCD and FESS. The strengths of the study include independence from commercial conflicts, use of several validated outcome tools, low attrition rate, and long follow-up. However, the study does not provide sufficient data to suggest equivalency of BCD and Draf I procedures. As noted by Ahmed and colleagues,[38] the study did not perform a pretrial power analysis, thus the group sizes may have not been large enough to discern a true difference in the frontal radiologic scores . The study also suffers from a selective reporting bias, failing to conduct a between-group analysis for CT, VAS, RSDI, and polyp scores, which would have facilitated direct comparison. Often, statistical significance was reported, although confidence intervals and *P*-values were omitted. Given the hybrid nature of the surgical procedures, the ability to differentiate the direct impact of the frontal intervention from concurrent ethmoidectomy is limited.

Balloon Dilation in the Office Setting

Two studies to date have reported on office-based BCD for frontal ostial stenosis in the office setting.[32,33]

BCD in the office setting: multicenter case series
Luong and colleagues[32] reported a multi-institutional case series on BCD for frontal sinus ostial stenosis in the office setting. Six adult patients underwent a total of 7 BCD with change of ostia size from 1 to 2 mm to 5 to 7 mm immediately after treatment. All procedures were performed using topical anesthesia without any complications. One frontal sinus ostia contracted more than 50%, requiring revision BCD in the office. All frontal ostia were patent with follow-up ranging from 4 to 9 months, with no patients requiring formal surgical revision in the operating room.

BCD in the office setting: surgery after Draf I and II
Eloy and colleagues[33] performed in-office BCD in 5 patients developing frontal stenosis after Draf I and II surgery. All procedures were well tolerated with use of topical and injected local anesthesia. All procedures were deemed successful, with improvement of frontal headaches and establishment of a patent drainage pathway at a mean follow-up of 5 months. Both studies provide proof of concept of the potential usefulness of balloon technology in the office setting. It may provide the ability to temporize sinus ostia stenosis in a subset of patients without the need for formal surgical revision in the operative suite. This potential application merits further investigation with accrual of additional patients and longer-term follow-up.

Balloon Dilation in the ICU Setting

Wittkopf and colleagues[34] reported on the usefulness of BCD in the management of acute rhinosinusitis in 5 critically ill patients in the ICU setting. Four of 5 patients were immunocompromised, 3 were leukopenic, and 4 were thrombocytopenic. All patients had focal findings on CT with a mean Lund-McKay score of 7. All patients underwent BCD because they were thought to be poor candidates for traditional FESS, although surgical indications were not clarified. BCD was performed without complications and with minimal blood loss. All patients returned to baseline health and met discharge criteria 3 days to 6 weeks after surgery. Thus, BCD may have a diagnostic role in obtaining cultures, and possibly a therapeutic role in the ventilation and drainage of opacified sinuses in critically ill patients. This application represents another potential of BCD that merits additional study; the impact of BCD on return to baseline health is unclear, especially because only 1 of the intraoperative cultures was positive.

WHAT DOES THE EVIDENCE TELL US?

The accrued evidence to date has reported on the usefulness of BCD on a variety of indications, including adult and pediatric CRS, limited CRS, and frontal sinusitis. Studies have also explored the use of the technology in alternate practice settings, including the office and ICU. The current database suggests that balloon technology is safe; BCD provides the ability to dilate frontal, sphenoid, and maxillary sinuses and to achieve patency in a large number of these cases for up to 2 years. However, limitations to the current evidence preclude meaningful recommendations on how to apply BCD in the treatment schema of CRS. Most of the data are comprised by uncontrolled, retrospective studies with poorly characterized patient cohorts lacking a matched control group, which seriously hinders the ability to make any comparative efficacy claims relative to FESS. **Table 2** highlights the grade of evidence available for several applications of BCD. The overall grade of the data is C, given that all available studies, except for 1 study qualifying for level 2b evidence,[30] comprise level 4 evidence. Given the widespread adoption of BCD, this underscores the importance of timely randomized clinical trials, preferably with inclusion of appropriately matched controls and validated outcome measures that make it possible to discern the impact of BCD, relative to FESS, on the underlying disease process.

CRITICAL POINTS

- Numerous studies have evaluated the usefulness of balloon catheter technology for surgical management of adult CRS, with overarching existing data deemed to be level 4.
- Three studies assessing BCD for pediatric CRS are graded level 4; they are confounded by concurrent adenoidectomy in a significant number of the children, precluding the ability to discern the impact of each intervention.
- Two studies have evaluated the use of transantral BCD for limited sinus disease, with both studies being graded level 4 evidence.

Table 2
Grade of recommendation for potential indications of balloon catheter technology for paranasal sinus inflammatory disease

Indication	Recommendation Grade
Disease Specific	
Adult medically refractory CRS	C
Pediatric medically refractory CRS	C
Minimal disease (CRS or RARS)	C
Specific Sinus	
Frontal sinus disease	C
Alternate Practice Site	
Office setting (ARS, RARS; CRS)	C
ICU setting (ARS)	D

Abbreviation: ARS, acute rhinosinusitis.

- Most studies reporting the use of BCD for frontal sinus disease are level 4, although 1 study provides level 2b evidence, suggesting possible usefulness of the technology for this indication.
- Level 4 evidence is available for the use of BCD in the office and ICU setting, although both may represent potentially important applications of balloon devices.
- The overall recommendation is grade C for the use of BCD for paranasal sinus inflammatory disease, with a higher level being reserved until well-controlled randomized trials are available.
- Most studies on balloon catheter dilation (BCD) for pediatric chronic rhinosinusitis are graded level 4, confounded by concurrent adenoidectomy in a significant number of study participants.

REFERENCES

1. Benninger MS, Ferguson BJ, Hadley JA, et al. Adult chronic rhinosinusitis: definitions, diagnosis, epidemiology, and pathophysiology. Otolaryngol Head Neck Surg 2003;129(Suppl 3):S1–32.
2. Fokkens W, Lund V, Mullol J. European position paper on rhinosinusitis and nasal polyps 2007. Rhinol Suppl 2007;20:1–136.
3. Slavin RG. Management of sinusitis. J Am Geriatr Soc 1991;39(2):212–7.
4. Cohen M, Kofonow J, Nayak JV. Biofilms in chronic rhinosinusitis: a review. Am J Rhinol Allergy 2009;23(3):255–60.
5. Senior BA, Glaze C, Benninger MS. Use of the rhinosinusitis disability index (RSDI) in rhinologic disease. Am J Rhinol 2001;15(1):15–20.
6. Smith TL, Batra PS, Seiden AM, et al. Evidence supporting endoscopic sinus surgery in the management of adult chronic rhinosinusitis: a systematic review. Am J Rhinol 2005;19(6):537–43.
7. Smith TL, Kern RC, Palmer JN, et al. Medical therapy vs surgery for chronic rhinosinusitis: a prospective, multi-institutional study. Int Forum Allergy Rhinol 2011; 1(4):235–41.
8. Lanza DC. Postoperative care and avoiding frontal recess stenosis. In: Abstracts of the International Advanced Sinus Symposium. Philadelphia; 1993.
9. Vaughan WC. Review of balloon sinuplasty. Curr Opin Otolaryngol Head Neck Surg 2008;16(1):2–9.
10. Batra PS, Ryan MW, Sindwani R, et al. Balloon catheter technology in rhinology: reviewing the evidence. Laryngoscope 2011;121(1):226–32.
11. Bolger WE, Vaughan WC. Catheter-based dilation of the sinus ostia: initial safety and feasibility analysis in a cadaver model. Am J Rhinol 2006;20(3):290–4.
12. Brown CL, Bolger WE. Safety and feasibility of balloon catheter dilation of paranasal sinus ostia: a preliminary investigation. Ann Otol Rhinol Laryngol 2006; 115(4):293–9.
13. Tao S, Meyer DR, Simon JW, et al. Success of balloon catheter dilatation as a primary or secondary procedure for congenital nasolacrimal duct obstruction. Ophthalmology 2002;109(11):2108–11.
14. Citardi MJ, Kanowitz SJ. A cadaveric model for balloon-assisted endoscopic paranasal sinus dissection without fluoroscopy. Am J Rhinol 2007;21(5):579–83.
15. Stankiewicz J, Tami T, Truitt T, et al. Transantral, endoscopically guided balloon dilatation of the ostiomeatal complex for chronic rhinosinusitis under local anesthesia. Am J Rhinol Allergy 2009;23(3):321–7.
16. Stankiewicz J, Truitt T, Atkins J Jr. One-year results: transantral balloon dilation of the ethmoid infundibulum. Ear Nose Throat J 2010;89(2):72–7.

17. Bolger WE, Brown CL, Church CA, et al. Safety and outcomes of balloon catheter technology: a multicenter 24-week analysis of 115 patients. Otolaryngol Head Neck Surg 2007;37(1):10–20.
18. Kuhn FA, Church CA, Goldberg AN, et al. Balloon catheter sinusotomy: one-year follow-up – outcomes and role of in functional endoscopic sinus surgery. Otolaryngol Head Neck Surg 2008;139(3 Suppl 3):S27–37.
19. Weiss RL, Church CA, Kuhn FA, et al. Long-term outcome analysis of balloon catheter sinusotomy: two-year follow-up. Otolaryngol Head Neck Surg 2008; 139(3 Suppl 3):S38–46.
20. Levine HL, Sertich AP II, Hoisington DR, et al. Multicenter registry of balloon catheter sinusotomy. Outcomes for 1,036 patients. Ann Otol Rhinol Laryngol 2008; 117(4):263–70.
21. Friedman M, Schalch P, Lin HC, et al. Functional endoscopic dilatation of the sinuses: patient satisfaction, postoperative pain, and cost. Am J Rhinol 2008; 22(2):204–9.
22. Ramadan HH. Safety and feasibility of balloon sinuplasty for treatment of chronic rhinosinusitis in children. Ann Otol Rhinol Laryngol 2009;118(3):161–5.
23. Ramadan HH, McLaughlin K, Josephson G, et al. Balloon catheter sinuplasty in young children. Am J Rhinol Allergy 2010;24(1):e54–6.
24. Ramadan HH, Terrell AM. Balloon catheter sinuplasty and adenoidectomy in children with chronic rhinosinusitis. Ann Otol Rhinol Laryngol 2010;119(9):578–82.
25. Catalano PJ, Payne SC. Balloon dilation of the frontal recess in patients with chronic frontal sinusitis and advanced sinus disease: an initial report. Ann Otol Rhinol Laryngol 2009;118(2):107–12.
26. Khalid AN, Smith TL, Anderson JC, et al. Fracture of bony lamellae within the frontal recess after balloon catheter dilatation. Am J Rhinol Allergy 2010;24(1):55–9.
27. Heimgartner S, Eckardt J, Simmen D, et al. Limitations of balloon sinuplasty in frontal sinus surgery. Eur Arch Otorhinolaryngol 2011;268(10):1463–7.
28. Hopkins C, Noon E, Roberts D. Balloon sinuplasty in acute frontal sinusitis. Rhinology 2009;47(4):375–8.
29. Wycherly BJ, Manes RP, Mikula SK. Initial clinical experience with balloon dilation in revision frontal sinus surgery. Ann Otol Rhinol Laryngol 2010;119(7):468–71.
30. Plaza G, Eisenberg G, Montojo J, et al. Balloon dilation of the frontal recess: a randomized clinical trial. Ann Otol Rhinol Laryngol 2011;120(8):511–8.
31. Andrews JN, Weitzel EK, Eller R, et al. Unsuccessful frontal balloon sinuplasty for recurrent sinus barotrauma. Aviat Space Environ Med 2010;81(5):514–6.
32. Luong A, Batra PS, Fakhri S, et al. Balloon catheter dilatation for frontal sinus ostium stenosis in the office setting. Am J Rhinol 2008;22(6):621–4.
33. Eloy JA, Friedel ME, Eloy JD, et al. In-office balloon dilation of the failed frontal sinusotomy. Otolaryngol Head Neck Surg 2012;146:320–2.
34. Wittkopf ML, Becker SS, Duncavage JA, et al. Balloon sinuplasty for the surgical management of immunocompromised and critically ill patients with acute rhinosinusitis. Otolaryngol Head Neck Surg 2009;140(4):596–8.
35. Marple BF, Stringer SP, Batra PS, et al. Going to the next level: health care's evolving expectations for evidence. Otolaryngol Head Neck Surg 2009;141:551–4.
36. Shin KS, Cho SH, Kim KR, et al. The role of adenoids in pediatric rhinosinusitis. Int J Pediatr Otorhinolaryngol 2008;72:1643–50.
37. Brietzke SE, Brigger MT. Adenoidectomy outcomes in pediatric rhinosinusitis: a meta-analysis. Int J Pediatr Otorhinolaryngol 2008;72:1541–5.
38. Ahmed J, Pal S, Hopkins C, et al. Functional endoscopic balloon dilation of sinus ostia for chronic rhinosinusitis. Cochrane Database Syst Rev 2011;(7):CD008515.

Epistaxis: A Contemporary Evidence Based Approach

M.L. Barnes, FRCS-ORL(Ed), MD*, P.M. Spielmann, FRCS-ORL(Ed), P.S. White, FRACS, FRCS(Ed), MBChB

KEYWORDS

- Epistaxis • Evidence • Emergency ENT

KEY POINTS

- Epistaxis is the second most common cause for ear/nose/throat emergency admission.
- Given this fact, there are surprisingly few studies or guidelines, and management is usually based on experience rather than high level evidence. A stepwise approach to epistaxis management is advocated: initial management, direct therapy, tamponade, and vascular intervention.
- There is a changing emphasis in epistaxis management, with a move away from the traditional approaches of prolonged admissions and reliance on extensive nasal packing.
- Arterial ligation procedures are increasingly commonly used, offering higher success rates and much reduced morbidity.
- A protocol is provided for clinical guidance and as a framework for future studies.

INTRODUCTION

Epistaxis is the second most common cause for emergency admission to ear/nose/throat services (following sore throat). In 2009/2010, there were more than 21,000 emergency admissions in England with a mean inpatient stay of 1.9 days. The majority of admissions are aged 60 to 70 years,[1] but there is a bimodal age incidence, with an earlier peak in childhood.[2]

Death due to epistaxis is rare. In 2005 in the United States, 7 epistaxis-related deaths were recorded, all from the population 75 years or older[3]; an approximate incidence in that age group of 1:2,500,000, and an overall incidence of 2:100 million. The epidemiology of epistaxis in Scotland has been well reviewed,[4] and readers are referred here for more details.

Despite the heavy caseload there are no national or consensus guidelines to inform management decisions, and the most junior members of staff are often the main

Department of Otolaryngology, Ward 26, Ninewells Hospital & Medical School, Dundee DD1 9SY, United Kingdom
* Corresponding author.
E-mail address: mr.mlbarnes@gmail.com

Otolaryngol Clin N Am 45 (2012) 1005–1017
http://dx.doi.org/10.1016/j.otc.2012.06.018
oto.theclinics.com

caregivers.[5] Across different centers, investigation profiles and treatment preferences vary. There are areas of controversy, and non-standardized practice exists. This situation needs to be addressed in an evidence-based fashion. The purpose of this article, therefore, is to review the literature concerning the management of epistaxis and to make recommendations (evidence-based where available) for treatment.

METHODS

A literature review was performed in July 2011. PubMed was searched using the term "Epistaxis"[Majr], limited to reviews within the last 10 years. Relevant articles were identified and obtained, as well as important ancestor references. Further specific searches were conducted without limits, to address each theme within the review, for example, "Epistaxis"[Majr] AND "Blood Coagulation Disorders"[Mesh]. More than 200 articles were reviewed, although few provided primary evidence beyond expert opinion to guide the development of an overall management protocol.

A MANAGEMENT PATHWAY
Management of Epistaxis

A stepwise approach to epistaxis management is advocated. In order, this should be initial management, followed by direct therapy, tamponade, and vascular intervention. When control of bleeding is not achieved, timely progression through the management steps is essential (**Fig. 1**).

Pathway Progression: Uncontrolled Epistaxis

Direct therapy or tamponade will almost invariably reduce bleeding, but sometimes control is not absolute, and intermittent or minor ongoing bleeding may occur. In such cases, a clinical decision must be made as to whether to progress with further management as per uncontrolled epistaxis, or to observe the patient. Such is not uncommon in cases of coagulopathy, where bleeding times may be significantly prolonged. The decision must be based on the ongoing rate of bleeding and the patient's risks. In some cases, a little further air in a tamponade balloon (often required within the hour after initial insertion), or applying a procoagulant dressing to an oozing cautery site (eg, Surgicel absorbable hemostat, Ethicon Inc, Somerville, NJ; or Algosteril Alginate Fiber Absorbable Hemostat, Smith & Nephew PLC, London, UK) may be helpful. Patients must not, however, sit for prolonged periods with poor control, multiple nasal packs, and no further intervention. These patients must receive a pack or vascular intervention if required.

Protocol Completion: Treated Epistaxis

Where possible, epistaxis should only be considered adequately treated when a topical therapy or vascular intervention has been used, although when a thorough examination has not identified a bleeding site, and simple vasoconstriction or tamponade has led to initial control, longer-term resolution may be achieved through normal hemostatic and tissue repair mechanisms in some cases.

Step 1. Initial management of epistaxis
Immediate management includes an Advanced Life Support–type ABC assessment (Airway, Breathing, Circulation) and resuscitation. Epistaxis is not usually an immediate airway threat but patients should be sat upright, and encouraged to lean forward and clear any clots from their pharynx. An assessment of blood loss (eg, volume, time, number of tissues, towels, or bowls) and the degree of any hypovolemic shock should

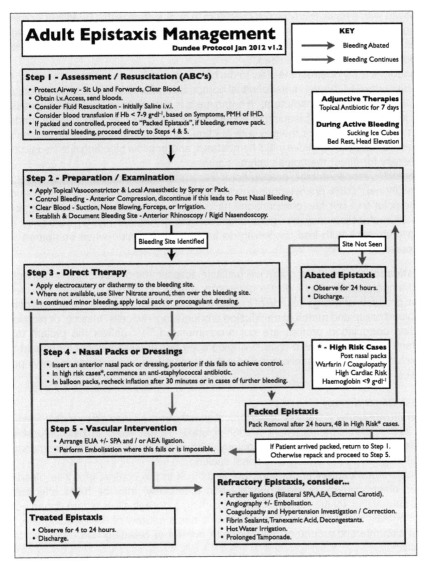

Fig. 1. Adult epistaxis management pathway. BID, twice a day; EUA, examination under anesthesia; IHD, ischemic heart disease; AEA, anterior ethmoid artery; SPA, sphenopalatine artery.

be made, while establishing venous access and fluid resuscitation where indicated. Gloves, gowns, and goggles are essential to protect both clinician and patient. A medical and drug history may elucidate precipitants. The side of bleeding as well as whether it is predominantly anterior or posterior should be determined.

In exceptional circumstances, postnasal bleeding may be so heavy as to warrant an immediate balloon pack (eg, Foley catheter and anterior pack) to prevent further blood loss, with arrangements for transfer to theater. In general, however, the first priority is to visualize the bleeding area through initial hemostatic measures and examination. Depending on the bleeding site, and local skills and facilities, this may be best achieved with a nasal thudicum or speculum in conjunction with a headlight or mirror, an auroscope, microscope, or endoscope, noting that each approach has its limitations. Nasoendoscopy facilities, above all others, are essential; identifying 80% of bleeding sites not otherwise seen.[6]

Blood will likely obstruct the view to the bleeding site. In anterior nasal bleeding, this can be controlled through anterior nasal compression for 10 to 60 minutes in conjunction with topical vasoconstrictors.[7] If hemostasis is not achieved or nasal compression only leads to postnasal bleeding, it should be discontinued, and an attempt made to clear blood and visualize the site with suction, forceps, irrigation,[8] or nose blowing. These methods may achieve initial hemostasis, and/or allow bleeding site visualization necessary for direct therapies such as cautery.

Topical vasoconstrictor preparations recommended include 1:1000 adrenalin (epinephrine),[9] 0.5% phenylephrine hydrochloride,[10] 4% cocaine, or 0.05% oxymetazoline solution,[7] but few comparisons have been conducted. One study suggested that oxymetazoline may be more effective than 1:100,000 (dilute) adrenalin, and equally effective with less propensity to induce hypertension when compared with 4% cocaine.[11]

Investigations A full blood count will facilitate assessment of blood loss and shock. A biochemistry profile may indicate circulatory effects on renal function or the breakdown products of a large volume of ingested blood. A sample should be sent to establish blood group and match of transfusion products (eg, red cells, plasma, or platelets). Routine coagulation profiles are not recommended,[12–14] unless the patient takes warfarin or is admitted as a child.[15] Angiography has an essential but infrequent role in excluding potentially fatal carotid aneurysms in trauma and in cases of heavy postsurgical bleeding.

Step 2. Direct therapy
Silver nitrate cautery Cautery using topical anesthetic is advocated by most investigators as the optimal management in adult epistaxis. Nonetheless, in 1993 only 24% of cases referred to specialist otolaryngology units in the United Kingdom were managed in this way, with 76% undergoing nasal packing.[5]

Silver nitrate cautery is common but is difficult in the context of active bleeding, where electrocautery or electrocoagulation (diathermy) may be more effective. A local cauterizing solution is achieved by touching a dry salt silver nitrate tipped applicator against moist mucosa. The objective is direct cautery of the bleeding site, but initial circumferential contact may facilitate control of bleeding and more definitive results.[8]

Silver nitrate is available in 75% and 95% preparations. A histopathological study comparing the two found that 95% silver nitrate caused twice the depth of burn, which it was thought might increase the risk of complications including septal perforation.[16] It is believed that bilateral cautery may also increase the risk of septal perforation,[17] with a 4- to 6-week interval being advocated between sides,[18] although Link and colleagues[19] found this not to be the case using silver nitrate (n = 46).

Silver nitrate ($AgNO_3$) can cause black staining, which may be addressed by application of saline (NaCl) to form silver chloride (AgCl) and sodium nitrate ($NaNO_3$)[20]; both are white crystals, and the latter is readily soluble in water. Stains usually resolve over a period of weeks,[21] but permanent mucosal tattooing has been reported.[22–24]

Electrocautery and electrocoagulation (diathermy) Toner and Walby[25] compared routine use of hot-wire electrocautery with use of silver nitrate, finding no difference in the rates of recurrent bleeding at 2 months, although the confidence interval (CI) was broad, with some trend toward greater benefit with electrocautery (95% CI −11%–24%).

Although specialist equipment is required, electrocautery (hot wire) or diathermy may have advantages over silver nitrate, which can be difficult to apply to the site in cases of uncontrolled bleeding. No further electrocautery or electrocoagulation studies were identified.

After direct therapy, in some cases of minor ongoing bleeding, the addition of a hemostatic dressing such as Surgicel (Ethicon) or Kaltostat (ConvaTec Ltd, Skillman, NJ), or the use of a very localized pack over the bleeding site, may help to prevent further pathway progression.

Step 3. Nasal packs or dressings
If local therapy fails, control of bleeding can be achieved by tamponade, using a variety of nasal packs, or by promotion of hemostasis through nasal dressings. Modern nasal packs are easily and relatively comfortably inserted by practitioners not specialized in otorhinolaryngology, for example, in the emergency department, ambulance, or family practice. As a consequence, many patients now arrive at the authors' department with packs inserted. However, this does prevent immediate direct therapy, which might otherwise allow a treated patient to be sent home. Once a pack is inserted, it is usually recommended that it is left in place for 24 hours, necessitating admission, although care at home with packs has been described.[10]

A variety of nasal packing materials is available. Examples include polyvinyl acetal polymer sponges (eg, Merocel, Medtronic Inc, Minneapolis, MN), nasal balloons (eg, the Rapid Rhino Balloon pack with a self-lubricating hydrocolloid fabric covering, ArthroCare Corp, Austin, TX), nasal dressings (eg, Kaltostat calcium alginate, ConvaTec Ltd), and traditional ribbon packs, for example, BIPP (Bismuth, Iodoform, Paraffin Paste) or petroleum jelly–coated ribbon gauze. Each of these packs is illustrated in **Fig. 2**. Some (eg, Rapid Rhino, Kaltostat) are reported to provide procoagulant surfaces, which may be helpful in coagulopathic patients, most commonly those on warfarin.

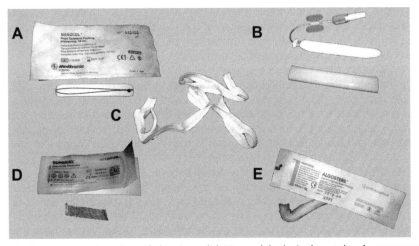

Fig. 2. Common nasal packs and dressings. (*A*) Merocel (polyvinyl acetal polymer sponge pack); (*B*) Rapid Rhino (self-lubricating hydrocolloid covered balloon pack); (*C*) a traditional ribbon pack, in this case BIPP (Bismuth Iodoform Paraffin Paste); (*D*) Surgicel (oxidized regenerated cellulose absorbable hemostat); (*E*) Algosteril (alginate fiber absorbable hemostat).

A nasopharyngeal pack may be placed in posterior epistaxis (approximately 5% of cases[26]), especially when initial anterior packs fail. Traditional postnasal packs were rolled gauze attached to tapes passed out through the nose and mouth to secure.[26] More recently, Brighton or Foley catheters have been used, inflated with saline and secured transnasally with an anterior clamp, for example, an umbilical clip.

Postnasal packs are extremely uncomfortable and are prone to cause significant hypoxia.[27] Hospitalization, oxygen therapy via face mask, and in some cases sedation are required; a combination that increases the risks of hypoxia and aspiration. Other complications of nasal packs (especially nasopharyngeal) include displacement with airway obstruction, pressure necrosis of the palate, alar or columellar skin, and sinus infection or toxic shock syndrome. The latter is caused by staphylococcal exotoxin TSST-1, and presents with fever, diarrhea, hypotension, and a rash.[26] *Staphylococcus aureus* can be isolated in one-third of patients, of which 30% produce the exotoxin.[28] Therefore, prolonged packing should be avoided and anti-staphylococcal antibiotics prescribed if a pack is to remain in situ for more than 24 hours[8] (see discussion on high-risk cases).

Balloon packs may deflate over time,[29] so should be checked after the first hour or if bleeding recommences. Some minor ongoing bleeding is not uncommon immediately following pack insertion, and may resolve given careful observation.

Following pack removal it is imperative to examine the nasal cavity, to exclude underlying abnormality and to identify and manage the bleeding source if possible.

Step 4. Ligation/embolization
Surgery In a 1993 United Kingdom national survey of practice, 9.3% of epistaxis patients referred to an otolaryngologist required a posterior nasal pack (commonly a Foley catheter). A general anesthetic was required in 5.6% to control bleeding, and fewer than 1% had a formal arterial ligation (ethmoid, maxillary, or external carotid).[5]

In the authors' own center, with 593 acute admissions for epistaxis over the last 2 years, 47% had hospital stays of 1 day or less. Of the 317 longer-term cases, 7% were taken to theater and underwent arterial ligation: 21 of the sphenopalatine artery (SPA) and 2 of the anterior ethmoid artery (AEA). In some cases, the theater equipment and anesthetic will facilitate visualization of the bleeding site, bleeding control, and direct cautery. Where this remains impossible, or uncertainty is present about the control established, arterial ligation is performed.

In the past, ligation was commonly of the maxillary artery or the external carotid artery. Although the distribution of these arteries is wider, recent studies suggest that SPA ligation is more successful, possibly because of difficulties completing the other procedures, or a failure to address more distal collateral circulation.[30] SPA ligation is associated with minor complications such as nasal crusting, decreased lacrimation, and paresthesia of the palate or nose.[31] Septal perforation and inferior turbinate necrosis have also been reported.[32,33]

By contrast, ligation of the maxillary artery through a canine fossa approach can be complicated by dental or nasolacrimal duct injury, facial and gum numbness, or oroantral fistula.[34] Ligation of the external carotid artery is associated with a small risk of injury to the hypoglossal and vagus nerves, and a lower success rate.[30]

When compared with traditional packing techniques, SPA ligation has been shown to enable a reduced inpatient stay, improved patient satisfaction, and cost reductions.[35] Feusi and colleagues.[36] reviewed SPA ligation efficacy studies in 2005: 13 investigators reported 264 patients with 1-year success rates of between 70% and 100%. More recent studies with longer-term follow-up (15–25 months) reported success rates of between 75% and 100%.[37–40] Ligation of all[41] SPA branches is essential.[42]

AEA ligation has an essential role in traumatic or postsurgical epistaxis, in which nasal or ethmoid bony injury leads to bleeding beyond the SPA distribution. Recent attempts have been made to avoid the external scar, performing AEA ligation by endonasal or transcaruncular approaches. The endonasal approach, first described by Woolford and Jones,[43] requires either an artery within a mesentery[44] or an approach to the artery through the lamina papyracea.[45] The former was feasible in 20% or fewer of cases.[44] The latter, performed through the lamina, appears to be safe and feasible in most cases,[45,46] although this is likely an approach best left to expert hands. In both cases, preoperative or intraoperative computed tomography scans and image guidance are advised.

A transcaruncular approach is an appealing alternative. Morera and colleagues[47] report a case series of 9 patients in which all were successful with no reported complications. For now, however, a pragmatic approach may be to use an endoscope in a conventional external approach, allowing the scar to be minimized.[48]

The choice of surgical ligation type is a clinical decision, which must be based on the history and examination findings. Epistaxis traditionally has been defined as anterior or posterior, with posterior bleeds considered to relate to the Woodruff plexus. The definitions have been inconsistent, however,[49] and the relevance of the Woodruff plexus recently questioned.[50]

An understanding of the anatomy is essential for both surgeons and interventional radiologists. To this end, the reader is referred to excellent texts by Lee and colleagues[42] and Biswas and colleagues.[51]

Interventional radiology: embolization Selective embolization of the maxillary or facial arteries should be considered in cases where surgical ligation fails, or is impossible because of anesthetic concerns. A variety of materials have been used including metal coils, Gelfoam, and cyanoacrylate glue. Success rates between 79% and 96% are reported,[52] but complications are not uncommon: cerebrovascular accident, arterial dissection, facial skin necrosis, facial numbness, and groin hematoma can occur, with historic rates of up to 47% but only 6% in larger, more recent series.[53]

Percutaneous angiography is performed to identify the vascular anatomy. Extravasation may suggest the site of epistaxis, but is not often seen. Radiopaque nasal packing (such as BIPP) must be removed. Selective embolization of the relevant arterial supply, typically the internal maxillary artery, reduces the hydrostatic pressure of blood to the nasal cavity, allowing hemostasis, which must be balanced against devascularizing the facial soft tissues. Embolization of the ethmoidal arteries is not possible; cannulation of the ophthalmic arteries carries a high risk of blindness.

Refractory Acute Epistaxis

Occasionally bleeding will continue (usually slowly or intermittently), despite all conservative measures, good nasal packs, examination under anesthetic, and even arterial ligations. In such cases, it is important to reconsider questions regarding anatomy and physiology.

For anatomy

Which side is it bleeding? Is it passing through a perforation, or around the choana? Has a competent practitioner visualized the area of bleeding directly? In cases with a history of trauma, is there an anterior ethmoid laceration, or a carotid aneurysm? Is there a role for further ligations of the bilateral sphenopalatine, or anterior and posterior ethmoid arteries? Will a maxillary artery or external carotid ligation add anything (eg, minor contributions from the facial and greater palatine branches)? Will angiography be informative and potentially therapeutic?

For physiology

Is the patient coagulopathic? Are they bleeding diffusely? Have measures been taken to reverse any drug-induced coagulopathy? If they have bled extensively, have their clotting factors been replaced? Has hypertension been addressed? Will tranexamic acid,[54] topical hemostatics,[55] or fibrin sealants[56,57] help?

Adjunctive Treatments

Topical treatments

For the purposes of the current protocol, regarding epistaxis requiring admission, topical treatments are considered to be inappropriate as sole therapy. However, topical agents may have a role as an adjunct and, noting their efficacy in minor recurrent epistaxis, especially in childhood,[58] the authors recommend them in all cases. Options include Naseptin cream (0.1% chlorhexidine dihydrochloride with 0.5% neomycin sulfate), petroleum jelly, Bactroban, triamcinolone 0.025%,[59] and others.[60]

Ice packs

Ice packs are a tradition on many of our wards. When ice cubes are sucked, there is a measurable reduction in nasal blood flow assessed by nasal laser Doppler flowmetry.[61] However, no change is seen when ice is applied to the forehead or neck.[62]

Preventing Epistaxis Deaths

In 1961, Quinn[63] wrote of his own experience and reviewed previous cases of fatal epistaxes, recognizing the groups at risk; those with significant comorbidity (eg, ischemic heart disease, coagulopathy) and endonasal tumors, or following head and facial trauma or surgery. He advocated angiography following trauma, as well as "adequate blood replacement and an informed attitude toward surgical interruption of the blood supply." He also reported the association of anterior ethmoid bleeding with trauma, the use of ferrous sulfate, and the association of cranial nerve signs with internal carotid laceration or aneurism. His observations seem just as relevant today as then, and still address the most important issues; in particular, the recognition of high-risk groups and the need in such cases for early and relatively aggressive fluid resuscitation to prevent complications and deaths, most commonly in elderly patients with ischemic heart disease.

Quinn[63] recognized the difficulty of balancing the need to transfuse anemic epistaxis patients against the risks, noting the possible contribution of a blood transfusion to the death of at least one patient. Prolonged admissions with nasal packs and poorly controlled bleeding will exacerbate this risk, and for these reasons Kotecha and colleagues[5] recommended earlier surgical intervention in some elderly patients with compromised respiratory or cardiovascular systems.

In the current protocol, the authors recommend a transfusion threshold of 7 to 9 g/dL. This figure is based primarily on a study in critically unwell patients in which a restrictive policy (transfusion indicated if hemoglobin <8 g/dL cf <10 g/dL) was shown to improve survival outcomes, particularly in the young (<55 years) and those relatively less unwell.[64]

Although rare, death in association with epistaxis has also been reported to occur through airway obstruction. Again, significant comorbidity (eg, neurologic impairment caused by preexisting disease or head injury) may be present. Airway obstruction secondary to nasal packing is a risk, attributable to either pack or clot dislodgment.[65]

In some patients, nasal obstruction itself can lead to significant arterial oxygen desaturation.[27] Again, an awareness of these potential scenarios with appropriate measures to prepare the patient, protect the airway, and monitor oxygenation is important to prevent fatal complications.

The most common case report of death secondary to epistaxis relates to rupture of an internal carotid aneurysm, often of traumatic or surgical origin. In torrential bleeds of this nature, only early suspicion with angiography, coil occlusion, stenting, or surgical ligation of the aneurysm or the internal carotid in the neck will prevent death.[66] In the operative context, Valentine and colleagues[67] recently compared several measures for initial hemostasis in carotid injury, concluding that crushed muscle hemostasis followed by U-clip repair was the most effective, achieving primary hemostasis while maintaining vascular patency in all cases.

LITERATURE REVIEW ON EPISTAXIS

In reviewing the epistaxis literature, one is confronted with a wealth of expert opinion and descriptive articles. Few primary research studies are conducted, and those available focus on management techniques rather than on pathway decisions. Without placing the patients in the context of a management pathway, these studies may lack transferability; one's own patients may represent a different population at a different point in the pathway. It is for these reasons that a management pathway must be defined, and as a starting point the authors advocate the protocol described herein.

In developing a contemporary protocol, one must recognize the changing emphasis of epistaxis management with a move away from traditional approaches of prolonged admissions and reliance on extensive nasal packing. Refined arterial ligation procedures are increasingly commonly used, offering higher success rates and less morbidity. These procedures have facilitated shorter admissions, with happier patients as well as hospital managers.

The current protocol excludes contexts such as coagulopathy, hereditary hemorrhagic telangiectasia (HHT), and children, although useful generalizations can be made. Of admitted epistaxis patients, 62% have an iatrogenic coagulopathy (21% warfarin, 41% antiplatelet). This group requires longer inpatient stays and more aggressive management.[68,69] Although management follows the same principles, the coagulopathy itself must be addressed, and care must be taken not to cause further trauma through aggressive cautery, nasal packing, or vascular intervention. Procoagulant dressings may be helpful. The authors hope to provide further guidance on the management of this group in a later article.

The authors are aware of several different approaches to epistaxis that have not been recommended in this guideline, from simple vasoconstrictor treatments[70] to hot-water irrigation[71–73] or cryotherapy.[74] Although efficacy studies are reported, few if any comparisons have been performed against conventional techniques in the context of a defined management protocol. It is hoped that this article will facilitate future scientific comparisons to allow the best timing of such interventions to be established.

As always, further research in the field is needed. Despite the frequency of epistaxis as a presentation, little formal research has been conducted. The authors recommend that any interventional studies place themselves in the context of the overall pathway of patient management, as well as tightly defining patient flow (stepwise by protocol) and demographics; for example, age, sex, blood pressure, anticoagulant use, other medications (including herbal), HHT, prior episodes, trauma or operative history, and so forth. The authors are developing an epistaxis admission data set, optically captured from an admission pro forma, and would be happy to hear from any other interested centers.

REFERENCES

1. The Information Centre for Health and Social Care. 2011. Available at: http://www. hesonline.nhs.uk Accessed May 2011.
2. Juselius H. Epistaxis. A clinical study of 1,724 patients. J Laryngol Otol 1974;88: 317–27.
3. Centers for Disease Control and Prevention. National center for health statistics. Vitalstats; 2005. Available at: http://www.cdc.gov/nchs/vitalstats.htm. Accessed July 31, 2011.
4. Walker TW, Macfarlane TV, McGarry GW. The epidemiology and chronobiology of epistaxis: an investigation of Scottish hospital admissions 1995-2004. Clin Otolaryngol 2007;32:361–5.
5. Kotecha B, Fowler S, Harkness P, et al. Management of epistaxis: a national survey. Ann R Coll Surg Engl 1996;78:444–6.
6. McGarry GW. Nasal endoscope in posterior epistaxis: a preliminary evaluation. J Laryngol Otol 1991;105:428–31.
7. Kucik CJ, Clenney T. Management of epistaxis. Am Fam Physician 2005;71: 305–11.
8. Viehweg TL, Roberson JB, Hudson JW. Epistaxis: diagnosis and treatment. J Oral Maxillofac Surg 2006;64:511–8.
9. Middleton PM. Epistaxis. Emerg Med Australas 2004;16:428–40.
10. Upile T, Jerjes W, Sipaul F, et al. A change in UK epistaxis management. Eur Arch Otorhinolaryngol 2008;265:1349–54.
11. Katz RI, Hovagim AR, Finkelstein HS, et al. A comparison of cocaine, lidocaine with epinephrine, and oxymetazoline for prevention of epistaxis on nasotracheal intubation. J Clin Anesth 1990;2:16–20.
12. Supriya M, Shakeel M, Veitch D, et al. Epistaxis: prospective evaluation of bleeding site and its impact on patient outcome. J Laryngol Otol 2010;124: 744–9.
13. Thaha MA, Nilssen EL, Holland S, et al. Routine coagulation screening in the management of emergency admission for epistaxis—is it necessary? J Laryngol Otol 2000;114:38–40.
14. Padgham N. Epistaxis: anatomical and clinical correlates. J Laryngol Otol 1990; 104:308–11.
15. Sandoval C, Dong S, Visintainer P, et al. Clinical and laboratory features of 178 children with recurrent epistaxis. J Pediatr Hematol Oncol 2002;24:47–9.
16. Amin M, Glynn F, Phelan S, et al. Silver nitrate cauterisation, does concentration matter? Clin Otolaryngol 2007;32:197–9.
17. Lanier B, Kai G, Marple B, et al. Pathophysiology and progression of nasal septal perforation. Ann Allergy Asthma Immunol 2007;99:473–9 [quiz: 480–1, 521].
18. Schlosser RJ. Clinical practice. Epistaxis. N Engl J Med 2009;360:784–9.
19. Link TR, Conley SF, Flanary V, et al. Bilateral epistaxis in children: efficacy of bilateral septal cauterization with silver nitrate. Int J Pediatr Otorhinolaryngol 2006;70: 1439–42.
20. Maitra S, Gupta D. A simple technique to avoid staining of skin around nasal vestibule following cautery. Clin Otolaryngol 2007;32:74.

21. Oxford Hands-on Science (H-Sci) Project: Chemical Safety Database. Chemical safety data: Silver nitrate; Available at: http://cartwright.chem.ox.ac.uk/hsci/chemicals/silver_nitrate.html. Accessed August 17, 2011.
22. Kayarkar R, Parker AJ, Goepel JR. The Sheffield nose—an occupational disease? Rhinology 2003;41(2):125–6.
23. Mayall F, Wild D. A silver tattoo of the nasal mucosa after silver nitrate cautery. J Laryngol Otol 1996;110:609–10.
24. Nguyen RC, Leclerc JE, Nantel A, et al. Argyremia in septal cauterization with silver nitrate. J Otolaryngol 1999;28:211–6.
25. Toner JG, Walby AP. Comparison of electro and chemical cautery in the treatment of anterior epistaxis. J Laryngol Otol 1990;104:617–8.
26. Tan LK, Calhoun KH. Epistaxis. Med Clin North Am 1999;83:43–56.
27. Lin YT, Orkin LR. Arterial hypoxemia in patients with anterior and posterior nasal packings. Laryngoscope 1979;89:140–4.
28. Breda SD, Jacobs JB, Lebowitz AS, et al. Toxic shock syndrome in nasal surgery: a physiochemical and microbiologic evaluation of Merocel and Nugauze nasal packing. Laryngoscope 1987;97:1388–91.
29. Ong CC, Patel KS. A study comparing rates of deflation of nasal balloons used in epistaxis. Acta Otorhinolaryngol Belg 1996;50:33–5.
30. Srinivasan V, Sherman IW, O'Sullivan G. Surgical management of intractable epistaxis: Audit of results. J Laryngol Otol 2000;114:697–700.
31. Snyderman CH, Goldman SA, Carrau RL, et al. Endoscopic sphenopalatine artery ligation is an effective method of treatment for posterior epistaxis. Am J Rhinol 1999;13:137–40.
32. Gifford TO, Orlandi RR. Epistaxis. Otolaryngol Clin North Am 2008;41:525–36, viii.
33. Moorthy R, Anand R, Prior M, et al. Inferior turbinate necrosis following endoscopic sphenopalatine artery ligation. Otolaryngol Head Neck Surg 2003;129: 159–60.
34. Schaitkin B, Strauss M, Houck JR. Epistaxis: medical versus surgical therapy: a comparison of efficacy, complications, and economic considerations. Laryngoscope 1987;97:1392–6.
35. Moshaver A, Harris JR, Liu R, et al. Early operative intervention versus conventional treatment in epistaxis: randomized prospective trial. J Otolaryngol 2004; 33:185–8.
36. Feusi B, Holzmann D, Steurer J. Posterior epistaxis: systematic review on the effectiveness of surgical therapies. Rhinology 2005;43:300–4.
37. Harvinder S, Rosalind S, Gurdeep S. Endoscopic cauterization of the sphenopalatine artery in persistent epistaxis. Med J Malaysia 2008;63:377–8.
38. Nouraei SA, Maani T, Hajioff D, et al. Outcome of endoscopic sphenopalatine artery occlusion for intractable epistaxis: a 10-year experience. Laryngoscope 2007;117:1452–6.
39. Asanau A, Timoshenko AP, Vercherin P, et al. Sphenopalatine and anterior ethmoidal artery ligation for severe epistaxis. Ann Otol Rhinol Laryngol 2009; 118:639–44.
40. Abdelkader M, Leong SC, White PS. Endoscopic control of the sphenopalatine artery for epistaxis: long-term results. J Laryngol Otol 2007;121:759–62.
41. Holzmann D, Kaufmann T, Pedrini P, et al. Posterior epistaxis: endonasal exposure and occlusion of the branches of the sphenopalatine artery. Eur Arch Otorhinolaryngol 2003;260:425–8.
42. Lee HY, Kim HU, Kim SS, et al. Surgical anatomy of the sphenopalatine artery in lateral nasal wall. Laryngoscope 2002;112:1813–8.

43. Woolford TJ, Jones NS. Endoscopic ligation of anterior ethmoidal artery in treatment of epistaxis. J Laryngol Otol 2000;114:858–60.

44. Solares CA, Luong A, Batra PS. Technical feasibility of transnasal endoscopic anterior ethmoid artery ligation: assessment with intraoperative CT imaging. Am J Rhinol Allergy 2009;23:619–21.

45. Pletcher SD, Metson R. Endoscopic ligation of the anterior ethmoid artery. Laryngoscope 2007;117:378–81.

46. Camp AA, Dutton JM, Caldarelli DD. Endoscopic transnasal transethmoid ligation of the anterior ethmoid artery. Am J Rhinol Allergy 2009;23:200–2.

47. Morera E, Artigas C, Trobat F, et al. Transcaruncular electrocoagulation of anterior ethmoidal artery for the treatment of severe epistaxis. Laryngoscope 2011;121: 446–50.

48. Douglas SA, Gupta D. Endoscopic assisted external approach anterior ethmoidal artery ligation for the management of epistaxis. J Laryngol Otol 2003;117:132–3.

49. McGarry GW. Epistaxis. In: Gleeson M, Browning GG, Burton MJ, et al, editors. Scott-Brown's otorhinolaryngology, head and neck surgery. London: Hodder Arnold; 2008. p. 1596–608.

50. Chiu TW, McGarry GW. Prospective clinical study of bleeding sites in idiopathic adult posterior epistaxis. Otolaryngol Head Neck Surg 2007;137:390–3.

51. Biswas D, Ross SK, Sama A, et al. Non-sphenopalatine dominant arterial supply of the nasal cavity: an unusual anatomical variation. J Laryngol Otol 2009;123: 689–91.

52. Smith TP. Embolization in the external carotid artery. J Vasc Interv Radiol 2006;17: 1897–912 [quiz: 1913].

53. Elahi MM, Parnes LS, Fox AJ, et al. Therapeutic embolization in the treatment of intractable epistaxis. Arch Otolaryngol Head Neck Surg 1995;121:65–9.

54. Sabbà C, Gallitelli M, Palasciano G. Efficacy of unusually high doses of tranexamic acid for the treatment of epistaxis in hereditary hemorrhagic telangiectasia. N Engl J Med 2001;345:926.

55. Shinkwin CA, Beasley N, Simo R, et al. Evaluation of Surgicel Nu-Knit, Merocel and Vaseline gauze nasal packs: a randomized trial. Rhinology 1996;34:41–3.

56. Walshe P, Harkin C, Murphy S, et al. The use of fibrin glue in refractory coagulopathic epistaxis. Clin Otolaryngol Allied Sci 2001;26:284–5.

57. Walshe P. The use of fibrin glue to arrest epistaxis in the presence of a coagulopathy. Laryngoscope 2002;112:1126–8.

58. Kubba H, MacAndie C, Botma M, et al. A prospective, single-blind, randomized controlled trial of antiseptic cream for recurrent epistaxis in childhood. Clin Otolaryngol Allied Sci 2001;26:465–8.

59. London SD, Lindsey WH. A reliable medical treatment for recurrent mild anterior epistaxis. Laryngoscope 1999;109:1535–7.

60. Kara N, Spinou C, Gardiner Q. Topical management of anterior epistaxis: A national survey. J Laryngol Otol 2009;123:91–5.

61. Porter MJ. A comparison between the effect of ice packs on the forehead and ice cubes in the mouth on nasal submucosal temperature. Rhinology 1991;29: 11–5.

62. Teymoortash A, Sesterhenn A, Kress R, et al. Efficacy of ice packs in the management of epistaxis. Clin Otolaryngol Allied Sci 2003;28:545–7.

63. Quinn FB. Fatal epistaxis. Calif Med 1961;94:88–92.

64. Hébert PC, Wells G, Blajchman MA, et al. A multicenter, randomized, controlled clinical trial of transfusion requirements in critical care. N Engl J Med 1999;340: 409–17.

65. Williams M, Onslow J. Airway difficulties associated with severe epistaxis. Anaesthesia 1999;54:812–3.
66. Lehmann P, Saliou G, Page C, et al. Epistaxis revealing the rupture of a carotid aneurysm of the cavernous sinus extending into the sphenoid: treatment using an uncovered stent and coils. Review of literature. Eur Arch Otorhinolaryngol 2009;266:767–72.
67. Valentine R, Boase S, Jervis-Bardy J, et al. The efficacy of hemostatic techniques in the sheep model of carotid artery injury. Int Forum Allergy Rhinol 2011;1: 118–22.
68. Smith J, Siddiq S, Dyer C, et al. Epistaxis in patients taking oral anticoagulant and antiplatelet medication: prospective cohort study. J Laryngol Otol 2011;125: 38–42.
69. Soyka MB, Rufibach K, Huber A, et al. Is severe epistaxis associated with acetylsalicylic acid intake? Laryngoscope 2010;120:200–7.
70. Doo G, Johnson DS. Oxymetazoline in the treatment of posterior epistaxis. Hawaii Med J 1999;58:210–2.
71. Stangerup SE, Thomsen HK. Histological changes in the nasal mucosa after hot-water irrigation. An animal experimental study. Rhinology 1996;34:14–7.
72. Stangerup SE, Dommerby H, Lau T. Hot-water irrigation as a treatment of posterior epistaxis. Rhinology 1996;34:18–20.
73. Stangerup SE, Dommerby H, Siim C, et al. New modification of hot-water irrigation in the treatment of posterior epistaxis. Arch Otolaryngol Head Neck Surg 1999;125:686–90.
74. Hicks JN, Norris JW. Office treatment by cryotherapy for severe posterior nasal epistaxis–update. Laryngoscope 1983;93:876–9.

Evidence-Based Practice
Postoperative Care in Endoscopic Sinus Surgery

Luke Rudmik, MD[a],*, Timothy L. Smith, MD, MPH[b]

KEYWORDS

- Endoscopic sinus surgery • Chronic rhinosinusitis • Sinusitis • Postoperative care
- Nasal irrigations • Debridement • Topical steroids • Sinus stent

KEY POINTS

The following points present level of evidence as based on grading by the Oxford Centre for Evidence-Based Medicine.

- Postoperative care following endoscopic sinus surgery (ESS) is important to optimize clinical outcomes.
- Nasal saline irrigations should be used following ESS (Grade: B).
- In-office endoscopic sinus cavity debridement after ESS improves both short-term and long-term clinical outcomes (Grade: B).
- Topical steroid therapy is integral for control of postoperative mucosal inflammation and should be started following ESS (Grade: A).
- Off-label topical steroid solutions may be considered in cases with severe mucosal inflammation (Grade: D).
- Perioperative systemic corticosteroids improve endoscopic outcomes following ESS in patients with nasal polyposis (Grade: not available; 1 level 1b study).
- Systemic antibiotics improve short-term symptoms and reduce crusting following ESS (Grade: B).
- Drug-eluting middle meatal spacers and stents improve endoscopic outcomes in patients with nasal polyposis (Grade: A).

OVERVIEW

Chronic rhinosinusitis (CRS) is a disabling inflammatory condition of the sinonasal mucosa that produces symptoms of nasal congestion, discharge, facial pressure, and olfactory dysfunction.[1] Furthermore, several studies have demonstrated that CRS produces a significant reduction in both disease-specific symptoms and general

Conflict of interest: There are no conflicts of interest.
[a] Rhinology and Sinus Surgery, Division of Otolaryngology – Head and Neck Surgery, Department of Surgery, University of Calgary, Calgary, Alberta, Canada; [b] Rhinology and Endoscopic Sinus-Skull Base Surgery, Department of Otolaryngology – Head and Neck Surgery, Oregon Health & Science University, Portland, OR, USA
* Corresponding author. Division of Otolaryngology – Head and Neck Surgery, Foothills Medical Centre, Suite 602 South Tower, 1403 – 29th Street Northwest, Calgary, Alberta T2N 2T9, Canada.
E-mail address: lukerudmik@gmail.com

quality of life (QoL).[2–4] Management of CRS is focused on reducing mucosal inflammation and improving sinonasal function. The use of topical and systemic medical therapy remains the mainstay of treatment; however, a subset of patients will have persistent symptoms despite best medical efforts, and become candidates for endoscopic sinus surgery (ESS). Several studies have demonstrated the positive impact of ESS on both symptom-related and health-related QoL (HRQoL) outcomes in patients with medically refractory CRS.[1,5–8] With more than 250,000 ESS procedures performed in the United States every year, it is important for the surgeon to optimize factors that improve postoperative success, which can produce positive long-term clinical outcomes.[9] Although there are several minor technical variations, the fundamentals of ESS are to preserve mucosal lining while removing diseased tissue, creating an accessible sinus cavity, and ventilating the natural draining sinus pathways.[10]

The primary goals of early postoperative care are to reduce mucosal inflammation and infection, improve short-term patient symptoms, promote early return of ciliary function, and prevent complications. Optimizing these goals should incur the best chance to maintain long-term HRQoL improvement and minimize the need for revision ESS. There is no standardized approach to postoperative care and, because of numerous reported strategies, there remains a debate regarding what constitutes the optimal postoperative care protocol. The most commonly described postoperative care modalities include: nasal saline irrigations, in-office sinus cavity debridement, topical nasal steroid sprays, off-label topical steroids, short-course systemic steroids, systemic antibiotics, and middle meatal drug-eluting spacers and stents (**Box 1**).

Following a successful ESS procedure, an open and accessible sinus cavity will allow for continued topical medical therapy, which is critical for long-term success by minimizing mucosal inflammation. This article discusses the evidence pertaining to the different postoperative care strategies, and provides an evidence-based approach to postoperative care following ESS.

EVIDENCE-BASED CLINICAL ASSESSMENT

Following ESS, the milieu of old blood, exposed bone, unresorbed packing, and retained secretions can predispose to infection and inflammation, and provide a potential framework for scarring and early disease recurrence. Although there may be

---

Box 1
Common ESS postoperative care interventions

- Nasal Saline Irrigations
  - Low-volume
  - High-volume
- Endoscopic nasal and sinus cavity debridement
- Topical corticosteroid therapies
  - Sprays
  - Drops
  - Irrigations
- Systemic corticosteroid therapy
- Systemic antibiotic therapy
- Middle meatal drug-eluting spacers
- Middle meatal drug-eluting stents

a minority of surgeons who believe postoperative care following ESS is un-necessary,[11] most experts believe that despite careful patient selection and meticulous surgery, a failure of dedicated postoperative care likely predisposes to potentially avoidable complications,[12–14] such as synechiae, middle turbinate lateralization, ostial stenosis, and rapid polyp recurrence (**Fig. 1**). The return of normal mucosal histology and ciliary function often takes longer than 12 weeks following surgery, therefore, postoperative follow-up is often recommended to ensure an adequate healing sinus cavity.[15]

In a recent multi-institutional evidence-based review with recommendations article by Rudmik and colleagues,[16] the recommended postoperative care treatments were: nasal saline irrigations, in-office sinus cavity debridement, and topical nasal steroid sprays. Because of a relative balance of harm and benefit, options were made for systemic steroids, systemic antibiotics, and drug-eluting spacers. Because of increased pain and the risk of rhinitis medicamentosa, the only recommendation against was for the routine use of topical decongestants. To further refine the optimal postoperative care strategy, further research is needed to confirm the evidence-based protocol that is proposed and elucidate the ideal frequency and timing of postoperative follow-up visits. The following sections discuss the different postoperative care strategies and present the evidence for each topic.

EVIDENCE-BASED MANAGEMENT
Nasal Saline Irrigations

Nasal douching with saline solutions has been well established as a treatment adjunct in CRS.[17–19] However, the role of saline irrigations in the early postoperative period remains controversial. Advocates for early postoperative nasal saline irrigations hypothesize that nasal douching aids with debris removal and softens crusting, which may produce improved mucociliary clearance and potentially easier in-office debridement. There is significant variation is the delivery mode, volume, and frequency of saline irrigations:

- Delivery modes include squeeze bottles, atomization sprays, and electrical fluid delivery devices.
- The volume of saline douching varies from atomized 2 mL to 240 mL and the frequency varies from once daily to 4 times daily.

There are no studies that evaluate the optimal postoperative saline irrigation protocol. Although saline irrigations are safe and well tolerated, potential adverse effects include local irritation, epistaxis, nasal burning, headaches, ear plugging, and unexpected nasal drainage.

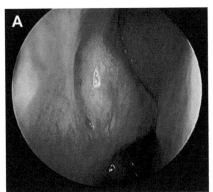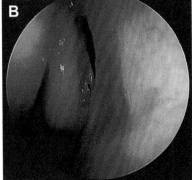

Fig. 1. (*A*) Complete right middle turbinate lateralization. (*B*) Synechiae between left middle turbinate and lateral nasal wall.

Nasal saline irrigation studies

Six randomized studies have evaluated the impact of saline irrigations on clinical outcomes following ESS.[20–25] All study methodologies were heterogeneous, as they used different postoperative care protocols with different saline irrigation volumes and frequencies. Two studies evaluated low-volume postoperative nasal saline irrigations.

- A randomized trial (level 2b) by Freeman and colleagues[23] demonstrated that the benefits of postoperative saline irrigations were limited to early endoscopic appearance, specifically a reduction in discharge and crusting, while they failed to demonstrate any long-term endoscopic improvement such as a reduction in synechiae or adhesions. However, one criticism of this study was the low-volume saline irrigation protocol (2 mL atomization 3 times a day), which questions whether it provided a strong enough mechanical debridement to make a difference.
- Another randomized (level 2b) trial by Pinto and colleagues[21] evaluated 3 postoperative patient groups (no irrigations, normal saline irrigations, hypertonic saline irrigations), which irrigated 30 mL 4 times a day following ESS. The results demonstrated that hypertonic saline produced increased postoperative pain scores whereas the normal saline irrigations did not offer any additional benefit compared with the control group. Again, this study used a low-volume irrigation protocol (30 mL), making it difficult to draw conclusions about the commonly used large-volume (240 mL) irrigation strategy.
- One randomized (level 1b) trial by Liang and colleagues[24] evaluated a large-volume (240 mL daily) saline irrigation protocol and demonstrated that the benefits were limited to patients with mild CRS, with those patients with moderate to severe CRS failing to demonstrate a difference in symptoms and endoscopic appearance. This finding may suggest that patients with moderate to severe CRS often require additional postoperative medical therapy to control inflammation and reduce symptoms.

Despite some controversy in the literature, most experts agree that there is a preponderance of benefit over harm, and nasal saline irrigations should be started within the early postoperative period, usually 24 to 48 hours after ESS. Although large volume saline irrigation has been demonstrated to be superior to low volume saline irrigation in the management of CRS,[26] the effects of saline volume in the early postoperative period have not yet been evaluated.

Postoperative In-Office Sinus Cavity Debridement

The sinus cavity following ESS often has a large amount of crusting, old blood, unresorbed dissolvable packing, and retained secretions. This postoperative local environment is thought to provide a framework for scarring, ostial stenosis, and middle turbinate lateralization. Debridement of the postoperative sinus cavity is thought to optimize early mucosal healing by reducing the inflammatory load and lowering the risk of infection. Debridement technique often includes a rigid nasal endoscope scope for visualization, and the use of a suction instrument for soft debris and endoscopic graspers for harder crusts. Most surgeons agree that postoperative sinus debridement is a useful adjunct to maximizing long-term ESS outcomes. Arguments against debridement include exposing patients to increased pain, potential for mucosal stripping, and other rare adverse events such as epistaxis and syncope.

Postoperative debridement studies

There have been 4 randomized trials evaluating the role of postoperative debridement after ESS.

- An early pilot study (level 2b) by Nilssen and colleagues failed to demonstrate a clinical benefit of sinus debridement; however, it had several limitations including being underpowered.[27]
- A recent randomized trial (level 1b) by Bugten and colleagues[28] demonstrated that early postoperative sinus cavity debridement resulted in reduced crust and middle meatal adhesion rates at 3 months follow-up, and their long-term follow-up study in 2008 reported that the initial short-term improvements were stable after a mean of 56 weeks.[29]

Although most experts agree that postoperative debridement is a useful adjunct to optimizing ESS outcomes, the timing and frequency of debridement is somewhat controversial.

- A study by Kuhnel and colleagues[30] demonstrated that early crust debridement was associated with underlying mucosal avulsion in 23% of cases, although this risk was negligible after 2 weeks.
- Two subsequent level 1b randomized trials have demonstrated that the optimal timing for the first postoperative debridement is 1 week following the ESS procedure.[31,32]
- The randomized trial (level 1b) by Lee and Byun[30] demonstrated that patients who received multiple debridements within the first week received similar short-term (4 weeks) and long-term (6 months) symptom outcomes compared with patients with debridement(s) at 1-week intervals. Furthermore, the patients who received multiple debridements within the first week after ESS reported the greatest disturbances in socioeconomic activities and had the highest rate of omitting postoperative clinic visits.
- The randomized trial (Level 1b) by Kemppainen and colleagues[29] demonstrated that patients who received 3 sinus cavity debridements within the first week after ESS had reduced nasal discharge scores compared with patients who received a debridement at 1 week after ESS.

When evaluating the evidence, the most accepted practice would include a sinus cavity debridement at 1 week after ESS, while subsequent debridements are often surgeon dependent and based on the degree of crusting and inflammation (**Figs. 2** and **3**).

Topical Nasal Steroids

Topical nasal corticosteroid therapy is an integral component of anti-inflammatory CRS medical therapy. Application techniques include nasal sprays, atomizers, drops, and irrigations. Common CRS approved topical nasal steroid sprays include fluticasone, mometasone, and budesonide, while common off-label solutions include budesonide irrigations (0.5 mg/2 mL or 1 mg/2 mL mixed into 240 mL of saline), prednisolone 1% ophthalmic drops, dexamethasone 0.1% ophthalmic drops, and ciprofloxacin/dexamethasone 0.3%/0.1% otic drops (**Table 1**). Although these higher-potency off-label formulations provide increased concentrations of local steroid therapy, the major disadvantage is the unknown systemic absorption profile with potential for adrenal suppression and other long-term systemic steroid effects. Standard first-line therapy typically uses approved nasal steroid sprays while reserving the off-label formulations for cases of severe postoperative mucosal inflammation. Furthermore, nasal sprays tend to provide more "nasal" coverage, whereas irrigations and drops tend to provide improved "sinus" penetration and may be a better postoperative topical therapy delivery technique.[33] Unlike the use of systemic steroids, standard nasal steroid sprays have minimal systemic effects and therefore can be used as long-term corticosteroid therapy.

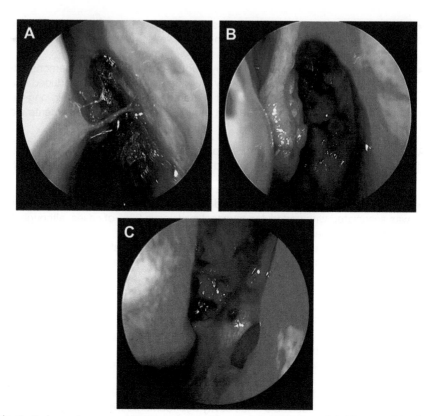

Fig. 2. Endoscopic appearance at postoperative week 1. (*A*) Before debridement. (*B*) After debridement. (*C*) Post-debridement maxillary antrostomy.

Topical nasal steroid studies

There have been 4 randomized, double-blind, placebo-controlled trials (level 1b) evaluating topical nasal sprays in the early postoperative period.[34–37]

- Only one study failed to demonstrate a clinical improvement in postoperative polyp recurrence and symptoms.[37]

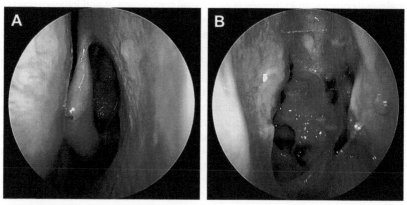

Fig. 3. Endoscopic appearance at postoperative week 3. (*A*) Middle meatus view. (*B*) Ethmoid cavity with view of sphenoidotomy.

Table 1
Options for postoperative topical corticosteroid therapy

Approved nasal sprays	Fluticasone propionate (50 µg per spray): 2 sprays each nostril once a day Mometasone furoate (50 µg per spray): 2 sprays each nostril once a day Budesonide aqua (32 µg per spray): 1 spray each nostril once a day
Off-label nasal drops	Prednisolone 1% ophthalmic drops Dexamethasone 0.1% ophthalmic drops Ciprofloxacin/dexamethasone 0.3%/0.1% otic drops
Off-label nasal irrigations	Budesonide saline irrigations (0.5 mg/2 mL or 1 mg/2 mL mixed into 240 mL of saline)

- The 3 most recent level 1b trials evaluating postoperative topical steroid sprays demonstrated a significant clinical improvement following ESS.

Patients with nasal polyps appear to receive the most benefit as polyp recurrence rate was reduced and time to polyp recurrence was lengthened. The timing for when to start topical nasal steroid spray therapy is poorly defined; however, each study reported starting therapy in the period between 2 and 6 weeks after ESS. Although there are no major drawbacks associated with earlier topical steroid spray therapy (before 2 weeks after ESS), the limited accessibility as a result of old blood and crusts would often negate any clinical benefit. Potential adverse effects are rare and include local irritation, epistaxis, cough, and headache.[38]

- A retrospective study by Del Guadio and Wise[39] evaluated 3 postoperative off-label nasal steroid solutions (dexamethasone ophthalmic drops, prednisolone ophthalmic drops, and ciprofloxacin/dexamethasone otic drops) in patients undergoing revision ESS who were at high risk for both ostial stenosis and oral steroid rescue courses. The results demonstrated that off-label steroid drops may lower the risk of revision sinus surgery and ostial stenosis while reducing the number of oral steroid rescue episodes. In this study only 1 patient of 36 required discontinuation of medication, because of a reduction in morning cortisol level.
- A study by Bhalla and colleagues[40] demonstrated a lack of significant adrenal suppression with the use of budesonide irrigations.
- Another recent study by Welch and colleagues[41] demonstrated that budesonide nasal irrigations (1 mg/2 mL in 240 mL saline) following ESS did not alter the serum cortisol or 24-hour urine cortisol levels.

Despite evidence for the short-term safety of off-label steroid solutions, future controlled studies will need to elucidate their benefits and long-term safety profile.

Most experts would agree that starting a topical nasal steroid spray between the first 2 and 6 weeks following ESS is necessary to optimize clinical outcomes by minimizing mucosal inflammation. Off-label high-concentration topical steroid solutions may reduce the risk of ostial stenosis and the need for an oral steroid rescue, and therefore may be considered in high-risk patients with severe postoperative mucosal inflammation.

Systemic Steroids

Patients undergoing ESS for medically recalcitrant CRS typically have significant underlying mucosal inflammation, and experts believe that controlling this inflammation in the perioperative period is necessary to optimize clinical outcomes. Although systemic steroids provide excellent improvement in CRS clinical status, the challenge remains balancing the benefits with the potential for harm. Potential adverse effects associated with systemic steroid therapy are listed in **Box 2**.[42]

Box 2
List of potential complications of short-course systemic steroids

- Elevated blood sugars
- Raised intraocular pressure
- Mood changes
- Insomnia
- Avascular necrosis of the hip
- Adrenal insufficiency
- Decreased bone mineral density[43] and cardiovascular disease[44] as a result of cumulative steroid dose over a lifetime

---

To minimize the risk of adverse events, most experts use short-course protocols such as durations between 7 and 14 days with moderate doses of 30 to 40 mg. The use of a tapering dose schedule is controversial, while some experts believe that therapy limited to less than 14 days does not require a taper. The authors' short-course steroid protocol is as follows:

Prednisone
- 30 mg × 4 days
- Then 20 mg × 4 days
- Then 10 mg × 4 days
- Total duration = 12 days, cumulative dose = 240 mg

Alternatively, in a level 1b study on perioperative systemic steroids, Wright and Agrawal[45] used a nontapering short-course protocol of prednisone 30 mg starting 5 days before ESS and continuing for 9 days after ESS (total duration 14 days, cumulative dose = 420 mg).

Systemic steroids studies

A randomized, double-blind, placebo-controlled trial (level 1b) by Wright and Agrawal[45] evaluated the role of perioperative prednisone on endoscopic appearance in patients with nasal polyposis. The study protocol started patients on 30 mg of prednisone 5 days before ESS and continued therapy for 9 days after ESS, without a taper. In addition to improved ease of surgery, the results demonstrated significant postoperative improvement in endoscopic appearance, which was most evident at the 2-week post-ESS time point. The study did not report any significant adverse events. Despite convincing evidence from this study, the potential side effects of short-term systemic steroid use must be balanced with the proven benefit in postoperative endoscopic appearance.

Because of the potential for serious adverse effects, the routine use of postoperative systemic steroids is controversial. Most experts would reserve this strategy for patients with moderate to severe CRS and nasal polyposis who are at high risk for postoperative complications. After careful patient selection and discussion of the potential risks, a short course of postoperative systemic steroids could be considered to minimize mucosal inflammation during the healing period and prevent complications related to excess mucosal edema and crusting.

Postoperative Antibiotics

Following ESS, the local environment of retained secretions, old blood, temporary ciliary dysfunction, and incomplete remucosalization all predispose to the development of a postoperative infection. Furthermore, the paranasal sinuses of patients with CRS tend to be colonized with bacteria and biofilm, which may predispose them to postoperative infection.[46,47] Potential sequelae include increased nasal crusting, discharge, and worse short-term symptoms. Traditionally, a course of postoperative antibiotics (7–10 days) has been recommended[12,48]; however, the literature regarding their use is conflicting.

Three randomized studies evaluated the role of postoperative antibiotics on ESS clinical outcomes.

- An early randomized, double-blind, placebo-controlled trial (level 1b) by Annys and colleagues[49] evaluated a very short course of postoperative antibiotics (2 days) and demonstrated it had no effect on outcomes.
- A recent randomized trial (level 2b) by Jiang and colleagues[50] evaluated a longer course of postoperative antibiotics (amoxicillin/clavulanate 375 mg 3 times per day × 3 weeks) and demonstrated no difference in endoscopic appearance at the 3-week follow-up period. The disadvantages of this study were a failure to use a placebo and performing the endoscopic evaluation at 3 weeks, which would have missed the early postoperative period when antibiotics would have their greatest benefit.
- The most recent randomized, double-blind, placebo-controlled trial (level 1b) by Albu and colleagues[51] evaluated a long postoperative antibiotic protocol (amoxicillin-clavulanate 625 mg twice a day × 2 weeks). The results from this study demonstrate that postoperative antibiotics improve patient symptoms within the first 5 days and endoscopic appearance at the 12-day period. In addition, there was a significant reduction in sinonasal crust formation.

When using the 2 aforementioned level 1b studies, most experts would agree that postoperative antibiotics, following ESS, function to optimize early clinical outcomes. The benefits appear to be limited to the early post-ESS period, as symptoms were improved at 5 days and endoscopic appearance improved at 12 days. Although the optimal duration is poorly defined, the evidence suggests that a short 2-day course has no effect whereas a longer course up to 14 days provides a clinical response. Antibiotic choice must take into account common sinonasal pathogens, and usually involves the use of a penicillin-based agent or macrolide. Future studies need to elucidate the ideal duration of postoperative antibiotics after ESS.

Drug-Eluting Middle Meatal Spacers

Nasal crusting, retained secretions, and mucosal edema can limit early topical therapy following ESS. To improve local drug delivery in the early postoperative period, surgeons have developed off-label drug-eluting middle meatal spacers to provide a slow release of continuous topical therapy while removing the potential for patient noncompliance. Current off-label drug-eluting spacers are produced by the treating surgeon, who determines the type and dosage of steroid. Therefore, the major disadvantage is unknown drug release and limited data on systemic absorption. The ideal dose and safety profile must be evaluated before they can be recommended for routine use.

Three studies evaluated the role of drug-eluting spacers after ESS.[52–54]

- The studies by Kang and colleagues[52] (level 2b) and Cote and Wright[53] (level 1b) evaluated postoperative ethmoid cavity packing soaked with topical triamcinolone in CRS patients with nasal polyps. The studies demonstrated significant improvements in the endoscopic appearance at both early and late postoperative periods, as well as reduced polyp recurrence.

- The specific protocol used in the level 1b study by Cote and Wright[53] included a triamcinolone-soaked Nasopore spacer (Stryker Canada, Hamilton, ON, Canada) placed within the ethmoid cavity at the completion of ESS and removed at the week-1 debridement.

A recent level 1b study by Rudmik et al, utilized an off-label mixture of carboxymethylcellulose (CMC) foam and dexamethasone (4 ml of 4mg/ml) in patients who underwent ESS for medically refractory CRS without nasal polyposis.[54] The results failed to demonstrate an advantage of the steroid eluting spacer compared to placebo, however, the outcomes must be taken in context of the authors postoperative care protocol which utilized a short dose of systemic steroids and large volume saline irrigations.

Drug-Eluting Middle Meatal Stents

Drug-eluting stents are being developed for CRS, and they may have significant benefit in the treatment of this chronic inflammatory disease.[55] Potential drawbacks of stents include[51]:

- Risk of inducing inflammation as a foreign material
- Potential for unintended systemic absorption of the medication[56]

The Propel Sinus Implant (Intersect ENT, Palo Alto, CA, USA) has recently received approval from the Food and Drug Administration for use in patients with medically refractory CRS who have undergone ESS. The Propel implant is a dissolvable mometasone furoate–eluting stent, which is placed into a dissected ethmoid cavity and expands to contact the mucosa (**Fig. 4**). The stent eludes 370 µg of mometasone over 30 days and dissolves over 30 to 45 days.

Sinus implant/stent studies

A recent randomized, double-blind, placebo-controlled trial (level 1b) by Murr and colleagues evaluated the Propel sinus implant following ESS. The study evaluated 43 medically refractory CRS patients with and without nasal polyposis who elected ESS.[57] To prevent confounding effects, patients were not permitted to use either topical or systemic steroids for 30 days following ESS. Overall, the results demonstrated

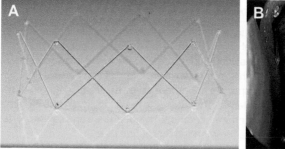
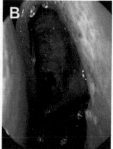

Fig. 4. The Propel Sinus Implant (Intersect ENT, Palo Alto, CA, USA). (*A*) Expanded ex vivo. (*B*) Expanded in an ethmoid cavity following ESS. (*Courtesy of* Intersect ENT, Palo Alto, CA; with permission.)

a significant reduction in polyp recurrence, adhesions, and mucosal inflammation on postoperative days 21 and 45. Furthermore, there was no evidence of adrenal suppression.

There have been 2 subsequent randomized trials (level 1b) evaluating the Propel stent, both of which demonstrated a reduction in the need for postoperative interventions, lysis of adhesions, and courses of oral steroid, as well as a reduction in polyp recurrence.[58,59]

A recent meta-analysis (level 1a) by Han and colleagues[54] demonstrated that drug-eluting stents reduced the need for postoperative interventions by 35% ($P = .008$), lysis of adhesions by 51% ($P = .0016$), and oral steroid need by 40% ($P = .0023$).[60]

Drug-eluting stents have shown promising initial results and may play an integral role in postoperative care following ESS for medically refractory CRS. However, all studies have primarily evaluated their impact in patients with nasal polyposis and have not fully evaluated their impact on patients' symptoms or HRQoL. Future studies need to evaluate the role of drug-eluting spacers/stents in patients with CRS without nasal polyposis, as well as HRQoL outcomes.

THE BOTTOM LINE: WHAT DOES THE EVIDENCE TELL US?

The evidence suggests that a strong postoperative care protocol would involve using nasal saline irrigations beginning 24 to 48 hours after ESS, performing an in-office debridement at 1 week after ESS, and starting a topical nasal steroid spray in the first 1 to 2 weeks after ESS. The need for multiple in-office debridements is often case dependent, and the surgeon must translate the clinical assessment of healing into the need for a debridement. For CRS cases with severe mucosal inflammation, the use of higher-concentration off-label topical steroid solutions, short-course systemic corticosteroids, or systemic antibiotics may improve clinical outcomes. Recent level 1a evidence demonstrates that middle meatal drug-eluting stents may significantly improve endoscopic outcomes for medically refractory CRS with nasal polyposis.

REFERENCES

1. Soler ZM, Mace J, Smith TL. Symptom-based presentation of chronic rhinosinusitis and symptom-specific outcomes after endoscopic sinus surgery. Am J Rhinol 2008;22:297–301.
2. Alobid I, Bernal-Sprekelsen M, Mullol J. Chronic rhinosinusitis and nasal polyps: the role of generic and specific questionnaires on assessing its impact on patient's quality of life. Allergy 2008;63:1267–79.
3. Alobid I, Guilemany JM, Mullol J. The impact of chronic rhinosinusitis and nasal polyposis in quality of life. Front Biosci (Elite Ed) 2009;1:269–76.
4. Birch DS, Saleh HA, Wodehouse T, et al. Assessing the quality of life for patients with chronic rhinosinusitis using the "Rhinosinusitis Disability Index". Rhinology 2001;39:191–6.
5. Smith TL, Litvack JR, Hwang PH, et al. Determinants of outcomes of sinus surgery: a multi-institutional prospective cohort study. Otolaryngol Head Neck Surg 2010;142:55–63.
6. Smith TL, Batra PS, Seiden AM, et al. Evidence supporting endoscopic sinus surgery in the management of adult chronic rhinosinusitis: a systematic review. Am J Rhinol 2005;19:537–43.
7. Bhattacharyya N. Clinical outcomes after endoscopic sinus surgery. Curr Opin Allergy Clin Immunol 2006;6:167–71.
8. Soler ZM, Smith TL. Quality of life outcomes after functional endoscopic sinus surgery. Otolaryngol Clin North Am 2010;43:605–12, x.

9. Bhattacharyya N. Ambulatory sinus and nasal surgery in the United States: demographics and perioperative outcomes. Laryngoscope 2010;120:635–8.

10. Kennedy DW. Functional endoscopic sinus surgery. Technique. Arch Otolaryngol 1985;111:643–9.

11. Fernandes SV. Postoperative care in functional endoscopic sinus surgery? Laryngoscope 1999;109:945–8.

12. Kennedy DW. Prognostic factors, outcomes and staging in ethmoid sinus surgery. Laryngoscope 1992;102:1–18.

13. Lund VJ, MacKay IS. Outcome assessment of endoscopic sinus surgery. J R Soc Med 1994;87:70–2.

14. Stammberger H. Endoscopic endonasal surgery—concepts in treatment of recurring rhinosinusitis. Part I. Anatomic and pathophysiologic considerations. Otolaryngol Head Neck Surg 1986;94:143–7.

15. Inanli S, Tutkun A, Batman C, et al. The effect of endoscopic sinus surgery on mucociliary activity and healing of maxillary sinus mucosa. Rhinology 2000;38:120–3.

16. Rudmik L, Soler Z, Orlandi R, et al. Early post-operative care following endoscopic sinus surgery: an evidence-based review with recommendations. Int Forum Allergy Rhinol 2011;1(6):417–30.

17. Harvey R, Hannan SA, Badia L, et al. Nasal saline irrigations for the symptoms of chronic rhinosinusitis. Cochrane Database Syst Rev 2007;3:CD006394.

18. Heatley DG, McConnell KE, Kille TL, et al. Nasal irrigation for the alleviation of sinonasal symptoms. Otolaryngol Head Neck Surg 2001;125:44–8.

19. Tomooka LT, Murphy C, Davidson TM. Clinical study and literature review of nasal irrigation. Laryngoscope 2000;110:1189–93.

20. Pigret D, Jankowski R. Management of post-ethmoidectomy crust formation: randomized single-blind clinical trial comparing pressurized seawater versus antiseptic/mucolytic saline. Rhinology 1996;34:38–40.

21. Pinto JM, Elwany S, Baroody FM, et al. Effects of saline sprays on symptoms after endoscopic sinus surgery. Am J Rhinol 2006;20:191–6.

22. Fooanant S, Chaiyasate S, Roongrotwattanasiri K. Comparison on the efficacy of dexpanthenol in sea water and saline in postoperative endoscopic sinus surgery. J Med Assoc Thai 2008;91:1558–63.

23. Freeman SR, Sivayoham ES, Jepson K, et al. A preliminary randomised controlled trial evaluating the efficacy of saline douching following endoscopic sinus surgery. Clin Otolaryngol 2008;33:462–5.

24. Liang KL, Su MC, Tseng HC, et al. Impact of pulsatile nasal irrigation on the prognosis of functional endoscopic sinus surgery. J Otolaryngol Head Neck Surg 2008;37:148–53.

25. Staffieri A, Marino F, Staffieri C, et al. The effects of sulfurous-arsenical-ferruginous thermal water nasal irrigation in wound healing after functional endoscopic sinus surgery for chronic rhinosinusitis: a prospective randomized study. Am J Otolaryngol 2008;29:223–9.

26. Pynnonen MA, Mukerji SS, Kim HM, et al. Nasal saline for chronic sinonasal symptoms: a randomized controlled trial. Arch Otolaryngol Head Neck Surg 2007;133:1115–20.

27. Nilssen EL, Wardrop P, El-Hakim H, et al. A randomized control trial of post-operative care following endoscopic sinus surgery: debridement versus no debridement. J Laryngol Otol 2002;116:108–11.

28. Bugten V, Nordgard S, Steinsvag S. The effects of debridement after endoscopic sinus surgery. Laryngoscope 2006;116:2037–43.

29. Bugten V, Nordgard S, Steinsvag S. Long-term effects of postoperative measures after sinus surgery. Eur Arch Otorhinolaryngol 2008;265:531–7.

30. Kuhnel T, Hosemann W, Wagner W, et al. How traumatising is mechanical mucous membrane care after interventions on paranasal sinuses? A histological immuno-histochemical study. Laryngorhinootologie 1996;75:575–9 [in German].

31. Kemppainen T, Seppa J, Tuomilehto H, et al. Repeated early debridement does not provide significant symptomatic benefit after ESS. Rhinology 2008;46: 238–42.

32. Lee JY, Byun JY. Relationship between the frequency of postoperative debride-ment and patient discomfort, healing period, surgical outcomes, and compliance after endoscopic sinus surgery. Laryngoscope 2008;118:1868–72.

33. Harvey RJ, Debnath N, Srubiski A, et al. Fluid residuals and drug exposure in nasal irrigation. Otolaryngol Head Neck Surg 2009;141:757–61.

34. Rowe-Jones JM, Medcalf M, Durham SR, et al. Functional endoscopic sinus surgery: 5 year follow up and results of a prospective, randomised, stratified, double-blind, placebo controlled study of postoperative fluticasone propionate aqueous nasal spray. Rhinology 2005;43:2–10.

35. Jorissen M, Bachert C. Effect of corticosteroids on wound healing after endo-scopic sinus surgery. Rhinology 2009;47:280–6.

36. Stjarne P, Olsson P, Alenius M. Use of mometasone furoate to prevent polyp relapse after endoscopic sinus surgery. Arch Otolaryngol Head Neck Surg 2009;135:296–302.

37. Dijkstra MD, Ebbens FA, Poublon RM, et al. Fluticasone propionate aqueous nasal spray does not influence the recurrence rate of chronic rhinosinusitis and nasal polyps 1 year after functional endoscopic sinus surgery. Clin Exp Allergy 2004;34:1395–400.

38. Product information. 2010. Available at: http://www.spfiles.com/pinasonex.pdf. Accessed July 20, 2012.

39. Del Gaudio JM, Wise SK. Topical steroid drops for the treatment of sinus ostia stenosis in the postoperative period. Am J Rhinol 2006;20:563–7.

40. Bhalla RK, Payton K, Wright ED. Safety of budesonide in saline sinonasal irri-gations in the management of chronic rhinosinusitis with polyposis: lack of significant adrenal suppression. J Otolaryngol Head Neck Surg 2008;37: 821–5.

41. Welch KC, Thaler ER, Doghramji LL, et al. The effects of serum and urinary cortisol levels of topical intranasal irrigations with budesonide added to saline in patients with recurrent polyposis after endoscopic sinus surgery. Am J Rhinol Allergy 2010;24:26–8.

42. Poetker DM, Reh DD. A comprehensive review of the adverse effects of systemic corticosteroids. Otolaryngol Clin North Am 2010;43:753–68.

43. van Staa TP, Leufkens HG, Cooper C. The epidemiology of corticosteroid-induced osteoporosis: a meta-analysis. Osteoporos Int 2002;13:777–87.

44. Souverein PC, Berard A, Van Staa TP, et al. Use of oral glucocorticoids and risk of cardiovascular and cerebrovascular disease in a population based case-control study. Heart 2004;90:859–65.

45. Wright ED, Agrawal S. Impact of perioperative systemic steroids on surgical outcomes in patients with chronic rhinosinusitis with polyposis: evaluation with the novel Perioperative Sinus Endoscopy (POSE) scoring system. Laryngoscope 2007;117:1–28.

46. Zhang Z, Han D, Zhang S, et al. Biofilms and mucosal healing in postsurgical patients with chronic rhinosinusitis. Am J Rhinol Allergy 2009;23:506–11.

47. Jervis-Bardy J, Foreman A, Field J, et al. Impaired mucosal healing and infection associated with *Staphylococcus aureus* after endoscopic sinus surgery. Am J Rhinol Allergy 2009;23:549–52.

48. Stammberger H, Posawetz W. Functional endoscopic sinus surgery. Concept, indications and results of the Messerklinger technique. Eur Arch Otorhinolaryngol 1990;247:63–76.

49. Annys E, Jorissen M. Short term effects of antibiotics (Zinnat) after endoscopic sinus surgery. Acta Otorhinolaryngol Belg 2000;54:23–8.

50. Jiang RS, Liang KL, Yang KY, et al. Postoperative antibiotic care after functional endoscopic sinus surgery. Am J Rhinol 2008;22:608–12.

51. Albu S, Lucaciu R. Prophylactic antibiotics in endoscopic sinus surgery: A short follow-up study. Am J Rhinol Allergy 2010;24:306–9.

52. Cote DW, Wright ED. Triamcinolone-impregnated nasal dressing following endoscopic sinus surgery: a randomized, double-blind, placebo-controlled study. Laryngoscope 2010;120:1269–73.

53. Kang IG, Yoon BK, Jung JH, et al. The effect of high-dose topical corticosteroid therapy on prevention of recurrent nasal polyps after revision endoscopic sinus surgery. Am J Rhinol 2008;22:497–501.

54. Rudmik L, Mace J, Mechor B. Effect of a dexamethasone Sinu-Foam(TM) middle meatal spacer on endoscopic sinus surgery outcomes: A randomized, double-blind, placebo-controlled trial. Int Forum Allergy Rhinol 2012;2:248–51.

55. Bednarski KA, Kuhn FA. Stents and drug-eluting stents. Otolaryngol Clin North Am 2009;42:857–66, x.

56. Valentine R, Wormald PJ. Are routine dissolvable nasal dressings necessary following endoscopic sinus surgery? Laryngoscope 2010;120:1920–1.

57. Murr AH, Smith TL, Hwang PH, et al. Safety and efficacy of a novel bioabsorbable, steroid-eluting sinus stent. Int Forum Allergy Rhinol 2011;1:23–32.

58. Marple BF, Smith TL, Han JK, et al. Advance II: A Prospective, Randomized Study Assessing Safety and Efficacy of Bioabsorbable Steroid-Releasing Sinus Implants. Otolaryngol Head Neck Surg 2012;146:1004–11.

59. Forwith KD, Chandra RK, Yun PT, Miller SK, Jampel HD, et al. ADVANCE: a multisite trial of bioabsorbable steroid-eluting sinus implants. Laryngoscope 2011; 121:2473–80.

60. Han JK, Marple BF, Smith TL, et al. Effect of steroid-releasing sinus implants on postoperative medical and surgical interventions: an efficacy meta-analysis. Int Forum Allergy Rhinol 2012.

Evidence-Based Practice
Functional Rhinoplasty

Daniel E. Cannon, MD*, John S. Rhee, MD, MPH

KEYWORDS

- Functional rhinoplasty • Evidence-based medicine • Nasal valve
- Systematic review

KEY POINTS

- Subjective patient-reported measures have an important role in the evaluation of nasal obstruction. Of these measures, the Nasal Obstruction Symptom Evaluation and visual analog scales are the most applicable to nasal valve compromise (NVC).
- Several objective measures for nasal obstruction exist, although none of them are widely accepted as the gold standard. New methods for evaluating nasal physiology, such as computational fluid dynamics, may prove valuable in the evaluation and treatment of NVC.
- In general, there is weak correlation between existing subjective and objective measures of nasal obstruction and controversy over which are most important in evaluating the efficacy of treatment.
- Surgical treatment of NVC consists of a wide variety of techniques, with evidence for their efficacy, although better study designs and outcome measures are needed.

PROBLEM/OVERVIEW

Nasal obstruction is a complaint frequently encountered in otolaryngology. This obstruction can occur as a result of underlying inflammatory or anatomic pathologic conditions. Inflammatory pathologic conditions include allergic rhinitis, nasal polyposis, and chronic rhinosinusitis. Among the anatomic causes are septal deviation, turbinate hypertrophy, and nasal valve compromise (NVC). The nasal valve was first described by Mink in the early twentieth century[1] but has received increasing attention recently. It is the narrowest portion of the nasal airway and, therefore, where the most resistance to airflow occurs.[2] It can be divided into external and internal portions (Fig. 1).[3] The external nasal valve is the area in the nasal vestibule formed by the alar rim, nasal sill, caudal septum, and medial crus of the lower lateral cartilage. The

Financial disclosures/conflicts of interest: The authors have nothing to disclose.
Department of Otolaryngology and Communication Sciences, Medical College of Wisconsin, 9200 West Wisconsin Avenue, Milwaukee, WI 53226, USA
* Corresponding author.
E-mail address: dcannon@mcw.edu

Otolaryngol Clin N Am 45 (2012) 1033–1043
http://dx.doi.org/10.1016/j.otc.2012.06.007
0030-6665/12/$ – see front matter © 2012 Published by Elsevier Inc.

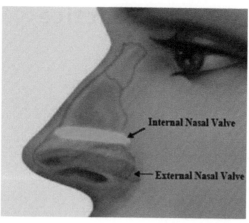

Fig. 1. Locations and components of internal and external nasal valves.

internal nasal valve is the area bound by the caudal edge of the upper lateral cartilage, nasal septum, head of the inferior turbinate, and nasal sill (**Fig. 2**) and is located approximately 1.3 cm from the nares.[2] It is proposed that the nasal valve serves as a regulator to prevent airflow from exceeding the capacity of the nose to warm and humidify inspired air.[4,5]

Problems with nasal airflow occurring at the nasal valve exhibit both static and dynamic properties. There can be fixed anatomic obstruction caused by abnormalities of any of the structures that contribute to the makeup of the nasal valve, including the septum, turbinates, and nasal cartilages. These abnormalities can exist as a result of traumatic, congenital, or iatrogenic causes.[6] There can also be a dynamic component to NVC. Bernoulli's principle states that air flowing into narrowed segments accelerates, leading to a decrease in intraluminal pressure. This phenomenon can contribute to dynamic collapse of the lateral nasal wall during inspiration, leading to further compromise of the nasal valve region resulting in obstruction of nasal airflow.[2,7] The difficulty in evaluating patients with NVC is determining whether the problem is the small diameter of the nasal valve causing fixed obstruction or whether the lack of rigidity of the lateral nasal wall leading to dynamic collapse is the issue because the surgical approach may differ depending on the underlying problem.

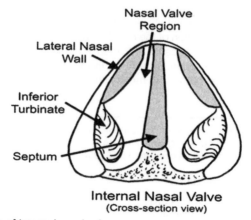

Fig. 2. Components of internal nasal valve.

Functional rhinoplasty has emerged in the literature as a collective term for procedures that address nasal obstruction occurring at the nasal valve.[8] This term serves to differentiate procedures directed at correcting nasal obstruction from those that address the cosmetic appearance of the nose and includes techniques that target the nasal septum (dorsal and caudal portions), lateral nasal wall, and the soft tissue nasal vestibule. However, in reality, the structure and function of the nose are intimately related. Therefore, procedures performed with the intent to change the cosmetic appearance of the nose can also affect its function and vice versa.[3,9–11] One must be cognizant of this relationship when counseling patients and undertaking nasal surgery for either cosmetic or functional purposes. Functional rhinoplasty and nasal valve repair are commonly used as synonymous terms and, thus, are used interchangeably for the purposes of this article.

EVIDENCE-BASED CLINICAL ASSESSMENT
History and Physical Examination

The main symptom of NVC is decreased nasal airflow. However, there are a myriad of conditions that can present with nasal obstruction. These conditions include infectious, inflammatory, and neoplastic conditions, and the treatment varies depending on the underlying cause. Therefore, a detailed history should include the timing, onset, seasonal variation, laterality, prior history of nasal trauma or surgery, and exacerbating or alleviating factors of nasal obstruction. It is also important to determine the presence or absence of associated symptoms, such as epistaxis, anosmia, rhinorrhea, or postnasal drainage. This differentiation can help identify or rule out causes of nasal obstruction that are not attributable to pathologic conditions of the nasal valve.

There is currently no gold standard objective test to diagnose NVC[2]; it remains a clinical diagnosis. A general assessment of the external appearance of the nose can identify problems with the potential to cause nasal obstruction, such as nasal tip ptosis, a narrow midvault, an inverted-V deformity, or narrowed nostrils. Additional physical examination techniques can identify abnormalities of the lateral nasal wall related to weak or malformed upper and/or lower lateral cartilages. Specifically, findings on physical examination suggestive of NVC include visible inspiratory collapse of the lateral nasal wall or alar rim. Also, subjective and audible improvement in nasal airflow during a Cottle maneuver (lateral retraction of the cheek) or modified Cottle maneuver (intranasal lateralization of the lateral nasal wall) is consistent with NVC.

Anterior rhinoscopy is an adequate intranasal evaluation of the nasal valve region and will provide information about the position of the septum and size of the turbinates. Nasal endoscopy can be useful to rule out other causes of nasal obstruction not attributable to NVC if the diagnosis is uncertain but is not routinely indicated. If surgery is being planned or considered, preoperative photography can be helpful for patient counseling, preoperative planning, and documentation, even in cases when the surgical intent is purely functional, but this is especially true if surgery is being undertaken for both functional and cosmetic purposes.

In patients with NVC, it can be difficult to determine which components of the nasal valve to address because there are several anatomic structures that contribute. However, identifying the problematic area can help guide the surgeon in deciding which procedure is likely to provide the most benefit. In general, functional rhinoplasty techniques target a specific area or component of the nasal valve. Also, determining whether obstruction is resulting more from fixed or dynamic obstruction can help the surgeon decide between a procedure intended to increase the actual diameter of the nasal valve or one that aims to strengthen a weak lateral wall or alar rim.

Subjective Measures of Nasal Obstruction

Traditionally, a common method of assessing nasal obstruction and reporting outcomes of functional nasal surgery is subjective patient-reported measures. For assessing the efficacy of a surgical intervention, a comparison of preoperative and postoperative results is often used. In addition, there has been a trend in medicine toward evaluating quality of life (QOL) in the assessment of disease processes and the efficacy of treatment.[12] Generic health-related QOL can be measured using scales, such as the Medical Outcomes Study Short Forms (SF-12 and SF-36).[13–15] However, disease-specific QOL measures can be superior to generic QOL instruments because they may be more sensitive for the detection and quantification of small changes.[16] There are validated QOL instruments specific for rhinologic disease, such as the Rhinosinusitis Disability Index,[17,18] Rhinoconjunctivitis Quality of Life Questionnaire,[19,20] and the Sinonasal Outcomes Test,[21] each of which has been used in the past for evaluating septal or nasal valve pathologic conditions. These instruments all include nasal obstruction in their evaluation; however, their primary purpose is the evaluation of inflammatory nasal disease, which may secondarily result in nasal obstructive symptoms.

Nasal obstruction symptom evaluation scale

The QOL measure most relevant to structurally based nasal valve pathologic conditions is the Nasal Obstruction Symptom Evaluation scale, a disease-specific quality-of-life instrument developed for the assessment of nasal obstruction with evidence in support of its validity, reliability, and sensitivity.[22] With this instrument, patients are asked to rate the severity of several nasal symptoms and the results are summed and scaled. Its original use was in patients undergoing septoplasty who demonstrated an improvement in disease-specific QOL after surgery.[23] Subsequent studies using the NOSE scale in patients undergoing surgery for NVC also demonstrated statistically significant improvements in disease-specific QOL.[24,25]

Visual analog scales

Visual analog scales (VAS) are a common method of subjectively measuring symptoms in various conditions that have also been used as an evaluation method and outcome measure in nasal obstruction. In VAS, patients are asked to rate their experience of symptoms on a linear scale ranging from no obstruction to complete obstruction.[26] Multiple studies have shown improvement in VAS for nasal obstruction after nasal valve repair.[4,27] One potential advantage of VAS over other objective tests is that, for patients with unilateral symptoms, VAS for each side of the nasal cavity can be assessed separately. Several studies show better correlation between VAS for nasal obstruction and objective measurement techniques when unilateral VAS is used.[28–30]

Objective Measures of Nasal Obstruction

Aside from subjective measures, there is also interest in the development and implementation of validated objective measures to assist in preoperative evaluation and to better assess surgical outcomes. Several techniques have been developed and validated to date. Of these, rhinomanometry and acoustic rhinometry (AR) have been used most frequently.[4,27] Rhinomanometry allows the determination of nasal airway resistance by simultaneously measuring transnasal pressure drop and nasal airflow.[31] This technique has been used to objectively document changes in nasal resistance after nasal valve surgery. However, it is not in widespread use because of several limitations. These drawbacks include the inability to precisely locate the area of obstruction and the need for specialized equipment and a well-trained operator.[32]

AR for nasal obstruction

AR is a technique that uses the measurement of deflected sound waves to provide an estimate of the cross-sectional area (CSA) of the nasal cavity as a function of the distance from the nostrils.[33] AR is relatively easy to perform and is quick and noninvasive. It too has limitations, however. Similar to rhinomanometry, it does require specialized equipment and an experienced operator. Also, the results obtained are sensitive to variations in technique and testing conditions.[34] Another known limitation of AR is that it overestimates CSA in areas beyond 5 cm from the nostrils[35] or after constricted regions or areas of drastic changes in nasal anatomy.[36] The advantages of AR make it one of the most common objective methods used to evaluate nasal patency. However, it has not achieved widespread clinical use because of the limitations noted previously.

Imaging studies for nasal obstruction

Imaging studies, such as computed tomography (CT) or magnetic resonance imaging (MRI) scans, can have a role in the evaluation of nasal obstruction, with utility in evaluating infectious, inflammatory, or neoplastic disease, but have a limited role in the evaluation of nasal valve pathologic conditions specifically.[2] CT imaging can be used as a method of measuring the nasal valve angle (between the septum and upper lateral cartilage). When used for this purpose, the most accurate measures are obtained from views other than the traditional coronal view, which may underestimate the true nasal valve angle. Specifically, a modified view known as the nasal base view, which uses slices oriented perpendicular to the approximated acoustic axis of the nose, provides the most accurate information about the nasal valve angle.[37] This technique has not been adopted for widespread use because there is subjectivity in the selection of the acoustic axis and the need to reformat CT images into a nonstandard view. There is also a lack of evidence in regard to its reproducibility, although studies comparing this method with AR-derived data show good correlation in the measurement of the nasal valve area.[38]

Computational fluid dynamics for nasal obstruction

Computational fluid dynamics (CFD) is emerging as a new method to evaluate nasal airflow and resistance as well as other physiologic parameters important to the function of the nose, including particle deposition and air conditioning. CFD is a technology used widely in engineering as a way to model the motion of fluids. For this technique, anatomically accurate 3-dimensional computational models of patients' nasal cavities are generated from imaging data captured by CT or MRI (**Fig. 3**). CFD software programs can then be used to obtain computed measures of airflow, resistance, heat transfer, and air humidification.

The ability to study multiple parameters of interest under different simulated conditions with minimal cost or inconvenience to patients makes CFD an attractive method to investigate nasal function. A further benefit of CFD over other objective measures of nasal function is the ability to determine airflow and other factors of interest at precise anatomic locations rather than in the nasal cavity as a whole as is done with other methods. Another exciting extension of CFD technology is the ability to do simulated surgery on the digital models. The computed nasal geometry can be virtually modified in a manner reflecting surgical techniques, and, subsequently, new patterns of airflow and heat and water vapor transport can be calculated.[39,40]

There are also limitations with current CFD technology. There is additional cost to obtain the necessary imaging studies. Also, at present, the process of producing the digital models is time and labor intensive, although as technology has advanced,

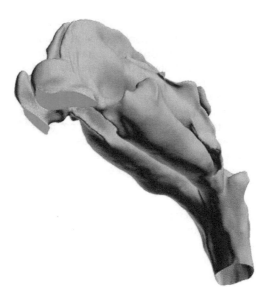

Fig. 3. Digital nasal airway model for use in CFD analysis.

the cost and time to build models has declined and is expected to continue to do so. Further, although models can be built from either CT or MRI scans, the models based on CT imaging give better results because of better resolution, thus subjecting patients to radiation exposure that they would otherwise not receive. CFD also makes assumptions that are reasonable in many cases but may not always hold true, such as laminar flow of air within the nasal cavity, fixed and rigid nasal cavity walls, and steady-state airflow.[31]

CFD analysis with respect to nasal function is still in its early stages and most studies are limited in scope and number. Further studies are needed to fully validate the method and elucidate the correlation between CFD-derived parameters and actual clinical and patient-reported data. However, this exciting technology holds great promise and may prove to be a valuable resource in objective preoperative evaluation, surgical planning, and analysis of surgical outcomes for surgeons performing functional rhinoplasty.

Controversy in Outcome Measures

An area of conflict in many medical conditions is the relationship between what patients subjectively report and what is objectively observed by physicians or measured by objective tests.[26] This point is especially true in the area of nasal obstruction. This issue is complex and is not explained by nasal resistance and airflow alone. Nasal sensation also plays a large role, as demonstrated by studies whereby nasal sensation has been blocked with local anesthetics in the nasal cavity or vestibule, with studies reporting both increases and decreases in perceived nasal airflow without any measured effect on nasal resistance.[41] This finding suggests that the sensation of nasal airflow may, under certain circumstances, be independent of any objectively measurable change in nasal resistance. Therefore, some investigators have made the argument that subjective patient-reported measures are the most important factor when evaluating nasal obstruction.[2,41,42]

Ideally, a gold standard objective test would be quantifiable, reproducible, and have a strong correlation with subjective measures of nasal airflow.[26,31] As described earlier, such a test has not been reported to date. Independently, subjective and objective tests have shown validity and reproducibility but there is weak correlation when compared side by side.[26,41,43] It has been proposed that the different methods of assessment are capturing different aspects of the nasal airway and, therefore, may be complementary.[26] Although an ideal test of nasal patency remains elusive, it may prove to be the case in the future that a combination of testing methods with both subjective and objective components best approaches the conditions mentioned earlier. In the meantime, the debate is ongoing regarding the role of subjective and objective measures in the evaluation of nasal obstruction.

EVIDENCE-BASED SURGICAL TECHNIQUE

With respect to evidence for the efficacy of functional rhinoplasty, there have been 3 important contributions to the literature in recent years: 2 systematic reviews and 1 clinical consensus statement.

In 2008, Rhee and colleagues[27] conducted a systematic review of the existing literature on the efficacy of modern-day rhinoplasty techniques for the treatment of NVC. Their review spanned a 25-year period, from 1982 to 2007. Forty-four articles met their inclusion criteria and were each assigned a level of evidence.

- Only 2 of the studies, both cohort studies that compared one surgical technique to another, achieved level 2b evidence.
- The remaining 42 studies were all level 4 evidence and were of varying quality.
- Procedures performed in the reviewed studies included spreader grafts, butterfly onlay grafts, alar batten grafts, dorsal onlay grafts, alar cartilage relocation, alar rim grafts, suture suspension, flaring sutures, columellar struts, and onlay grafts.
- All of the included articles were in support of the efficacy of functional rhinoplasty techniques for the treatment of NVC, with reported effectiveness ranging from 65% to 100%.
- Of the articles, only 6 (14%) reported outcomes using validated patient-reported questionnaires and 12 (27%) used objective measures, the most common objective measurement being rhinomanometry.
- In 75% of the studies, adjunctive surgical procedures were performed in combination with nasal valve surgery, including septoplasty, turbinate reduction, functional endoscopic sinus surgery, and orthognathic surgery, which diluted the ability to measure the efficacy of the functional rhinoplasty component alone.
- In all, the investigators assigned the evidence an aggregate grade C recommendation in support of functional rhinoplasty as a treatment of NVC.

An additional corroborating systematic review conducted by Spielmann and colleagues[4] was published in 2009.

- The authors noted that there seemed to be a move toward the use of stronger outcome measures because most of the articles that used validated objective or subjective measures were published after 2004.
- The investigators also noted that much of the published literature on functional rhinoplasty is more concerned with technical descriptions of surgical technique rather than establishing evidence of a long-term benefit.
- The investigators concluded, similarly to the Rhee and colleagues review aforementioned, that the evidence was generally in favor of the efficacy of functional rhinoplasty. Again, this finding would correlate to an overall grade C recommendation.

The American Academy of Otolaryngology-Head and Neck Surgery's Consensus Statement

As a reflection of the lack of cohesiveness among clinicians regarding the diagnosis and management of pathologic conditions involving the nasal valve as well as the relative lack of strong evidence in the literature, the American Academy of Otolaryngology-Head and Neck Surgery, in 2010, endorsed a clinical consensus statement aimed at addressing the ambiguities and disparities that exist regarding NVC.[2] It was thought that a consensus statement was more appropriate as opposed to a clinical practice guideline based on the lack of strong evidence available. The panel members, all experts in functional nasal surgery, reviewed the existing literature on NVC, including the 2 reviews previously mentioned. With regard to the literature, the panel noted that much of the difficulty in analyzing the evidence for nasal valve repair lies in the wide variety of techniques that were reported as well as the additional procedures (ie, septoplasty, turbinate reduction, or endoscopic sinus surgery) that are often done in conjunction with rhinoplasty, making it difficult to determine how much of the benefit might be attributable to these other interventions. However, they did note a consistent finding of beneficial effects of nasal valve surgery in all reviewed studies. Regarding outcome measures, there was a near consensus regarding the relative importance of patient-reported outcome measures versus objective measures in measuring the success of an intervention. The general conclusion was that patient-oriented outcomes are more important than objective outcomes.

Nonsurgical Management

Patients who have NVC and coexisting allergic or inflammatory symptoms or findings on physical examination suggestive of rhinitis may benefit from treatment of these conditions or a trial of medical therapy, such as intranasal steroids, before considering surgical intervention. However, in absence of these symptoms or findings, there is no role for medical therapy.[2] There are additional nonsurgical options that may be considered, including nasal dilator strips or stents.[44–47] The ability of patients to adhere to these treatments in the long term is unknown. However, these alternatives may be a good option for patients who do not wish to pursue surgery or are not good candidates for surgery because of medical comorbidities.

BOTTOM LINE: WHAT DOES THE EVIDENCE TELL US?

Although the gold standard in evidence-based medicine is the randomized controlled trial,[48] this is often not a possibility in surgical research because of the ethical and practical difficulties of randomizing patients to different surgical procedures in a blinded fashion. Therefore, surgical outcome studies often rely on retrospective and observational studies (ie, level 2b evidence) at best, with a preponderance of level 4 and 5 evidence.[49] To date, most functional rhinoplasty studies are uncontrolled studies (level 4 evidence) of varying quality. The heterogeneity of study designs and outcome measures does not allow pooling of studies to strengthen the existing evidence. Additionally, many of the studies include simultaneous procedures aimed to correct nasal obstruction (ie, septoplasty, turbinate reduction), adding another level of complexity in analyzing the evidence because it is impossible to determine how much benefit was a result of nasal valve repair itself.

However, it is important to make the distinction between weak evidence and lack of evidence for efficacy.[2] Although the existing evidence is relatively weak, it does show a consistent benefit of nasal valve repair (grade C recommendation). The reported efficacy ranges from 65% to 100%[4,27]; there are no studies reporting that functional rhinoplasty is ineffective. Studies with improved design, including comparison cohorts and using validated outcome measures, would better establish the efficacy of functional rhinoplasty for the correction of NVC.[27,42]

REFERENCES

1. Yarlagadda BB, Dolan RW. Nasal valve dysfunction: diagnosis and treatment. Curr Opin Otolaryngol Head Neck Surg 2011;19(1):25–9.
2. Rhee JS, Weaver EM, Park SS, et al. Clinical consensus statement: diagnosis and management of nasal valve compromise. Otolaryngol Head Neck Surg 2010; 143(1):48–59.
3. Ballert JA, Park SS. Functional rhinoplasty: treatment of the dysfunctional nasal sidewall. Facial Plast Surg 2006;22(1):49–54.
4. Spielmann PM, White PS, Hussain SS. Surgical techniques for the treatment of nasal valve collapse: a systematic review. Laryngoscope 2009;119(7):1281–90.
5. Kim DW, Rodriguez-Bruno K. Functional rhinoplasty. Facial Plast Surg Clin North Am 2009;17(1):115–31, vii.
6. Khosh MM, Jen A, Honrado C, et al. Nasal valve reconstruction: experience in 53 consecutive patients. Arch Facial Plast Surg 2004;6(3):167–71.
7. Wittkopf M, Wittkopf J, Ries WR. The diagnosis and treatment of nasal valve collapse. Curr Opin Otolaryngol Head Neck Surg 2008;16(1):10–3.
8. Most SP. Trends in functional rhinoplasty. Arch Facial Plast Surg 2008;10(6): 410–3.
9. Kim YH, Kim BJ, Jang TY. Use of porous high-density polyethylene (Medpor) for spreader or extended septal graft in rhinoplasty: aesthetics, functional outcomes, and long-term complications. Ann Plast Surg 2011;67(5):464–8.
10. Ballert JA, Park SS. Functional considerations in revision rhinoplasty. Facial Plast Surg 2008;24(3):348–57.
11. Gola R. Functional and esthetic rhinoplasty. Aesthetic Plast Surg 2003;27(5): 390–6.
12. Rhee JS, McMullin BT. Outcome measures in facial plastic surgery: patient-reported and clinical efficacy measures. Arch Facial Plast Surg 2008;10(3): 194–207.
13. Ware J Jr, Kosinski M, Keller SD. A 12-item short-form health survey: construction of scales and preliminary tests of reliability and validity. Med Care 1996;34(3):220–33.
14. McHorney CA, Ware JE Jr, Raczek AE. The MOS 36-item short-form health survey (SF-36): II. Psychometric and clinical tests of validity in measuring physical and mental health constructs. Med Care 1993;31(3):247–63.
15. Ware JE Jr, Sherbourne CD. The MOS 36-item short-form health survey (SF-36). I. Conceptual framework and item selection. Med Care 1992;30(6):473–83.
16. Patrick DL, Deyo RA. Generic and disease-specific measures in assessing health status and quality of life. Med Care 1989;27(Suppl 3):S217–32.
17. Benninger MS, Senior BA. The development of the rhinosinusitis disability index. Arch Otolaryngol Head Neck Surg 1997;123(11):1175–9.
18. Senior BA, Glaze C, Benninger MS. Use of the rhinosinusitis disability index (RSDI) in rhinologic disease. Am J Rhinol 2001;15(1):15–20.
19. Juniper EF, Guyatt GH. Development and testing of a new measure of health status for clinical trials in rhinoconjunctivitis. Clin Exp Allergy 1991;21(1):77–83.
20. Juniper EF, Guyatt GH, Andersson B, et al. Comparison of powder and aerosolized budesonide in perennial rhinitis: validation of rhinitis quality of life questionnaire. Ann Allergy 1993;70(3):225–30.

21. Hopkins C, Gillett S, Slack R, et al. Psychometric validity of the 22-item sinonasal outcome test. Clin Otolaryngol 2009;34(5):447–54.
22. Stewart MG, Witsell DL, Smith TL, et al. Development and validation of the Nasal Obstruction Symptom Evaluation (NOSE) scale. Otolaryngol Head Neck Surg 2004;130(2):157–63.
23. Stewart MG, Smith TL, Weaver EM, et al. Outcomes after nasal septoplasty: results from the Nasal Obstruction Septoplasty Effectiveness (NOSE) study. Otolaryngol Head Neck Surg 2004;130(3):283–90.
24. Rhee JS, Poetker DM, Smith TL, et al. Nasal valve surgery improves disease-specific quality of life. Laryngoscope 2005;115(3):437–40.
25. Most SP. Analysis of outcomes after functional rhinoplasty using a disease-specific quality-of-life instrument. Arch Facial Plast Surg 2006;8(5):306–9.
26. Lam DJ, James KT, Weaver EM. Comparison of anatomic, physiological, and subjective measures of the nasal airway. Am J Rhinol 2006;20(5):463–70.
27. Rhee JS, Arganbright JM, McMullin BT, et al. Evidence supporting functional rhinoplasty or nasal valve repair: a 25-year systematic review. Otolaryngol Head Neck Surg 2008;139(1):10–20.
28. Clarke JD, Hopkins ML, Eccles R. Evidence for correlation of objective and subjective measures of nasal airflow in patients with common cold. Clin Otolaryngol 2005;30(1):35–8.
29. Sipila J, Suonpaa J, Silvoniemi P, et al. Correlations between subjective sensation of nasal patency and rhinomanometry in both unilateral and total nasal assessment. ORL J Otorhinolaryngol Relat Spec 1995;57(5):260–3.
30. Hirschberg A, Rezek O. Correlation between objective and subjective assessments of nasal patency. ORL J Otorhinolaryngol Relat Spec 1998;60(4):206–11.
31. Pawar SS, Garcia GJ, Kimbell JS, et al. Objective measures in aesthetic and functional nasal surgery: perspectives on nasal form and function. Facial Plast Surg 2010;26(4):320–7.
32. Chandra RK, Patadia MO, Raviv J. Diagnosis of nasal airway obstruction. Otolaryngol Clin North Am 2009;42(2):207–25, vii.
33. Hilberg O, Jackson AC, Swift DL, et al. Acoustic rhinometry: evaluation of nasal cavity geometry by acoustic reflection. J Appl Physiol 1989;66(1):295–303.
34. Clement PA, Gordts F. Standardisation Committee on Objective Assessment of the Nasal Airway, IRS, and ERS. Consensus report on acoustic rhinometry and rhinomanometry. Rhinology 2005;43(3):169–79.
35. Terheyden H, Maune S, Mertens J, et al. Acoustic rhinometry: validation by three-dimensionally reconstructed computer tomographic scans. J Appl Physiol 2000;89(3):1013–21.
36. Cakmak O, Celik H, Ergin T, et al. Accuracy of acoustic rhinometry measurements. Laryngoscope 2001;111(4 Pt 1):587–94.
37. Poetker DM, Rhee JS, Mocan BO, et al. Computed tomography technique for evaluation of the nasal valve. Arch Facial Plast Surg 2004;6(4):240–3.
38. Cakmak O, Coskun M, Celik H, et al. Value of acoustic rhinometry for measuring nasal valve area. Laryngoscope 2003;113(2):295–302.
39. Rhee JS, Pawar SS, Garcia GJ, et al. Toward personalized nasal surgery using computational fluid dynamics. Arch Facial Plast Surg 2011;13(5):305–10.
40. Garcia GJ, Rhee JS, Senior BA, et al. Septal deviation and nasal resistance: an investigation using virtual surgery and computational fluid dynamics. Am J Rhinol Allergy 2010;24(1):e46–53.

41. Andre RF, Vuyk HD, Ahmed A, et al. Correlation between subjective and objective evaluation of the nasal airway. A systematic review of the highest level of evidence. Clin Otolaryngol 2009;34(6):518–25.
42. Rhee JS. Measuring outcomes in nasal surgery: realities and possibilities. Arch Facial Plast Surg 2009;11(6):416–9.
43. Stewart MG, Smith TL. Objective versus subjective outcomes assessment in rhinology. Am J Rhinol 2005;19(5):529–35.
44. Kirkness JP, Wheatley JR, Amis TC. Nasal airflow dynamics: mechanisms and responses associated with an external nasal dilator strip. Eur Respir J 2000; 15(5):929–36.
45. Peltonen LI, Vento SI, Simola M, et al. Effects of the nasal strip and dilator on nasal breathing–a study with healthy subjects. Rhinology 2004;42(3):122–5.
46. Roithmann R, Chapnik J, Cole P, et al. Role of the external nasal dilator in the management of nasal obstruction. Laryngoscope 1998;108(5):712–5.
47. Ellegard E. Mechanical nasal alar dilators. Rhinology 2006;44(4):239–48.
48. McCarthy CM. Randomized controlled trials. Plast Reconstr Surg 2011;127(4): 1707–12.
49. Offer GJ, Perks AG. In search of evidence-based plastic surgery: the problems faced by the specialty. Br J Plast Surg 2000;53(5):427–33.

Evidence-Based Practice
Sublingual Immunotherapy for Allergic Rhinitis

Sarah K. Wise, MD, MSCR[a], Rodney J. Schlosser, MD[b],*

KEYWORDS

- Sublingual immunotherapy • Allergic rhinitis • Allergy • Antigen • Allergen • Safety
- Efficacy • Anaphylaxis

KEY POINTS

The following points provide the level of evidence based on the Oxford Center for Evidence-Based Medicine. Additional critical points are provided and the points here are expanded at the conclusion of this article.

- Sublingual immunotherapy (SLIT) reduces symptoms and medication use in allergic rhinitis. Subgroup analysis shows a benefit for seasonal and perennial antigens, adults and children, and higher antigen doses (evidence grade = 1a-).
- SLIT has shown a significant benefit for grass pollen and house dust mite antigens (evidence grade = 1a-).
- Recommended maintenance SLIT dosing for grass pollen is 15 to 25 μg major allergen per dose. Dosing for other antigens is not established (evidence grade = 1b).
- Most well-designed controlled SLIT trials have been performed with single-antigen therapy (evidence grade = 1b).
- The safety profile of SLIT for allergic rhinitis remains excellent (evidence grade = 1a-).

DISEASE OVERVIEW: ALLERGIC RHINITIS

Allergic rhinitis has a significant public health and quality-of-life impact in the United States. Using data extracted from the Agency for Healthcare Research and Quality 2007 Medical Expenditure Panel Survey, Bhattacharyya[1] recently reported that 17.8 million adults in the United States (7.9% of the US population) sought care for allergic rhinitis in 2007. In this report, patients with allergic rhinitis were older, were more commonly female, had 3 more physician office visits, filled 9 more prescriptions, and had an overall health care expenditure totaling $1492 per person annually over

[a] Otolaryngology-Head and Neck Surgery, Emory University, 550 Peachtree Street, MOT 9th Floor, Atlanta, GA 30308, USA; [b] Otolaryngology-Head and Neck Surgery, Medical University of South Carolina and Ralph H. Johnson VA Medical Center, 135 Rutledge Avenue, MSC 550, Charleston, SC 29425, USA
* Corresponding author.
E-mail address: schlossr@musc.edu

Otolaryngol Clin N Am 45 (2012) 1045–1054
http://dx.doi.org/10.1016/j.otc.2012.06.008
0030-6665/12/$ – see front matter Published by Elsevier Inc.

oto.theclinics.com

persons without allergic rhinitis.[1] Much of the increased health care expenditure for allergic rhinitis is allocated to pharmacotherapy, including antihistamines, decongestants, topical and oral corticosteroids, and others. Antigen avoidance measures are also advocated as an adjunct to the overall treatment plan for allergic rhinitis or perhaps as the sole treatment when a single-antigen trigger can be identified and avoided appropriately.

Antigen-specific immunotherapy is frequently used as part of the treatment paradigm for allergic rhinitis. Although sublingual immunotherapy (SLIT) was first reported in the United States in 1900, the primary modality of antigen-specific immunotherapy in the United States over the last century has been subcutaneous immunotherapy (SCIT).[2] The benefits of SCIT for seasonal allergic rhinitis[3] and perennial allergic asthma[4] have been demonstrated in numerous randomized controlled trials and recent Cochrane reviews. However, safety concerns with SCIT remain. Systemic reactions with SCIT have been reported in 0.05% to 3.2% of injections and 0.84% to 46.7% of patients, including 23 near-fatal (5.4 per 1 million injections) and 3.4 fatal events per year (1 per 2.5 million injections).[5–8] Concerns regarding systemic and fatal reactions with SCIT led the British Committee on the Safety of Medicines to question the safety of this immunotherapy modality in 1986.[9] A surge of interest in alternative methods of antigen-specific immunotherapy followed. Immunotherapy methods, such as intranasal, bronchial, and oral administration, were investigated but none of these were as promising as SLIT because of the intolerable side effects or lack of efficacy.

SLIT has been a predominant immunotherapy modality in Europe for several years. However, over the last decade, clinical interest in SLIT has been growing rapidly in the United States. This increased interest and use of SLIT in clinical practice worldwide has also been accompanied by numerous randomized clinical trials assessing the efficacy of SLIT. This article reviews the evidence behind diagnostic testing for allergic rhinitis, followed by a discussion of the current evidence supporting SLIT for allergic rhinitis.

EVIDENCE-BASED CLINICAL ASSESSMENT AND DIAGNOSTIC TESTING FOR ALLERGIC RHINITIS

Allergic rhinitis is preliminarily diagnosed based on

- History
- Symptom complex
- Physical examination

Common symptoms of allergic rhinitis include intermittent clear rhinorrhea, sneezing, and pruritus of the nose. These symptoms may be accompanied by nasal congestion or obstruction and associated itching of the eyes and throat, watery eyes, and skin or pulmonary symptoms, among others. In the assessment of patients suspected of having allergic rhinitis, it is important to evaluate potential triggers by inquiring about the seasonality of symptoms; exacerbating environments or situations; family history of allergy or asthma; and other associated diseases, like rhinosinusitis, otitis media, and dermatitis.

Risk Factors for Allergic Rhinitis

Certain risk factors for developing allergic rhinitis have been described and may provide useful information as part of an allergic rhinitis history. These risk factors include a family history of atopy, first-born child or only child, cigarette smoke exposure, higher socioeconomic status, and total immunoglobulin E (IgE) more than 100 IU/L before 6 years of age.[10] Physical examination findings of allergic rhinitis are relatively nonspecific and may also be seen with several other sinonasal conditions. Edema of the nasal mucosa, inferior and middle turbinate hypertrophy, and lymphoid hypertrophy of the Waldeyer ring may be seen with allergic rhinitis but may also be present in upper respiratory infections, rhinosinusitis, and nasal obstructive conditions. In short, physical examination findings may support the diagnosis of allergic rhinitis but should not be the sole diagnostic factor for this condition.

Patient History and Environmental Triggers for Allergic Rhinitis

It is important to remember that much of the initial assessment and treatment plan for patients with allergic rhinitis depends on patient history and environmental triggers even though items necessary for a complete allergy history and physical examination vary depending on the environment and geographic location in which patients with allergic rhinitis are being evaluated and treated. A thorough history and physical examination leading to a diagnosis of allergic rhinitis is often sufficient to guide initial avoidance measures and pharmacotherapy. However, if the diagnosis is in question, specific antigen reactivity information is desired, or allergen immunotherapy is being considered, skin or in vitro allergy testing should be undertaken.

Skin Testing for Allergic Rhinitis

Skin testing for inhalant allergy is based on the principle that once an antigen crosses the intact skin or mucosal barrier, the antigen will interact with mast cells in the tissue and cross-link adjacent specific IgE molecules.[11] Depolarization of the mast cell ensues, and histamine is released in a dose-dependent fashion with respect to the antigen administered. This histamine release results in the classic wheal and flare reaction characteristic of the allergy skin test. Measurement of the wheal size allows a partially quantitative assessment of allergen reactivity. In vitro testing for IgE-mediated allergy may be undertaken as an alternative to skin testing. The first in vitro test for specific IgE was the radioallergosorbent test, or RAST test, reported in *Lancet* in 1967.[12,13] Other examples of in vitro methods for the detection of allergen-specific IgE include ImmunoCAP and enzyme allergosorbent tests.[11,14] Although the specific techniques used in each of these in vitro methods vary to some degree, a common principle involves the exposure of patients' serum to typical antigens in the test assay. The patients' IgE binds to these antigens and is then quantified via labeling and detection techniques specific to the individual assay. Quantification of allergen-specific IgE is possible because of the techniques used for in vitro allergy testing.

In the late 1980s and early 1990s, several articles were published comparing the advantages and disadvantages of skin testing and in vitro testing for inhalant allergies. In 1988, Ownby[15] commented that the results of both skin an in vitro tests depend largely on the quality of the extracts used to perform the tests. Further, this article concluded that appropriately performed skin tests represent the best testing modality for the detection of allergen-specific IgE, whereas in vitro tests may be used in circumstances when the skin is not appropriate for testing, anaphylaxis is expected to occur with skin testing, or patients cannot discontinue medications that interfere with skin testing. With either skin or in vitro testing, the results of the test must be correlated with the patients' history before making a decision regarding treatment. Although in vitro allergy tests are noted to be less sensitive than skin testing methods, the use of in vitro test results for allergen-specific immunotherapy has been shown to be safe in large clinical series.[16] Further, although much of this literature dates back 20 or more years, many of the same arguments are used in comparisons of skin versus in vitro allergy testing today.

More recent evaluations of skin testing methods question certain aspects of testing protocols. In a 2008 review, Calabria and Hagan[17] reported that the available literature at that time indicated that when a skin prick test is negative, a positive intradermal skin test did not correlate well with in vitro and challenge test results, therefore providing little additional information for the overall diagnosis. However, these investigators note that a negative intradermal skin test result seems to have a high negative predictive value. Krouse and colleagues[18] generally agree that negative allergy screens by prick/puncture techniques are typically reliable with regard to the presence or absence of allergy. These investigators do note, however, that intradermal testing following a negative skin prick test may provide useful information if clinical suspicion for allergy remains high, especially in the case of mold antigens or unusual inhalant reactivity. Finally, special consideration should be given to skin testing for inhalant allergy when SLIT is planned. Because of the high safety profile associated with SLIT, in combination with short SLIT escalation protocols, quantification (or semiquantification) of allergy skin test reactivity is often unnecessary. Compared with skin testing for patients planning to undergo SCIT, in which intradermal dilutional testing is often performed to best determine patients' specific endpoint for each antigen and shorten the escalation period as much as possible, patients on SLIT will have short escalation protocols with all antigens typically starting at the same dilution, thus obviating extensive dilutional skin testing.

EVIDENCE-BASED MEDICAL MANAGEMENT: SLIT FOR ALLERGIC RHINITIS
Efficacy of SLIT

Beginning in 2006, multiple large, multicenter, randomized, double-blind, placebo-controlled trials of SLIT efficacy for seasonal allergic rhinitis have been published. The 2 most widely cited of these initial studies are those by Durham and colleagues[19] and Dahl and colleagues.[20]

- The 2006 study reported by Durham and colleagues[19] was a multinational, multicenter, randomized, double-blind, placebo-controlled study of SLIT in which 855 patients were randomized to 3 Timothy grass tablet dosing regimens or placebo. Seven-hundred ninety patients completed this trial, which used a preseasonal and coseasonal dosing schedule. The highest dose regimen (15 µg major allergen) resulted in a significant reduction of allergy symptoms and medication use. These benefits were seen over the season and the peak season.
- Likewise, Dahl and colleagues[20] published a multicenter, multinational, randomized, double-blind, placebo-controlled Timothy grass SLIT trial that included 634 randomized patients (546 completed). This study also showed a significant reduction in allergy symptoms and medication use and a significant increase in well days with SLIT, as compared with placebo.
- In 2010, Durham and colleagues[21] reported on the long-term effects of Timothy grass SLIT in patients with allergic rhinitis. In a double-blind, randomized, placebo-controlled trial of 257 participants, sustained significant benefit in symptom control and medication use were seen at the 1-year follow-up after 3 years of active SLIT treatment. Further, the sustained benefits were the same as during the active treatment phase.

Similar results have been seen for SLIT efficacy for seasonal allergic rhinitis in the pediatric population, a group in which SLIT is potentially attractive because of its safety, convenience, and avoidance of needles.

- A multicenter, randomized, double-blind, placebo-controlled study published by Bufe and colleagues[22] in 2009 included 253 children aged 5 to 16 years with grass pollen allergy. With preseasonal and coseasonal administration of Timothy grass tablets, there were significant reductions in allergic rhinitis symptom and medication scores and a significant reduction in asthma symptoms. Observed immunologic changes were similar to those seen in adults.
- Similarly, Wahn and colleagues[23] showed significant reduction in allergic rhinitis symptoms and medication use in 266 children aged 5 to 17 years with a 5-grass tablet in a multicenter, multinational, randomized, double-blind, placebo-controlled trial.

Based on the availability of well-conducted, randomized, placebo-controlled trials of SLIT efficacy, it is not surprising that meta-analyses have also been undertaken in this realm.

- The most recent Cochrane systematic review and meta-analysis of SLIT efficacy for allergic rhinitis was performed by Radulovic and colleagues in 2010[24] and is an update of the highly cited Wilson and colleagues Cochrane review and meta-analysis initially published in 2003.[25] This updated analysis pooled 49 randomized controlled trials of SLIT, involving 2333 actively treated and 2256 placebo participants. Using the standard mean difference (SMD) methodology, significant symptom reduction (SMD -0.49, $P<.00001$) and significant reduction in medication requirements (SMD -0.32, $P<.00001$) were noted, favoring SLIT over placebo. A subgroup analysis revealed a benefit for seasonal and perennial allergens as well as a significant benefit for pediatric and adult patients.
- In children, a meta-analysis of SLIT for seasonal allergic rhinitis was published in 2006 by Penagos and colleagues.[26] This analysis included 10 randomized double-blind placebo-controlled trials and a total of 484 participants. Significant reduction was seen for allergic rhinitis symptoms (SMD 0.56, $P = .02$) and medication use (SMD 0.76, $P = .03$) with SLIT treatment. Active treatment for greater than 18 months and treatment with pollen extracts showed a benefit in subgroup analyses.

With a plethora of randomized controlled SLIT trials available, meta-analyses have also been published for specific individual antigens. In these meta-analyses, significant benefit has been shown in allergic rhinitis symptom reduction and medication reduction for seasonal grass pollen[27] and house dust mite[28] SLIT treatment.

Although systematic reviews and meta-analyses are highly regarded as representing the highest levels of evidence, one should remember that many such meta-analyses have some degree of heterogeneity among the trials that are included. On reading any of these systematic reviews or meta-analyses, it is important for the reader to determine how meaningful this heterogeneity is and to what degree it should be considered in the overall interpretation of the study conclusions.

One aspect of SLIT efficacy that is often discussed is the treatment with a single antigen versus multiple antigens. Most controlled SLIT trials are performed with single-antigen therapy (ie, grass pollen, house dust mite, or birch only). This practice occurs for several reasons.

1. Compared with practices in the United States, there is a general tendency in European countries to test and treat with fewer antigens for allergic disease, and most of the available SLIT efficacy studies are performed in European countries.
2. To perform a well-designed clinical trial, it is important to control as many extraneous factors as possible. In this vein, a trial that treats only Timothy grass allergy with SLIT is able to measure Timothy grass pollen counts and correlate patient symptoms over the course of the season without the need to account for overlapping seasonal symptoms from other tree or weed antigens or year-round symptoms from perennial antigens.
3. Designing a clinical trial that incorporates multiple-antigen treatment requires all participants to have a similar antigen reactivity and symptom pattern for multiple antigens, which may lead to substantial problems with study enrollment.

The issues with single- versus multiple-antigen SLIT intuitively make sense when considering randomized placebo-controlled trial design, but translation to clinical practice in the United States is somewhat problematic. In the United States, general immunotherapy practice incorporates testing for a panel of at least 8 to 12 (and often more) common antigens. Treatment vials are then mixed according to the patients' individual pattern of reactivity, which most often incorporates multiple antigens. However, direct translation of single-antigen efficacy studies to multiple-antigen therapy is questioned. Few studies have evaluated the efficacy of SLIT with multiple antigens and even these are often limited to only 2 antigens rather than 10 antigens, which is the mean number included on an immunotherapy prescription in the United States.[29]

The few SLIT trials that have been performed with multiple antigens show conflicting results. For example, a 2009 US study by Amar and colleagues[30] was unable to demonstrate a significant benefit of multiple-antigen SLIT over single-antigen SLIT or placebo. In contrast, in a small open-label controlled study of 58 patients with grass and birch sensitization, Marogna and colleagues[31] found that patients treated with both grass and birch antigens had significant clinical improvement over those treated with a single antigen or placebo. Based on the current available evidence, treatment with multiple-antigen SLIT clearly needs additional investigation before solid clinical treatment recommendations can be made.

Safety of SLIT

SLIT has an extremely high safety profile. The safety of SLIT, which gives rise to its tendency to be dosed at home rather than in the physician's office, is one of the reasons this modality of allergy immunotherapy is so attractive for working individuals and children.

- Among 60 trials in the 2010 Cochrane systematic review and meta-analysis by Radulovic and colleagues,[24] no cases of anaphylaxis occurred and no patient required epinephrine for treatment of systemic reactions. In this meta-analysis, a total of 53 participants discontinued treatment because of adverse reactions (41 out of 824 patients undergoing SLIT and 12 out of 861 placebo patients), with treatment discontinuation for local reactions being the most common.
- In children, Penagos and colleagues[26] also reported no lethal or severe reactions in the 2006 meta-analysis of 10 pediatric SLIT studies for allergic rhinitis, with the exception of 3 patients with an onset of severe asthma that was thought to be caused by SLIT overdose.
- In the 2009 study by Bufe and colleagues,[22] 6 patients withdrew from the study because of a total of 15 adverse events. Two of these withdrawals were in the

placebo group and 3 in the active group were caused by local reactions without sequelae. There was one withdrawal caused by a serious systemic reaction that was judged as likely related to active treatment: tongue swelling and itching, shortness of breath, and tightness. This event did not require the administration of epinephrine.
- The pediatric SLIT study by Wahn and colleagues,[23] also published in 2009, reported no serious adverse events related to active treatment with the 5–grass pollen tablet, although 9 patients in the active treatment group withdrew from the study because of adverse events.

At this time, there are 11 cases of anaphylaxis reported during SLIT treatment.[32] Given available information, Calderon and colleagues[32] estimate that more than 1 billion SLIT doses have been taken since the year 2000 and calculate a risk of 1 case of anaphylaxis per 100 million SLIT doses. No deaths have been reported related to SLIT; nonetheless, practitioners prescribing SLIT should be aware of the potential for anaphylaxis with any form of immunotherapy. In reporting these episodes of SLIT-related anaphylaxis, some have speculated on the potential causes for the incitement of such severe reactions[32]:

- Prior systemic reaction or intolerance to immunotherapy
- Noncompliance and interruptions in immunotherapy treatment
- Severe or uncontrolled asthma
- High pollen counts
- Use of nonstandardized extracts
- Little to no escalation phase

Many of these possible causes for SLIT anaphylaxis have occurred in other research or clinical situations without leading to anaphylaxis, however. At this time, *the true cause for many of these cases of SLIT anaphylaxis is unknown*. Randomized blinded research is unethical in this realm and, therefore, we remain reliant on case reports and small case series to advise us of SLIT anaphylaxis potential.

SLIT Dosing

The most advantageous SLIT dose has not yet been determined for most antigens. The authors do have evidence to support an optimal SCIT maintenance dose of 5 to 20 µg of major allergen per injection, which is commonly defined as "the dose of an allergen vaccine inducing a clinically relevant effect in most patients without causing unacceptable side effects."[33,34] However, the desired SLIT maintenance dose to achieve an appropriate effect while remaining free of side effects has not been resolved, with the exception of grass pollen extract. As noted, the 2006 large-scale double-blind placebo-controlled trial of Timothy grass tablets by Durham and colleagues[19] identified the 15 µg dose to be the most efficacious in alleviating symptoms of allergic rhinitis and reducing medication use. Didier and colleagues[35] reported the optimum maintenance dose for a 5–grass pollen tablet to be somewhat higher at 25 µg major allergen per dose. These SLIT per-dose recommendations for grass pollen antigen are similar to the per-dose recommendation for SCIT. However, it should be noted that SLIT maintenance is commonly dosed daily, whereas SCIT maintenance injections are typically dosed monthly.

Aside from grass pollen, maintenance doses for SLIT antigens vary greatly and do not yet have strong supporting evidence. It is clear that SLIT maintenance doses are typically larger than SCIT maintenance doses, with SLIT maintenance doses being reported up to 500 times that of SCIT maintenance doses.[36] Because of differing maintenance dosing scheduled between SLIT (daily) and SCIT (monthly), it is best to compare the median monthly dose. Using this measure, the median monthly SLIT maintenance dose is distinctly higher at approximately 49 times the median monthly SCIT maintenance dose.

BOTTOM LINE: WHAT DOES THE EVIDENCE TELL US?

At this time, there is strong evidence to support certain aspects of allergic rhinitis diagnosis and SLIT treatment of allergic rhinitis. However, evidence is lacking in other aspects of this treatment paradigm.

First, available evidence supports the fact that allergic rhinitis has significant public health and economic impact, with nearly 8% of adults in the United States seeking care for allergic rhinitis and patients with allergic rhinitis spending nearly $1500 more in health care costs than those without.[1]

Secondly, when evaluating patients for possible allergic rhinitis, allergy skin testing is often undertaken in association with a thorough history and physical examination that guides the diagnosis. In proceeding through the allergy skin testing procedure, the practitioner should remain aware that with negative skin prick test results, a subsequent positive intradermal skin test does not correlate well with in vitro or challenge tests and provides little additional information in the diagnosis of allergy, whereas a negative intradermal skin test result has a high negative predictive value.[17]

Multiple large-scale single-antigen SLIT efficacy studies have been performed and show significant reduction in allergy symptoms and medication use.[19,20,22,23] These studies are largely well designed, randomized, double blind, and placebo controlled. In support of the SLIT efficacy evidence from individual randomized controlled trials, several systematic reviews and meta-analyses have also been performed. The evidence supporting SLIT for seasonal and perennial allergic rhinitis, and for adults and pediatric patients, is strong.[24,26] In addition, the clinical benefits of grass pollen SLIT beyond the active treatment period have been documented[21] as have appropriate dose ranges for grass pollen SLIT.[19,35] Less clear, however, is the translation of single-antigen SLIT efficacy results to clinical practice that incorporates multiple-antigen SLIT prescriptions as well as optimal dosing for antigens other than grass pollen. These areas deserve substantial future investigation before there is solid evidence to support clinical treatment decisions.

The safety of SLIT is well documented, with anaphylaxis risks distinctly lower than those historically quoted for SCIT. In addition, no lethal events have been reported related to SLIT. However, SLIT-related anaphylaxis events have been documented in case reports and small case series,[32] and we must remain vigilant of the safety concerns with any form of immunotherapy.

CRITICAL POINTS WITH EVIDENCE GRADE

- Allergic rhinitis is a major public health issue with significant health care costs[1] (evidence grade = 2c).
- With negative skin prick test results, intradermal skin tests provide little additional information for overall allergy diagnosis[17] (evidence grade = 4).
- SLIT reduces symptoms and medication use in allergic rhinitis. Subgroup analysis shows a benefit for seasonal and perennial antigens, adults and children, and higher antigen doses (evidence grade = 1a-).
- SLIT has shown a significant benefit for grass pollen and house dust mite antigens (evidence grade = 1a-).

- Recommended maintenance SLIT dosing for grass pollen is 15 to 25 μg major allergen per dose.[19,35] Dosing for other antigens is not established (evidence grade = 1b).
- Most well-designed controlled SLIT trials have been performed with single-antigen therapy (evidence grade = 1b). Controlled trials of multiple-antigen SLIT are lacking. Direct translation of single-antigen SLIT efficacy studies to multiple-antigen SLIT clinical practice is difficult.
- The safety profile of SLIT for allergic rhinitis remains excellent (evidence grade = 1a-).
- Anaphylaxis has been reported with SLIT (evidence grade = 5).

REFERENCES

1. Bhattacharyya N. Incremental healthcare utilization and expenditures for allergic rhinitis in the United States. Laryngoscope 2011;121:1830–3.
2. Curtis H. The immunizing cure of hayfever. Med News 1900;77:16–8.
3. Calderon M, Alves B, Jacobson M, et al. Allergen injection immunotherapy for seasonal allergic rhinitis. Cochrane Database Syst Rev 2007;(1):CD001936.
4. Abramson M, Puy R, Weiner J. Injection allergen immunotherapy for asthma. Cochrane Database Syst Rev 2010;(8):CD001186.
5. Cox L. Sublingual immunotherapy and allergic rhinitis. Curr Allergy Asthma Rep 2008;8:102–10.
6. Stewart G, Lockey R. Systemic reactions from allergen immunotherapy. J Allergy Clin Immunol 1992;90:567–78.
7. Amin H, Liss G, Bernstein D. Evaluation of near-fatal reactions to allergen immunotherapy injections. J Allergy Clin Immunol 2006;117:169–75.
8. Bernstein D, Wanner M, Borish L, et al. Twelve-year survey of fatal reactions to allergen injections and skin testing: 1990-2001. J Allergy Clin Immunol 2004; 113:1129–36.
9. Committee on the Safety of Medicines update: desensitizing vaccines. Br Med J 1986;293:948.
10. Skoner D. Allergic rhinitis: definition, epidemiology, pathophysiology, detection, and diagnosis. J Allergy Clin Immunol 2001;108:S2–8.
11. Shearer W. Specific diagnostic modalities: IgE, skin tests, and RAST. J Allergy Clin Immunol 1989;84:1112–6.
12. Wide L, Bennich H, Johansson S. Diagnosis of allergy by an in-vitro test for allergen antibodies. Lancet 1967;25:1105–7.
13. Kemeny D. Tests for immune reactivity in allergy. Curr Opin Immunol 1990;2:910–6.
14. Ewan P, Cooke D. Evaluation of a capsulated hydrophilic carrier polymer (the ImmunoCAP) for measurement of specific IgE antibodies. Allergy 1990;45:22–9.
15. Ownby D. Allergy testing: in vivo versus in vitro. Pediatr Clin North Am 1988; 35(5):995–1009.
16. Yeoh K, Wang D, Gordon B. Safety and efficacy of radioallergosorbent test-based allergen immunotherapy in treatment of perennial allergic rhinitis and asthma. Otolaryngol Head Neck Surg 2004;131:673–8.
17. Calabria C, Hagan L. The role of intradermal skin testing in inhalant allergy. Ann Allergy Asthma Immunol 2008;101:337–47.
18. Krouse J, Stachler R, Shah A. Current in vivo and in vitro screens for inhalant allergy. Otolaryngol Clin North Am 2003;36:855–68.
19. Durham S, Yang W, Pedersen M, et al. Sublingual immunotherapy with once-daily grass allergen tablets: a randomized controlled trial in seasonal allergic rhinoconjunctivitis. J Allergy Clin Immunol 2006;117:802–9.

20. Dahl R, Kapp A, Colombo G, et al. Efficacy and safety of sublingual immunotherapy with grass allergen tablets for seasonal allergic rhinoconjunctivitis. J Allergy Clin Immunol 2006;118:434–40.

21. Durham S, Emminger W, Capp A, et al. Long-term clinical efficacy in grass pollen-induced rhinoconjunctivitis after treatment with SQ-standardized grass allergy immunotherapy tablet. J Allergy Clin Immunol 2010;125:121–8.

22. Bufe A, Eberle P, Franke-Beckmann E, et al. Safety and efficacy in children of an SQ-standardized grass allergen tablet for sublingual immunotherapy. J Allergy Clin Immunol 2009;123:167–73.

23. Wahn U, Tabar A, Kuna P, et al. Efficacy and safety of 5-grass-pollen sublingual immunotherapy tablets in pediatric allergic rhinoconjunctivitis. J Allergy Clin Immunol 2009;123:160–6.

24. Radulovic S, Calderon M, Wilson D, et al. Sublingual immunotherapy for allergic rhinitis. Cochrane Database Syst Rev 2010;(12):CD002893.

25. Wilson D, Torres L, Durham S. Sublingual immunotherapy for allergic rhinitis. Cochrane Database Syst Rev 2003;(2):CD0002893.

26. Penagos M, Compalati E, Tarantini F, et al. Efficacy of sublingual immunotherapy in the treatment of allergic rhinitis in pediatric patients 3 to 18 years of age: a meta-analysis of randomized, placebo-controlled, double-blind trials. Ann Allergy Asthma Immunol 2006;97:141–8.

27. Di Bona D, Plaia A, Scafidi V, et al. Efficacy of sublingual immunotherapy with grass allergens for seasonal allergic rhinitis: a systematic review and meta-analysis. J Allergy Clin Immunol 2010;126:558–66.

28. Compalati E, Passalacqua G, Bonini M, et al. The efficacy of sublingual immunotherapy for house dust mites respiratory allergy: results of a GA2LEN meta-analysis. Allergy 2009;64:1570–9.

29. Nelson H. Multiantigen immunotherapy for allergic rhinitis and asthma. J Allergy Clin Immunol 2009;123:763–9.

30. Amar S, Harbeck R, Sills M, et al. Response to sublingual immunotherapy with grass pollen extract: monotherapy versus combination in a multiallergen extract. J Allergy Clin Immunol 2009;124:150–6.

31. Marogna M, Spadolini I, Massolo A, et al. Effects of sublingual immunotherapy for multiple or single allergens in polysensitized patients. Ann Allergy Asthma Immunol 2007;98:274–80.

32. Calderón M, Simons F, Malling H, et al. Sublingual allergen immunotherapy: mode of action and its relationship with the safety profile. Allergy 2012;67(3): 302–11.

33. van Rhee R. Indoor allergens: relevance of major allergen measurements and standardization. J Allergy Clin Immunol 2007;119:270–7.

34. Bousquet J, Lockey R, Malling H. Allergen immunotherapy: therapeutic vaccines for allergic diseases. A WHO position paper. J Allergy Clin Immunol 1998;102: 558–62.

35. Didier A, Malling H, Worm M, et al. Optimal dose, efficacy, and safety of once-daily sublingual immunotherapy with a 5-grass pollen tablet for seasonal allergic rhinitis. J Allergy Clin Immunol 2007;120:1338–45.

36. Cox L, Linnemann D, Nolte H, et al. Sublingual immunotherapy: a comprehensive review. J Allergy Clin Immunol 2006;117:1021–35.

Evidence-Based Practice
Pediatric Obstructive Sleep Apnea

Stacey L. Ishman, MD, MPH

KEYWORDS

- Pediatric • Children • Sleep-disordered breathing • Obstructive sleep apnea
- Tonsillectomy

KEY POINTS

- History and physical examination are not sufficient to differentiate between snoring and obstructive sleep apnea (OSA).
- Nocturnal in-laboratory polysomnography remains the gold standard for diagnosis of OSA.
- Adenotonsillectomy is the recommended initial treatment for OSA and sleep-disordered breathing for healthy children, even in those with risk factors associated with persistent pediatric OSA such as obesity.
- Efficacy data for partial tonsillectomy are limited despite multiple studies showing reduced postoperative bleeding and recovery time.
- Bariatric surgery is an option for extremely obese adolescents.
- Medical treatment may be a good option for mild OSA, either primary or persistent after adenotonsillectomy; although, more data are necessary.
- CPAP is an effective therapy in children, but similar to adults, adherence is a significant issue, and there may be facial side effects in children with long-term use.

OVERVIEW

Although obstructive sleep apnea (OSA) was described in literature as early as the 1700s, the first report of pediatric OSA was not published until 1976 in a case series of 8 children.[1] Since that time, much has been learned about OSA in children; however, there remain significant gaps in the understanding and evidence for the diagnosis, treatment, and management of pediatric OSA.

Disclosures. Funding sources: None.
Conflict of interest: Nothing.
Departments of Otolaryngology – Head and Neck Surgery, Pediatrics and Internal Medicine, Division of Pulmonary and Critical Care Medicine, Johns Hopkins School of Medicine, 601 North Caroline Street, Baltimore, MD 21287, USA
E-mail address: Sishman1@jhmi.edu

Otolaryngol Clin N Am 45 (2012) 1055–1069
http://dx.doi.org/10.1016/j.otc.2012.06.009
0030-6665/12/$ – see front matter © 2012 Elsevier Inc. All rights reserved.

oto.theclinics.com

Recent prospective general pediatric population studies using polysomnography (PSG) for diagnosis have found that the prevalence of pediatric OSA ranges from 1.2% to 5.7%.[2–4] These estimates are in keeping with previous estimates and similar to the estimates of symptomatic OSA in adults.[5] In addition, estimates of sleep-disordered breathing (SDB), which includes both OSA and snoring, are around 12%.[6]

Epidemiology

The epidemiology of OSA has also been investigated in a systematic review that suggests that there is a male predominance in pediatric OSA, especially in older boys;[7] although, several large studies have found no difference in the prevalence by sex.[8–10] It is also suggested that age is a mediator of this relationship, as those studies including older children were more likely to find an increased rate of SDB in boys.[7] In addition, minority status has been associated with increased prevalence of SDB, with multiple studies showing that black children are more likely to have SDB than white children.[2,11] Finally, comorbid factors such as obesity, craniofacial deformity, genetic syndrome status, and metabolic disease have also been associated with an increased incidence of SDB in children and adults (**Table 1**).

Sequelae to Pediatric Sleep Apnea

Most importantly, untreated OSA is associated with a number of sequelae, including cognitive deficits, hyperactivity, cardiovascular consequences, and inflammation.[12] Studies of neuropsychiatric function in children with SDB have almost universally found cognitive deficits in these children. Two representative prospective studies characterized these deficits and found lower general intelligence, learning, and memory results; decreased language and verbal skills; and diminished visual and auditory attention.[13,14] In addition, school performance has been shown to improve after treatment of SDB with adenotonsillectomy.[15]

Behavioral issues, and especially hyperactivity, have also been widely associated with SDB and OSA.[13,16] In these prospective studies, behavioral issues included attention-deficit/hyperactivity disorder (ADHD, as diagnosed by psychiatric interview),

Table 1	
Epidemiologic risk factors for pediatric obstructive sleep apnea syndrome	
Adenotonsillar Hypertrophy	Increased Airway Resistance
Obesity	Fatty infiltration of airway, abnormal ventilatory control
Race (African American)	Craniofacial structure, socioeconomic
Gender (male)	Slight male predominance in prepubertal children, which increases markedly after puberty
Prematurity	Neurologic impairment, adverse craniofacial growth, abnormal ventilatory control
Craniofacial dysmorphology	Increased airway resistance
Neurologic disorders	Abnormal motor control of the upper airway
Nasal/pharyngeal inflammation	Allergy or infection increasing airway resistance
Socioeconomic/environmental	Neighborhood disadvantage, passive cigarette smoke, indoor allergens, sleep quality (noise, stress)
Family history of OSAS	Heritable craniofacial structure, neuromuscular compensation, arousal threshold, ventilatory control

Abbreviation: OSAS, obstructive sleep apnea syndrome.
From Katz ES, D'Ambrosio CM. Pediatric obstructive sleep apnea. Clin Chest Med 2010;31:222; with permission.

depression, daytime sleepiness (by subjective report and objective multiple sleep latency testing), aggression, and oppositional and social problems. In addition, both behavioral issues and cognitive deficits were improved after adenotonsillectomy and were shown to have sustained improvement in a study that followed patients for 1 year after surgery.[16]

Comorbid medical conditions with pediatric sleep apnea
While the association between OSA and cardiovascular disease is well described in the adult literature, this association is not as well understood in children. Cardiac abnormalities of both the right and left ventricles have been reported and have been associated with postsurgical respiratory complications.[17] In addition, blood pressure elevations, both daytime and nighttime, have been correlated with OSA in children.[18] Autonomic dysfunction has also been reported in children with OSA during both wake and sleep.[19,20]

There is increasing recognition of the relationship between obesity and SDB and the risk of obesity in children after adenotonsillectomy. The traditional picture of children with OSA often included a population of children with failure to thrive. In these underweight children, the recognition that there was often a growth spurt after adenotonsillectomy was reported as a positive outcome of surgery. More recently, this same increase in weight after adenotonsillectomy has led to growing concern that normal weight and obese children are becoming overweight or more obese after surgery.[21]

Dissimilarities in child and adult sleep apnea
Differences between adult and pediatric SDB also include significant dissimilarities in respiratory events. As children are more likely to have hypopneas than discrete apneas, arousals are uncommon, and desaturations are less common than in adults. Children may also have long periods of flow-limited breathing that do not meet the definition of a respiratory event, but reflect partially obstructed breathing. In addition, children are more likely to have rapid eye movement (REM)-only disease than adults, which makes nap studies, either oximetry or polysomnography, problematic, as it will often not capture any significant REM sleep. Several large population studies have been performed to determine normative data for pediatric sleep and are reported in composite in **Table 2**.[22]

EVIDENCE-BASED CLINICAL ASSESSMENT
Clinical History

Multiple studies have looked at the effectiveness of history and physical examination in differentiating OSA from snoring and found that neither is effective in reliably separating the two.[23] An evaluation of clinical history in 480 patients who underwent concomitant home 16-channel polysomnography found that clinical symptoms, either solo or in combination, had a low sensitivity for diagnosis of OSA.[24] A smaller study of 83 patients with sleep study data found a statistically significant increase in the risk ratio (RR) for OSA when parents report the need to shake their children (RR = 1.94), the presence of witnessed apneas (RR = 1.63), and witnessed struggle to breathe (RR = 1.53), but none of these factors was found to be sufficient to predict OSA.[25] Additional measures, such as waist circumference and body mass index (BMI) z-score, have also been found to have a poor clinical correlation with symptoms of SDB.[26]

The use of surveys to screen for OSA has also been investigated with mixed results. The pediatric sleep questionnaire (PSQ) survey has shown reasonable sensitivity (78%) and specificity (72%) when compared with sleep study results and has been recommended as a screening tool with the caveat that subsequent definitive

Table 2	
Normal polysomnographic data for otherwise healthy children	
Sleep	
EEG arousal index (per h TST)	9 ± 3
Sleep efficiency (%)	89 ± 7
Stage 1 (% TST)	5 ± 3
Stage 2 (% TST)	42 ± 8
Slow wave sleep (% TST)	26 ± 8
REM sleep (% TST)	20 ± 5
REM cycles	4 ± 1
Periodic leg movement index (per h TST)	1 ± 1
Respiratory	
Obstructive apnea index (per h TST)	0.0 ± 0.1
Obstructive apnea/hypopnea index (per h TST)	0.1 ± 0.1
Central apnea index (per h TST)	0.5 ± 0.5
$P_{ET}CO_2 \geq 50$ mm Hg (% TST)	2.8 ± 11.3
Peak $P_{ET}CO_2$ (mm Hg)	46 ± 3
$S_oO_2 > 95\%$ (% TST)	99.6 ± 1
S_oO_2 90%–95% (% TST)	0.4 ± 1
$S_oO_2 < 90\%$ (% TST)	0.05 ± 0.2
Desaturation index ($\geq 4\%$/h TST)	0.4 ± 0.8
S_oO_2 Nadir (%)	93 ± 4

Data are presented as mean $\pm$ standard deviation.
Abbreviations: EEG, electroencephalograph; REM, rapid eye movement; TST, total sleep time.
From Katz ES, D'Ambrosio CM. Pediatric Obstructive Sleep Apnea. Clin Chest Med 2010;31: 221–34.

diagnostic testing would still be recommended if positive.[27] The OSA-18, a validated quality-of-life survey frequently used in pediatric otolaryngology, was also evaluated as a screening tool for moderate-to-severe OSA in 334 children and found to have poor sensitivity at 40%, with a negative predictive value of only 73%.[28]

Polysomnography

The gold standard for diagnosis is an attended, in-laboratory, nighttime polysomnogram.[6,23,29] The practice parameter for respiratory PSG indications published by the American Academy of Sleep Medicine (AASM) in 2011 reviewed 45 studies with PSG data before and after OSA treatment and found test–retest validity or improvement in PSG parameters to be robust in all 45 studies.[29]

Several studies have investigated the reliability of a single pediatric nocturnal sleep study[30–36] to determine if PSG has good test–retest reliability/consistency. This is important, as adult sleep study testing has found a first night effect, in which adults do not sleep as well during their first sleep study; thus sleep efficiency and architecture may underestimate OSA severity. In the pediatric studies, however, there were only minimal differences in measures of OSA severity, suggesting that a single night of PSG evaluation is adequate. However, while respiratory parameters were fairly constant, sleep architecture was significantly different between nights.

Additional validity measures have also been evaluated, including construct validity, a measure of whether the PSG is a true reflection of SDB, and convergent validity, which looks for evidence that 2 tests measuring the same problem move in the same direction (ie, the PSG and tests of outcomes like sleepiness and cognition). These evaluations have found that many measures change consistently when OSA is present, like sleepiness, neurocognitive outcomes, and quality of life.[12] Despite this, disease severity often does not correspond with degree of change in these outcomes.

Home sleep studies, also known as ambulatory PSGs, are approved for use in adults with high pretest probability of OSA, but they are not currently recommended for children by any of the current guidelines. There are few studies looking at home studies in children. The largest looked at 850 children between ages 8 and 11 years of age who underwent 4-channel ambulatory PSG, which included oximetry, heart rate, body position, and inductance plesmography. In this case, 94% of the home studies were found to be technically satisfactory.[11] The same study also had 55 patients who underwent in-laboratory 16-channel sleep studies; although, little is reported about this group. Based on these 55 patients, the study investigators reported that the home studies were sensitive at 88% and highly specific at 98% for an apnea–hypopnea index (AHI) greater than 5 events per hour as determined on the in-laboratory studies. Several other studies have investigated home studies in the sleep laboratory[37] or looked at a reduced number of channels from an in-laboratory study.[38] The first of these studies was performed on only 12 children ages 3 to 6 years and found to have poor specificity at 0%.[37] The second study looked at 30 children each with normal, mild/moderate OSA and severe OSA using only the oximetry and dual respiratory inductance plethysmography (RIP) bands and determined that there was correct classification of SDB category in 83% with a false-negative rate of only 8%.[38] It is unclear from the current data whether studies are feasible in children between 2 and 7 years of age, when tonsillar hypertrophy is most prominent.

In contrast, investigations of nap PSG have found that sensitivity ranged from 69% to 75%, while specificity ranged from 60% to 100%.[39–41] Because of this, the AASM does not recommend nap polysomnography as the sole method of diagnosis in children, as they are not as reliable as in-laboratory PSGs.[29] In addition, nap studies have been found to underestimate OSA severity, especially as they often do not include any significant REM sleep. For this reason, the American Academy of Pediatrics (AAP) suggests that nap polysomnography can be useful if it is positive for OSA, even if severity is inaccurate, but that negative studies should prompt a nocturnal PSG.[23]

Alternate Measures

Cardiovascular monitoring, including heart rate variability and pulse transit time, has also been evaluated for diagnosis of pediatric OSA with variable suboptimal rates of sensitivity and specificity.[42–44] One particular technique, peripheral arterial tonometry, appeared promising as a method to identify electroencephalographic arousals with sensitivity of 95% but was found to have poor specificity at 35%.[45] Refinement of these techniques is necessary before they can be considered for screening or diagnosis.

Audiotaping or videotaping, nocturnal oximetry, and nap polysomnography are all noted to be useful if they are positive for witnessed apneas, desaturations or obstructive events, but to have poor predictive value when the results are negative, leading to the suggestion that those who screen negative by these methods be referred for in-laboratory PSG.[23] In addition, determination of disease severity is limited or unable to be quantified by these techniques.

An initial study of nap oximetry found it to be an accurate screening tool for OSA in children in whom it was positive,[46] leading the AAP to state that positive nocturnal oximetry could be used to diagnose OSA. However, the practice guidelines went on to recommend that children with negative findings on this screening undergo further testing with a full PSG.[22] Since that time, 2 additional studies have compared oximetry and PSG results.[47,48] The first looked at 230 patients and concluded that nocturnal oximetry could be used to estimate disease severity in patients who screened positive, but 78% of the children in this study had normal or indeterminate studies and therefore went on to have a full PSG.

EVIDENCE-BASED MEDICAL MANAGEMENT OR SURGICAL TECHNIQUE
Adenotonsillectomy for Sleep Apnea

Consensus statements from the AAP[23] and American Academy of Otolaryngology – Head and Neck Surgery[49] agree that the primary treatment of OSA in healthy children over age 2 years is adenotonsillectomy. They exclude infants from these recommendations, because adenotonsillar hypertrophy is uncommon in this population. Additionally, the differential and treatment options for infants are significantly different than for older children. Additional exclusions include children with significant comorbidities such as craniofacial abnormalities, neuromuscular disease, genetic or metabolic syndromes, and cerebral palsy.

While adenotonsillectomy was previously assumed to resolve SDB in almost all healthy children, the most recent systematic review of adenotonsillectomy as treatment for OSA suggests that surgery may not be as curative as previously thought, with up to 34% of children found to have a respiratory disturbance index (RDI) of at least 5 after surgery.[50] In this same review, significant differences were seen in the resolution rates of SDB in uncomplicated children at 74% versus children with comorbidities (eg, morbid obesity, severe OSA, and age less than 3 years) at 39%. Children with craniofacial syndromes, trisomy 21, and neuromuscular disorders were not included in this systematic review.

There has been debate regarding the role of adenotonsillectomy in obese children. While there are not many studies measuring the effect of tonsil and adenoid removal in obese patients, multiple studies have found that obese children are more likely to have persistent pediatric OSA than nonobese children.[50] A meta-analysis of 4 studies and 110 obese children found that 51% had an AHI greater than 5 events per hour after adenotonsillectomy, about 15% higher than the rate of persistent OSA found in the systematic review mentioned previously.[50,51]

Complications associated with adenotonsillectomy include immediate and delayed bleeding, with rates of primary bleeding from 0.2% to 2.2% and secondary hemorrhage 0.1% to 3%.[52] Intraoperative complications include injury to teeth and surrounding tissues, difficulty with intubation, aspiration, airway fire, and cardiac arrest.[49] After surgery, complications frequently noted include nausea, vomiting, dehydration, pain, pain sounds redundant. Possibly ear pain, systematic pain, voice and swallowing issues, velopharyngeal insufficiency, and need for extended recovery or readmission. Less common complications include nasopharyngeal stenosis, postobstructive pulmonary edema, injury to surrounding arteries, Grisel syndrome (atlanto–axial subluxation), and Eagle syndrome (neck pain).[49] Mortality rates after adenotonsillectomy range from 1 death per 16,000 surgeries to 1 death per 35,000 surgeries.[53] A review of tonsillectomy malpractice claims found bleeding after surgery to be the most common complaint (34%), followed by anoxic injury (17%), functional deficits (16%), and medication issues leading to death.[54]

Partial Tonsillectomy for SDB

More limited treatment of SDB has also been reported using tonsillotomy or partial tonsillectomy and adenoidectomy alone. The rationale behind the use of partial tonsil removal is based on a desire to reduce the pain and bleeding rates associated with complete tonsil removal. Most studies of partial tonsillectomy focus on the effect on recovery and morbidity after the procedures, but few have reported sleep study results before and after surgery. A small series of 14 patients found 93% to have an AHI less than 1 after surgery.[55] A second compared 15 children, each undergoing partial versus complete tonsillectomy, but used multiple methods for quantification of SDB (overnight PSG versus nap PSG versus home studies) leading to significant methodological issues.[56] In this study, only 5 of 15 (33%) of the partial removal patients and 4 of 15 (27%) of complete removal patients had a postoperative AHI of greater than or equal to 5. While the residual OSA rates for both groups are higher than typically reported in other studies, the study investigators did find the results from the 2 methods to be equivalent. A large prospective study of tonsil bleeding rates in Austria looked at 9405 patients, including adults, and found that the bleeding rate for complete tonsillectomy was 15.0%, with 4.6% returning to the operating room, versus 2.3% for partial tonsillectomy and only 0.9% returning to the operating room.[57] Pain is also noted to be lower in most studies comparing tonsillectomy and partial tonsillectomy.[58,59]

In addition to the lack of efficacy data, partial tonsil removal carries a risk of tonsillar regrowth that has been reported to range from 0.5% to 17%.[60–62] Time to re-evaluation ranged from 1 to 18 months in the study with the highest regrowth rate (17%), 1.2 years in the lowest (0.5%), and 4 years for a study of 375 children with yearly evaluations (7.2%). In the latter study, 20 of 375 patients subsequently underwent completion tonsillectomy.[62] These studies suggest that the risk of tonsillar regrowth is high enough that children should be monitored for recurrence of OSA signs and symptoms.

Adenoidectomy

Similarly, there are no level 1 studies looking at the efficacy of adenoidectomy alone for the treatment of OSA or SDB. However, several studies have looked at follow-up after adenoidectomy performed without tonsillectomy. A retrospective survey of 206 parents of children who had undergone adenoidectomy alone was performed and found that symptomatic improvement was reported to be approximately 55% for shoring, 78% for nasal obstruction, and 82% for obstructed sleep.[63] Subsequently, 36 of these children were then evaluated in the office. Of the 16 with no improvement or worsening of symptoms, nasal pathology was most commonly seen, tonsil hypertrophy in 7/16. Adenoid hypertrophy seen in 15% to 25% of children regardless of symptoms. A second study looked at the likelihood of future tonsillectomy or revision adenoidectomy in 100 children, 48 of whom had SDB. They found that 38% of children with SDB subsequently underwent surgery, including tonsillectomy and/or revision adenoidectomy, versus 19% of those with nonobstructive symptoms.[64] Both of these studies suggest that adenoidectomy alone may be a viable option for a subset of children, but neither clearly delineates which children are best treated with adenoidectomy alone versus adenotonsillectomy. They also highlight the fact that regrowth of adenoids and obstructive symptoms can occur, especially in children who have their adenoids removed before 6 years of age.

Additional Sleep Surgery/Bariatric Surgery

Additional procedures have been reported to treat children with comorbidities such as Down syndrome, neurologic impairment, and obesity, in addition to children with persistent OSA after adenotonsillectomy. These include:

- Uvulopalatopharyngoplasty (UPPP)
- Nasal turbinate reduction

- Lingual tonsillectomy
- Hyoid myotomy and suspension
- Genioglossal advancement
- Partial midline glossectomy
- Tongue suspension suture

However, these reports are level 4 data, with case reports and case series often reported on children undergoing multiple procedures or with mixed cohorts of patients with limited polysomnographic data.[65–70]

Consideration of bariatric surgery for obese adolescents is also becoming common, and in 2011, the American Society for Metabolic and Bariatric Surgery published a best practice guideline that states that a "mounting body of evidence supports the use of modern surgical weight loss procedures for carefully selected, extremely obese adolescents."[71] Criteria for consideration included adolescents with:

- BMI >35 kg/m^2 with major comorbidities including type 2 diabetes, moderate-to-severe OSA (AHI≥15), pseudotumor cerebri, or severe nonalcoholic steatohepatitis
- BMI ≥40 kg/m^2 with comorbidities including hypertension, insulin resistance, glucose intolerance, substantially impaired quality of life or activities of daily living, dyslipidemia, and OSA with AHI of at least 5

A 2011 prospective randomized trial of 50 children ages 14 to 18 years with a BMI >35 kg/m^2 compared a medically supervised lifestyle to gastric banding with 2 years of follow-up.[72] Eighty-four percent of those with gastric banding and 12% of those with lifestyle changes lost more than 50% of the excess weight, with mean weight loss of 79% in the banding group and 13% in the lifestyle group. In addition, metabolic syndrome had resolved in all of those with gastric banding and 78% of those with lifestyle changes. Sleep was not directly measured in this study. A separate study of 10 children with OSA who underwent nocturnal polysomnography before and after bariatric surgery found a significant improvement in AHI.[73] BMI decreased from a mean of 60.8 (standard deviation [SD] 11.07) to 41.6 (SD 9.5), while the AHI decreased from 9.1 to 0.65 events per hour. Additional research is needed to determine the effect of bariatric surgery on sleep and sleep apnea in children.

Medical Treatment for Pediatric Sleep Apnea

While there are limited data regarding the efficacy of weight loss on OSA in children, weight loss has been shown to improve OSA disease severity in adults. In a meta-analysis of 342 adults, mean BMI was decreased by 17.9 kg/m^2 from a mean starting value of 55.3 kg/m^2, while the AHI decreased from 54.7 events per hour to 15.8 events per hour.[74] This represents a significant reduction in OSA disease severity, but still left a number of patients with moderate-to-severe OSA. An evaluation of a program that combines behavioral procedures with nutrition, exercise, and dietary education was performed in 61 children with 10 years follow-up.[75] They found that 34% of children had at least a 20% weight loss, and that 30% were no longer obese at 10 years in those with both parents and children involved in the education and counseling. This supports current recommendations that the most effective programs for pediatric weight loss are school-based programs that include behavioral counseling, dietary counseling, nutrition education, scheduled physical activity, and parental training and involvement.

Limited studies of medical therapy have looked at short courses of oral and nasal steroids. The single published trial of oral steroids for 5 days at 1mg/kg was not found to have any significant effect on SDB.[76] However, 3 studies have shown modest improvements in mild OSA with 26 weeks of nasal steroid therapy and improvement in the AHI ranging from 2 to 4 events per hour.[77–79]

In addition, studies of leukotrienes have been found in increased concentration in the tonsils and upper airway of children with OSA.[80] In light of this, a 16-week trial of monteleukast therapy was performed for 24 children with mild OSA and found a modest change in AHI from 3 to 2 events per hour.[81] A second trial of monteleukast in combination with nasal steroid therapy for 12 weeks found an improvement in AHI from 3.9 to 0.3 events per hour, with no changes seen in a control group.[82] These studies suggest that mild OSA, either after adenotonsillectomy or in lieu of adenotonsillectomy, may be reasonably treated with combined medial therapy. However, long-term results are not available, and it is not known if this improvement in AHI is durable or if it requires long-term medical therapy.

Oral Appliance Therapy/Rapid Maxillary Expansion

Adult studies of oral appliance therapy have found that they are most useful for non-obese patients with some degree of micrognathia or retrognathia. In addition, they are most often used in adults with mild-to-moderate OSA; however, there are few studies of oral appliances in children. One from 2004 looked at 20 children with mild-to-moderate OSA and found modest improvements in RDI from 7.9 to 3.7 events an hour after 6 months of use.[83]

Rapid maxillary expansion (RME) is intended to increase the width of the hard palate by opening up the midline palatal suture, and it is suggested for use only in children with maxillary constriction. It is used for 3 to 4 months duration and then left in place for a period of consolidation, usually 2 to 3 additional months, before removal (**Fig. 1**). A study of 31 nonobese children with maxillary constriction, no adenoidal hypertrophy, and OSA found an improvement of AHI from 12.2 to less than 1 event per hour in all 31 children.[84] Another study of 14 children found an improvement of AHI from 5.8 to 1.5 events per hour with a parallel reduction in snoring, sleepiness, tiredness, and oral breathing.[85] In this study, researchers screened 260 children presenting to an orthodontic clinic and found 35 eligible patients. Improvement in mean palatal expansion was 3.7 plus or minus 0.7 mm for the intercanine area and 5.0 plus or minus 2.2 mm for the inter-premolar measurement. A follow-up study by the same group on

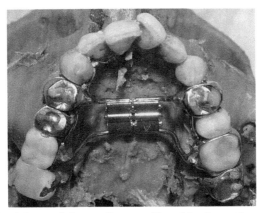

Fig. 1. Photograph of the tooth-borne distractor (Hyrax) in situ on the anatomic specimen. (*From* Koudstaal MJ, Smeets JB, Kleinrensink GJ, et al. Relapse and stability of surgically assisted rapid maxillary expansion: an anatomic biomechanical study. J Oral Maxillofac Surg 2009;67:10–4; with permission.)

10 of the 14 children with sleep studies at 12 and 24 months found no significant decrement in AHI or clinical symptoms.[86]

Continuous Positive Airway Pressure

A multicenter study of 29 children with a mean age of 10.5 years using continuous positive airway pressure (CPAP) or bi-level pressure (BiPAP) found that it improved AHI, sleepiness, and snoring during the 6 months of the study.[87] However, 8 of 29 children (28%) dropped out before the end of the study, and for those remaining in the trial, positive airway pressure (PAP) use was significantly overestimated by parents by a mean of 1.8 hours. Actual nightly use by compliance monitoring was 5.3 plus or minus 2.5 hours per night. Additional studies of CPAP in children have reported similar levels of adherence at 70%, such as a retrospective review of 46 children with OSA, with a mean age of 13.6 years.[88] However, compliance readings were only available in 27 children (59%), and only 19 were using CPAP at least 4 hours a night for at least 5 days a week. If it is assumed that only 19 of 46 children were using CPAP adequately at the end of the study period, the final adherence rate may have been as low as 41%. In addition, these studies are in older children and do not address CPAP use in younger patients.

A single retrospective study of facial side effects of PAP therapy was performed in 40 children from 2002 and 2003 with a median duration of PAP use of 15 months and median age of 10 years. The authors found a significant rate of skin injury (48%) including erythema and skin necrosis, global facial flattening (68%), and maxillary retrusion (37%).[89] However, this was not a longitudinal evaluation of bony facial changes, and the skeletal findings may be a greater reflection of the underlying pathology requiring PAP than the effect of the PAP mask itself.

BOTTOM LINE: WHAT DOES THE EVIDENCE TELL?

- History and physical examination are not sufficient to differentiate between snoring and obstructive sleep apnea (evidence grade B).
- Nocturnal in-laboratory polysomnography remains the gold standard for diagnosis of OSA (evidence grade A).
- Adenotonsillectomy is the recommended initial treatment for OSA and SDB for healthy children, even in those with risk factors associated with persistent pediatric OSA such as obesity (evidence grade B).
- Efficacy data for partial tonsillectomy are limited despite multiple studies showing reduced postoperative bleeding and recovery time (evidence grade C).
- Bariatric surgery is an option for extremely obese adolescents (evidence grade C).
- Medical treatment may be a good option for mild OSA, either primary or persistent after adenotonsillectomy, although more data are necessary (evidence grade C).
- CPAP is an effective therapy in children, but similar to adults, adherence is a significant issue. Additionally, there may be facial side effects in children with long-term use (evidence grade C).

REFERENCES

1. Guilleminault C, Eldridge FL, Simmons FB, et al. Sleep apnea in eight children. Pediatrics 1976;58:23–30.
2. Bixler EO, Vgontzas AN, Lin HM, et al. Sleep-disordered breathing in children in a general population sample: prevalence and risk factors. Sleep 2009;32:731–6.
3. Li AM, So HK, Au CT, et al. Epidemiology of obstructive sleep apnoea syndrome in Chinese children: a two-phase community study. Thorax 2010;65:991–7.

4. O'Brien LM, Holbrook CR, Mervis CB, et al. Sleep and neurobehavioral characteristics of 5- to 7-year-old children with parentally reported symptoms of attention-deficit/hyperactivity disorder. Pediatrics 2003;111(3):554–63.

5. Young T, Evans L, Finn L, et al. Estimation of the clinically diagnosed proportion of sleep apnea syndrome in middle-aged men and women. Sleep 1997;20(9):705–6.

6. Roland PS, Rosenfeld RM, Brooks LJ, et al. Clinical practice guideline: polysomnography for sleep-disordered breathing prior to tonsillectomy in children. Otolaryngol Head Neck Surg 2011;145(Suppl 1):s1–15.

7. Lumeng JC, Chervin RD. Epidemiology of pediatric obstructive sleep apnea. Proc Am Thorac Soc 2008;5(2):242–52.

8. Sogut A, Altin R, Uzun L, et al. Prevalence of obstructive sleep apnea syndrome and associated symptoms in 3–11-year-old Turkish children. Pediatr Pulmonol 2005;39:251–6.

9. Wing YK, Hui SH, Pak WM, et al. A controlled study of sleep related disordered breathing in obese children. Arch Dis Child 2003;88:1043–7.

10. Sánchez-Armengol A, Fuentes-Pradera MA, Capote-Gil F, et al. Sleep-related breathing disorders in adolescents aged 12 to 16 years: clinical and polygraphic findings. Chest 2001;119(5):1393–400.

11. Rosen CL, Larkin EK, Kirchner HL, et al. Prevalence and risk factors for sleep-disordered breathing in 8- to 11-year-old children: association with race and prematurity. J Pediatr 2003;142(4):383–9.

12. Gozal D. Sleep, sleep disorders and inflammation in children. Sleep Med 2009; 10(Suppl 1):S12–6.

13. O'Brien LM, Mervis CB, Holbrook CR, et al. Neurobehavioral implications of habitual snoring in children. Pediatrics 2004;114(1):44–9.

14. Surratt PM, Barth JT, Diamond R, et al. Reduced time in bed and obstructive sleep-disordered breathing in children are associated with cognitive impairment. Pediatrics 2007;119(2):320–9.

15. Chervin RD, Ruzicka DL, Giordani BJ, et al. Sleep-disordered breathing, behavior, and cognition in children before and after adenotonsillectomy. Pediatrics 2006;117(4):e769–78.

16. Kalra M, Kimball TR, Daniels SR, et al. Structural cardiac changes as a predictor of respiratory complications after adenotonsillectomy for obstructive breathing during sleep in children. Sleep Med 2005;6(3):241–5.

17. Li AM, Au CT, Sung RY, et al. Ambulatory blood pressure in children with obstructive sleep apnoea: a community based study. Thorax 2008;63(9):803–9.

18. Bonuck KA, Freeman K, Henderson J. Growth and growth biomarker changes after adenotonsillectomy: systematic review and meta-analysis. Arch Dis Child 2009;94(2):83–91.

19. Chaicharn J, Lin Z, Chen ML, et al. Model-based assessment of cardiovascular autonomic control in children with obstructive sleep apnea. Sleep 2009;32: 927–38.

20. Aljadeff G, Gozal D, Schechtman VL, et al. Heart rate variability in children with obstructive sleep apnea. Sleep 1997;20:151–7.

21. Gozal D. Sleep-disordered breathing and school performance in children. Pediatrics 1998;102(3 Pt 1):616–20.

22. Katz ES, D'Ambrosio CM. Pediatric obstructive sleep apnea. Clin Chest Med 2010;31:221–34.

23. American Academy of Pediatrics. Clinical practice guideline: diagnosis and management of childhood obstructive sleep apnea syndrome. Pediatrics 2002; 109(4):704–12.

24. Goodwin JL, Kaemingk KL, Mulvaney SA, et al. Clinical screening of school children for polysomnography to detect sleep-disordered breathing—the Tucson Children's Assessment of Sleep Apnea study (TuCASA). J Clin Sleep Med 2005;1(3):247–54.

25. Carroll JL, McColley SA, Marcus CL, et al. Inability of clinical history to distinguish primary snoring from obstructive sleep apnea syndrome in children. Chest 1995; 108(3):610–8.

26. Carotenuto M, Bruni O, Santoro N, et al. Waist circumference predicts the occurrence of sleep-disordered breathing in obese children and adolescents: a questionnaire-based study. Sleep Med 2006;7(4):357–61.

27. Chervin RD, Weatherly RA, Garetz SL, et al. Pediatric sleep questionnaire: prediction of sleep apnea and outcomes. Arch Otolaryngol Head Neck Surg 2007;133(3):216–22.

28. Constantin E, Tewfik TL, Brouillette RT. Can the OSA-18 quality-of-life questionnaire detect obstructive sleep apnea? Pediatrics 2010;125(1):e162–8.

29. Aurora RN, Zak RS, Karippot A, et al, American Academy of Sleep Medicine. Practice parameters for the respiratory indications for polysomnography in children. Sleep 2011;34(3):379–88.

30. Goodwin JL, Enright PL, Kaeming KL, et al. Feasibility of using unattended polysomnography in children for research–report of the Tucson Children's Assessment of Sleep Apnea study (TuCASA). Sleep 2001;24(8):937–44.

31. Katz ES, Greene MG, Carson KA, et al. Night-to-night variability of polysomnography in children with suspected obstructive sleep apnea. J Pediatr 2002;140(5): 589–94.

32. Li AM, Wing YK, Cheung A, et al. Is a 2-night polysomnographic study necessary in childhood sleep-related -disordered breathing? Chest 2004;126(5):1467–72.

33. Scholle S, Scholle HC, Kemper A, et al. First night effect in children and adolescents undergoing polysomnography for sleep-disordered breathing. Clin Neurophysiol 2003;114(11):2138–45.

34. Verhulst SL, Schrauwen N, De Backer WA, et al. First night effect for polysomnographic data in children and adolescents with suspected sleep disordered breathing. Arch Dis Child 2006;91(3):233–7.

35. Rebuffat E, Groswasser J, Kelmanson I, et al. Polygraphic evaluation of night-to-night variability in sleep characteristics and apneas in infants. Sleep 1994;17(4): 329–32.

36. Nieminen P, Tolonen U, Lopponen H. Snoring and obstructive sleep apnea in children: a 6-month follow-up study. Arch Otolaryngol Head Neck Surg 2000;126(4): 481–6.

37. Zucconi M, Calori G, Castonovo V, et al. Respiratory monitoring by means of an unattended device in children with suspected uncomplicated obstructive sleep apnea: a validation study. Chest 2003;124(2):602–7.

38. Mason DG, Iyer K, Terrill PI, et al. Pediatric obstructive sleep apnea assessment using pulse oximetry and dual RIP bands. Conf Proc IEEE Eng Med Biol Soc 2010;2010:6154–7.

39. Marcus CL, Keens TG, Ward SL. Comparison of nap and overnight polysomnography in children. Pediatr Pulmonol 1992;13(1):16–21.

40. Saeed MM, Keens TG, Stabile MW, et al. Should children with suspected obstructive sleep apnea syndrome and normal nap sleep studies have overnight sleep studies? Chest 2000;118(2):360–5.

41. Marcus CL, Keens TG, Bautista DB, et al. Obstructive sleep apnea in children with Down syndrome. Pediatrics 1991;88:132–9.

42. Noehren A, Brockmann PE, Urschitz MS, et al. Detection of respiratory events using pulse rate in children with and without obstructive sleep apnea. Pediatr Pulmonol 2010;45(5):459–68.

43. Katz ES, Lutz J, Black C, et al. Pulse transit time as a measure of arousal and respiratory effort in children with sleep-disordered breathing. Pediatr Res 2003; 53(4):580–8.

44. Foo JY, Bradley AP, Wilson SJ, et al. Screening of obstructive and central apnoea/hypopnoea in children using variability: a preliminary study. Acta Paediatr 2006; 95(5):561–4.

45. Tauman R, O'Brien LM, Mast BT, et al. Peripheral arterial tonometry events and electroencephalographic arousals in children. Sleep 2004;27(3):502–6.

46. Brouillette RT, Morielli A, Leimanis A, et al. Nocturnal pulse oximetry as an abbreviated testing modality for pediatric obstructive sleep apnea. Pediatrics 2000; 105(2):405–12.

47. Nixon GM, Kermack AS, Davis GM, et al. Planning adenotonsillectomy in children with obstructive sleep apnea: the role of overnight oximetry. Pediatrics 2004; 113(1 Pt 1):e19–25.

48. Kirk VG, Bohn SG, Flemons WW, et al. Comparison of home oximetry monitoring with laboratory polysomnography in children. Chest 2003;124(5):1702–8.

49. Baugh RF, Archer SM, Mitchell RB, et al. Clinical practice guideline: tonsillectomy in children. American Academy of Otolaryngology-Head and Neck Surgery Foundation. Otolaryngol Head Neck Surg 2011;144(Suppl 1):S1–30.

50. Friedman M, Wilson M, Lin HC, et al. Updated systematic review of tonsillectomy and adenoidectomy for treatment of pediatric obstructive sleep apnea/hypopnea syndrome. Otolaryngol Head Neck Surg 2009;140(6):800–8.

51. Costa DJ, Mitchell R. Adenotonsillectomy for obstructive sleep apnea in obese children: a meta-analysis. Otolaryngol Head Neck Surg 2009;140:455–60.

52. Windfuhr JP, Chen YS, Remmert S. Hemorrhage following tonsillectomy and adenoidectomy in 15,218 patients. Otolaryngol Head Neck Surg 2006;132:281–6.

53. Pratt LW, Gallagher RA. Tonsillectomy and adenoidectomy: incidence and mortality, 1968–1972. Otolaryngol Head Neck Surg 1979;87(2):159–66.

54. Stevenson AN, Myer CM 3rd, Shuler MD, et al. Complications and legal outcomes of tonsillectomy malpractice claims. Laryngoscope 2012;122(1):71–4 [Epub 2011 Nov 10].

55. Tunkel DE, Hotchkiss KS, Carson KA, et al. Efficacy of powered intracapsular tonsillectomy and adenoidectomy. Laryngoscope 2008;118(7):1295–302.

56. Mangiardi J, Graw-Panzer KD, Weedon J, et al. Polysomnography outcomes for partial intracapsular versus total tonsillectomy. Int J Pediatr Otorhinolaryngol 2010;74(12):1361–6.

57. Sarny S, Ossimitz G, Habermann W, et al. Hemorrhage following tonsil surgery: a multicenter prospective study. Laryngoscope 2011;121(12):2553–60.

58. Derkay CS, Darrow DH, Welch C, et al. Post-tonsillectomy morbidity and quality of life in pediatric patients with obstructive tonsils and adenoid: microdebrider vs electrocautery. Otolaryngol Head Neck Surg 2006;134(1):114–20.

59. Koltai PJ, Solares CA, Koempel JA, et al. Intracapsular tonsillar reduction (partial tonsillectomy): reviving a historical procedure for obstructive sleep disordered breathing in children. Otolaryngol Head Neck Surg 2003;129(5):532–8.

60. Celenk F, Bayazit YA, Yilmaz M, et al. Tonsillar regrowth following partial tonsillectomy with radiofrequency. Int J Pediatr Otorhinolaryngol 2008;72(1):19–22.

61. Zagolski O. Why do palatine tonsils grow back after partial tonsillectomy in children? Eur Arch Otorhinolaryngol 2010;267(10):1613–7.

62. Solares CA, Koempel JA, Hirose K, et al. Safety and efficacy of powered intracapsular tonsillectomy in children: a multi-center retrospective case series. Int J Pediatr Otorhinolaryngol 2005;69(1):21–6.

63. Joshua B, Bahar G, Sulkes J, et al. Adenoidectomy: long-term follow up. Otolaryngol Head Neck Surg 2006;135(4):576–80.

64. Brietzke SE, Gallagher D. The effectiveness of tonsillectomy and adenoidectomy in the treatment of pediatric obstructive sleep apnea/hypopnea syndrome: a meta-analysis. Otolaryngol Head Neck Surg 2006;134(6):979–84.

65. Kerschner JE, Lynch JB, Kleiner H, et al. Uvulopalatopharyngoplasty with tonsillectomy and adenoidectomy as a treatment for obstructive sleep apnea in neurologically impaired children. Int J Pediatr Otorhinolaryngol 2002;62(3):229–35.

66. Kosko JR, Derkay CS. Uvuloplatopharyngoplasty: treatment of obstructive sleep apnea in neurologically impaired pediatric patients. Int J Pediatr Otorhinolaryngol 1995;32(3):241–6.

67. Morita T, Kurata K, Hiratsuka Y, et al. A preoperative sleep study with nasal airway occlusion in pharyngeal flap surgery. Am J Otolaryngol 2004;25(5):334–8.

68. Sullivan S, Li K, Guilleminault C. Nasal obstruction in children with sleep-disordered breathing. Ann Acad Med Singapore 2008;37(8):645–8.

69. Miller FR, Watson D, Boseley M. The role of genial bone advancement trephine system in conjunction with uvulopalatopharyngoplasty in the multilevel management of obstructive sleep apnea. Otolaryngol Head Neck Surg 2004; 130(1):73–9.

70. Wootten CT, Shott SR. Evolving therapies to treat retroglossal and base-of-tongue obstruction in pediatric obstructive sleep apnea. Arch Otolaryngol Head Neck Surg 2010;136(10):983–7.

71. Michalsky M, Reichard K, Inge T, et al. ASMBS pediatric committee best practive guidelines. Surg Obes Relat Dis 2012;8(1):1–7 [Epub 2011 Sep 23].

72. O'Brien PE, Sawyer SM, Brown LC, et al. Laparoscopic adjustable gastric banding in severely obese adolescents: a randomized trial. JAMA 2010;303: 512–26.

73. Kalra M, Inge T, Garcia V. Obstructive sleep apnea in extremely overweight adolescents undergoing bariatric surgery. Obese Res 2005;13(7):1175–9.

74. Greenburg DL, Lettieri CJ, Eliasson AH. Effects of surgical weight loss on measures of obstructive sleep apnea: a meta-analysis. Am J Med 2009;122(6):535–42.

75. Epstein LH, Valoski A, Wing RR, et al. Ten-year follow-up of behavioral, family-based treatment for obese children. JAMA 1990;264(19):2519–23.

76. Al-Ghamdi SA, Manoukian JJ, Morielli A, et al. Do systemic corticosteroids effectively treat obstructive sleep apnea secondary to adenotonsillar hypertrophy? Laryngoscope 1997;107(10):1382–7.

77. Brouillette RT, Manoukian JJ, Ducharme FM, et al. Efficacy of fluticasone nasal spray for pediatric obstructive sleep apnea. J Pediatr 2001;138:838–44.

78. Kheirandish-Gozal L, Gozal D. Intranasal budesonide treatment for children with mild obstructive sleep apnea syndrome. Pediatrics 2008;122:e149–55.

79. Alexopoulos EI, Kaditis AG, Kalampouka E, et al. Nasal corticosteroids for children with snoring. Pediatr Pulmonol 2004;38:161–7.

80. Kaditis AG, Ioannou MG, Chaidas K, et al. Cysteinyl leukotriene receptors are expressed by tonsillar T cells of children with obstructive sleep apnea. Chest 2008;134:324–31.

81. Goldbart AD, Goldman JL, Veling MC, et al. Leukotriene modifier therapy for mild sleep–disordered breathing in children. Am J Respir Crit Care Med 2005;172: 364–70.

82. Kheirandish L, Goldbart AD, Gozal D. Intranasal steroids and oral leukotriene modifier therapy in residual sleep-disordered breathing after tonsillectomy and adenoidectomy in children. Pediatrics 2006;117:e61–6.
83. Cozza P, Polimeni A, Ballanti F. A modified monobloc for the treatment of obstructive sleep apnoea in paediatric patients. Eur J Orthod 2004;26(5):523–30.
84. Pirelli P, Saponara M, Guilleminault C. Rapid maxillary expansion in children with obstructive sleep apnea syndrome. Sleep 2004;27(4):761–6.
85. Villa MP, Malagola C, Pagani J, et al. Rapid maxillary expansion in children with obstructive sleep apnea syndrome: 12-month follow-up. Sleep Med 2007;8: 128–34.
86. Villa MP, Rizzoli A, Miano S, et al. Efficacy of rapid maxillary expansion in children with obstructive sleep apnea syndrome: 36 months of follow-up. Sleep Breath 2011;15(2):179–84.
87. Marcus CL, Rosen G, Ward SL, et al. Adherence to and effectiveness of positive airway pressure therapy in children with obstructive sleep apnea. Pediatrics 2006;117:e442–51.
88. Uong EC, Epperson M, Bathon SA, et al. Adherence to nasal positive airway pressure therapy among school-aged children and adolescents with obstructive sleep apnea syndrome. Pediatrics 2007;120(5):e1203–11.
89. Fauroux B, Lavis JF, Nicot F, et al. Facial side effects during noninvasive positive pressure ventilation in children. Intensive Care Med 2005;31(7):965–9.

Evidence-Based Practice
Pediatric Tonsillectomy

Karin P.Q. Oomen, MD, PhD[a], Vikash K. Modi, MD[a],*,
Michael G. Stewart, MD, MPH[b]

KEYWORDS

- Tonsillectomy • Children • Throat infections • Sleep-disordered breathing
- Evidence-based medicine

KEY POINTS

The following points are expanded at the conclusion of this article and additional critical points are presented.

- Gaps in knowledge about perioperative management for tonsillectomy in children remain.
- Outcome measures in sleep-disordered breathing and recurrent throat infections should focus on not only recurrence of disease but also quality of life and school performance as indicators of well-being.
- No consensus exists on indications for a preoperative polysomnogram in children without comorbidities. Currently, physicians are recommended to advocate for polysomnogram in patients with sleep-disordered breathing without comorbidities if the need for surgery is uncertain or in the presence of discordance between symptoms and physical examination.
- Reported success rates of tonsillectomy for sleep-disordered breathing in obese children are 10% to 20%; in normal-weight children they are 70% to 80%.
- Current guidelines do not recommend specific tonsillectomy techniques.
- The development of intracapsular tonsillectomy represents a different surgical strategy rather than a different instrumental technique that, with further study, could lead to new recommendations.

OVERVIEW

Tonsillectomy is one of the most common surgical procedures performed in children in the United States, with more than 530, 000 procedures performed annually.[1] Tonsillectomy is defined as a surgical procedure that removes the tonsil. Removal of the tonsil may be specified as complete, through dissecting the peritonsillar space between the

The authors have nothing to declare.
[a] Department of Otolaryngology-Head & Neck Surgery, Pediatric Otolaryngology-Head & Neck Surgery, Weill Cornell Medical College, 428 East 72nd Street, Suite 100, New York, NY 10021, USA; [b] Department of Otolaryngology, Head & Neck Surgery, Weill Cornell Medical College, 1305 York Avenue, 5th Floor, New York, NY 10021, USA
* Corresponding author.
E-mail address: Vkm2001@med.cornell.edu

Otolaryngol Clin N Am 45 (2012) 1071–1081
http://dx.doi.org/10.1016/j.otc.2012.06.010
0030-6665/12/$ – see front matter © 2012 Elsevier Inc. All rights reserved.

oto.theclinics.com

tonsil capsule and the muscular wall, or partial, through removing a varying amount of tonsillar tissue intracapsularly or subcapsularly.[2] Although tonsillectomy is a common procedure, it is associated with morbidity, including anesthesia risks, throat pain, and postoperative bleeding, which may result in admission for observation or further surgery to control bleeding. These and rarer complications have been well described and should be taken into account when considering surgery in children.[3]

This article provides an evidence-based perspective on perioperative clinical decision making and surgical technique for tonsillectomy.

EVIDENCE-BASED CLINICAL ASSESSMENT
Indications for Tonsillectomy

Indications for tonsillectomy are multiple, the most common and generally accepted of which are sleep-disordered breathing (SDB) and recurrent throat infections, with a gradual incidence shift toward SDB over the past 2 decades.[4]

SDB is now the single most common indication for tonsillectomy with or without adenoidectomy; SDB constitutes a range of disorders increasing in severity from snoring and restless sleep to obstructive sleep apnea (OSA).[5] SDB has a multifactorial etiology, and hypertrophic tonsils are usually a contributing factor. A recent meta-analysis has shown that tonsillectomy is effective for treating SDB in children with tonsillar hypertrophy,[6] and a recent clinical practice guideline recommends tonsillectomy in children with tonsil hypertrophy who have a polysomnography indicative of SDB.[2] Success rates are significantly lower for tonsillectomy in obese children with SDB.[7]

Throat infections are defined as episodes of sore throat caused by viral or bacterial infection of the pharynx, palatine tonsils, or both, and include a variety of terms, such as tonsillitis, pharyngitis, and strep throat.[2] Throat infections may be documented for each episode of sore throat with one or more of the following: temperature higher than 38.3°C, cervical adenopathy, tonsillar exudates, or positive test for group A β-hemolytic streptococci.

The actual benefit of tonsillectomy compared with observation in children with throat infections remains a subject of controversy. In 1984, a randomized controlled trial by Paradise and colleagues[8] showed a reduction in frequency and severity of infections in severely affected children with recurrent throat infections in the 2 years after tonsillectomy. In moderately affected children, the same group found only a modest benefit of tonsillectomy, which the authors believed was not sufficient to outweigh the risks, morbidity, and costs of surgery.[9] A recent clinical practice guideline recommended tonsillectomy in children with recurrent throat infections with a frequency of at least seven episodes in the prior year, at least five episodes per year in the prior 2 years, or at least three episodes per year in the prior 3 years.[2,8] Although the guideline recommended watchful waiting for recurrent throat infections with a lesser frequency, tonsillectomy is recommend in children with fewer throat infections if they exhibit modifying factors, such as multiple antibiotic allergy or intolerance, a combination of periodic fever, aphthous stomatitis, pharyngitis, and adenitis (PFAPA), or a history of peritonsillar abscess.[2]

Other rarer indications for surgery include orthodontic concerns, tonsiliths, halitosis, and chronic tonsillitis, all for which substantial evidence is currently not available or of lesser quality.[10–12]

Clinical Assessment of Tonsils

Careful history taking is vital and should include symptoms of

- Throat infections
- Snoring

- Apneas
- Restless sleep
- Nocturnal enuresis
- Somnolence
- Growth retardation
- Poor school performance
- Behavioral problems
- Attention deficit hyperactivity disorder

Physical examination should focus on the anatomy, which includes the size of the tonsils in relation to the position and size of the palate, tongue, and chin. Tonsil size is currently identified using a tonsil grading scale,[13,14] with tonsillar hypertrophy defined as 3+ or 4+. An important limitation of this grading system is that it does not provide a three-dimensional assessment of tonsil size, which would be more accurate in quantifying tonsillar hypertrophy. A previous study has shown that tonsillar size alone does not correlate with the severity of SDB,[10] but the combined volume of the tonsils and the adenoids do correlate more closely with SDB severity.[15]

Polysomnography

Unfortunately, neither history nor physical examination alone can reliably predict the presence or severity of SDB.[16] Currently, polysomnography is the gold standard for diagnosing and quantifying SDB in children, and can be a useful diagnostic tool before tonsillectomy.[17] Polysomnography is the electrical recording of physiologic variables during sleep, including gas exchange, respiratory effort, airflow, snoring, sleep stage, body position, limb movement, and heart rhythm. Not only does polysomnography identify the presence of SDB, it also helps define its severity and may serve as an aid in perioperative planning and assessing the risk of postoperative complications.

Since 2002, the American Academy of Pediatrics has recommended overnight polysomnography in all children with suspected SDB to confirm diagnosis.[17] A recent clinical practice guideline on polysomnography in children recommended referral for polysomnography in children with SDB before tonsillectomy if they exhibited one of the following comorbid conditions[5]:

- Obesity
- Down syndrome
- Craniofacial abnormalities
- Neuromuscular disorders
- Sickle cell disease
- Mucopolysaccharidosis

In these children, polysomnography helps determine the need for postoperative pulse oximetry and admission. The same guideline recommends polysomnography before tonsillectomy in children without any of the aforementioned comorbidities, but only if the need for surgery is uncertain or in the presence of discordance between the clinical history and/or tonsillar size on physical examination and the reported severity of SDB.

Polysomnography may be performed in a sleep laboratory or in an ambulatory setting, the latter being referred to as portable monitoring (PM). Because of the cost and inconvenience of laboratory-based polysomnography, several forms of PM have developed, but few devices have been tested in children, and substantial evidence for this method is lacking. Laboratory-based polysomnography is currently the gold standard for evaluation of SDB in children and is recommended in children for whom polysomnography is indicated to assess SDB before tonsillectomy.[5]

EVIDENCE-BASED SURGICAL TECHNIQUE FOR TONSILLECTOMY
Procedure

Total tonsillectomy via cold dissection
Traditional techniques for tonsillectomy consist of cold dissection with metal instruments including knife, scissor, or snare. These techniques involve complete removal of the tonsil with its capsule by dissecting the peritonsillar space, with hemostasis obtained through ligation of blood vessels during tonsil removal or cauterization of the wound bed. Complete dissection or total tonsillectomy (TT) with cold steel is still the technique against which effectiveness and safety of other techniques are compared.[2]

Total tonsillectomy via electrosurgery, cautery dissection, coblation, radiofrequency
In recent years, many new surgical approaches for TT have been explored to reduce perioperative morbidity. Electrosurgical or cautery dissection are common techniques used for complete tonsillectomy. Many newer techniques, including radiofrequency, coblation, harmonic scalpel, and PEAK PlasmaBlade, have been introduced to reduce postoperative pain and hemorrhage.

Outcomes of total tonsillectomy techniques
A recent systematic review has studied randomized controlled trials comparing TT performed using vessel sealing systems, harmonic scalpel, or coblation technique with conventional techniques of cold steel and/or cautery dissection.[18] No significant differences in postoperative pain were found in the coblation and/or harmonic scalpel method compared with the cold steel and/or cautery technique. Furthermore, several randomized controlled trials have compared traditional TT with other techniques, including coblation, cautery, and ultrasonic scalpel, without finding a significant difference in postoperative pain.[19–22]

Intracapsular tonsillectomy
A growing body of evidence suggests lower postoperative morbidity with a partial intracapsular tonsillectomy (IT) technique, in which most tonsillar tissue is removed, leaving a small amount of tonsillar tissue in the tonsillar fossa.[23–25] The belief is that the rim of tonsillar tissue left in the tonsillar fossa provides a buffer zone that prevents damage to the surrounding pharyngeal muscles, thereby reducing severity and duration of postoperative pain.[23,25] IT is also thought to reduce the amount of postoperative hemorrhage.[26] Several instruments have been used to perform IT, including the microdebrider, the coblator, and traditional cold steel. A study by Bitar and colleagues[25] compared the effects of microdebrider-assisted IT to electrocautery-assisted TT in children, showing no difference in surgical time or postoperative bleeding, but an earlier return to normal activity and reduced need for analgesics in the IT group. A study by Wilson and colleagues[23] compared microdebrider-assisted IT, coblator-assisted IT, and electrocautery-assisted TT and showed a significantly earlier return to normal diet and preoperative activity level, and reduction of days of pain in both IT groups. No significant differences were seen in occurrence of postoperative complications, such as hemorrhage. Chang[27] showed a significantly shorter postoperative recovery period for coblator-assisted IT compared with electrocautery-assisted TT in children.

A potential concern with IT might be regrowth of tonsillar tissue and need for revision surgery. Derkay and colleagues[26] showed a significantly higher incidence of residual tonsillar tissue in children who underwent microdebrider-assisted IT compared with those who had electrocautery-assisted TT. However, the incidence of recurrence of obstruction or infection in this group was unknown. Chan and colleagues[28] also showed a significantly higher incidence of residual tonsillar tissue, but no difference in recurrence of obstructive disease, pharyngitis, or antibiotic use. Ericsson and colleagues[24] and Bitar and colleagues[25] did not shown tonsillar regrowth at 12 and 20 months after IT, and no recurrence of symptoms after 3 years and 20 months, respectively. Irrespective of tonsillar regrowth, a retrospective chart review by Schmidt and colleagues[29] compared the efficacy of IT versus TT in treating recurrent tonsillitis and showed no difference in postoperative infection rates.

Postoperative Management of Tonsillectomy: Hospitalization

Several studies have established that pediatric tonsillectomy may be safely performed in an outpatient setting.[28,30,31] A previous clinical guideline recommends that children with complicated medical histories, including cardiac complications of OSA, neuro-muscular disorders, prematurity, obesity, failure to thrive, craniofacial anomalies, or a recent upper respiratory tract infection, should be admitted overnight because of a higher risk of postoperative respiratory complications.[17] SDB severity has also been identified as a risk factor for postoperative respiratory complications and is there-fore considered an indication for postoperative admission by many. Although tonsillec-tomy resolves or at least significantly improves OSA in most children, they may continue to experience upper airway obstruction and oxygen desaturation in the direct postoperative period.[32,33] An apnea-hypopnea index of 10 or more obstructive events per hour and/or oxygen saturation nadir less than 80% is currently considered the level of severity required for postoperative hospitalization with monitoring.[5,34] Admission after total tonsillectomy is also recommended for children younger than 3 years, regard-less of indication, because of postoperative pain resulting in poor oral intake.[35–37] With the advent of techniques such as IT, reduction of postoperative morbidity might lead to new insights on postoperative management. Bent and colleagues[38] compared children younger than 3 years with children aged 3 years or older undergoing IT for postopera-tive parameters such as pain, oral intake, or analgesic requirements. Because no signif-icant differences were found between the age groups, the investigators concluded that children younger than 3 years may undergo IT on an outpatient basis.

Postoperative Hemorrhage in Tonsillectomy

Postoperative hemorrhage is a well-known complication of tonsillectomy and may be categorized as primary or secondary. Primary hemorrhage is defined as bleeding within the first 24 hours after tonsillectomy, and occurs in 0.2% to 2.2% of patients.[2] Secondary hemorrhage occurs more than 24 hours after surgery, often between 5 and 10 days, because of sloughing of the primary eschar during healing of the tonsil bed. Rates of secondary hemorrhage for tonsillectomy range from 0.1% to 3%.[39] Clinicians who perform tonsillectomy are recommended to always inquire about bleeding after surgery, and determine their rate of primary and secondary posttonsillectomy hemor-rhage at least annually.[2]

Surgical technique can have an impact on postoperative bleeding. Several new tech-niques were recently introduced to reduce postoperative hemorrhage. Many previous studies have focused on comparison of "hot" (electrosurgery or electrocautery tech-niques) versus cold tonsillectomy with respect to postoperative bleeding, with similar unequivocal outcomes.[18–22] Several systematic reviews[18,40–43] have summarized randomized controlled trials on conventional cold steel tonsillectomy versus diathermy, monopolar cautery, coblation, or harmonic scalpel techniques, but none has shown a significant difference in postoperative hemorrhage rates among techniques.

Other studies have focused on comparison of IT and TT with respect to postoperative complications such as hemorrhage.[23,25,26,28,44–50] Three large retrospective case series have shown a significantly lower rate of postoperative bleeding for IT compared with TT.[44,47,49] However, most prospective trials fail to demonstrate a significant difference in postoperative hemorrhage between IT and TT,[23,25,26,28,45,46] although one trial reports a significantly lower intraoperative blood loss with IT.[45]

SDB and Other Postoperative Concerns in Tonsillectomy

With SDB being the most common indication for tonsillectomy, postoperative monitoring for possible residual SDB is an important consideration. Before surgery, caregivers must be counseled that tonsillectomy is not curative in all cases of SDB in children, especially in children with obesity, and further treatment may be required after surgery.[2] Clinical guidelines do not recommend routine polysomnography after tonsillectomy in children with SDB. When SDB or related comorbid conditions, such as growth retardation, poor school performance, enuresis, or behavioral problems, have been the indication for surgery, SDB is considered cured when the caregiver reports that symptoms are resolved postoperatively. In these cases, postoperative polysomnography is deemed unnecessary, but substantial evidence for this assumption is lacking. Any postoperative report of continuing symptoms of SDB should be taken seriously and indicates the need for further evaluation, including consideration of formal polysomnography.[2] A recent systematic review does recommend postoperative polysomnography for children with perioperative evidence of moderate to severe OSA, obesity, craniofacial anomalies, and neurologic disorders.[50]

WHAT THE EVIDENCE INDICATES

Tonsillectomy is a safe surgical procedure performed on a large scale, most commonly for SDB and recurrent throat infections. The positive effect of tonsillectomy has been established for severely affected children with recurrent throat infections in a randomized controlled trial but could not be shown for children who were less severely affected (grade B evidence).[8,9] A systematic review of cohort studies and a few case series found tonsillectomy to be an effective treatment for SDB (grade B–C evidence).[6]

Polysomnography is the gold standard for diagnosing SDB, but guidelines do not recommend that polysomnography be performed routinely preoperatively in children with suspected SDB and tonsil hypertrophy. Polysomnography is recommended in children with specific comorbidities based on results from observational studies (grade C evidence).[5] In children without comorbidities but an uncertain need for surgery or discordance between history and examination, preoperative polysomnography should be performed (grade C evidence).[5]

In an attempt to reduce postoperative hemorrhage rates, several tonsillectomy techniques have been developed, but systematic reviews of randomized controlled trials have thus far not provided evidence of such a reduction using any particular technique (grade A evidence).[40,41] Many randomized controlled trials have compared various newer and conventional TT techniques but could not demonstrate differences in postoperative pain (grade B evidence).[19–22]

Studies comparing TT and IT show faster recovery and pain reduction in patients treated with IT but no significantly lower risk of postoperative bleeding (grade B evidence).[23,25,26,28,45,46,48] Retrospective case series, however, do show a significantly lower postoperative bleeding rate for IT (grade C evidence).[44,47,49]

Evidence grades and conclusions are summarized in **Table 1**.

Table 1
Conclusions and grades of evidence for tonsillectomy

Category	References	Description	n	Level of Evidence	Evidence Grade	Conclusion
Effects of tonsillectomy	8	Parallel randomized and nonrandomized clinical trials	187	1b	B	Tonsillectomy reduces throat infections in severely affected children
	8,9	Parallel randomized and nonrandomized clinical trials	515	1b	B	Tonsillectomy does not reduce throat infections in less severely affected children
	6	Systematic review and meta-analysis of randomized controlled trials and observational studies	1097	2a	B–C	Tonsillectomy is an effective treatment for sleep-disordered breathing
Preoperative polysomnography	5	Clinical practice guideline–based observational studies	246	2b–3b	C	Polysomnography is recommended in children with specific comorbidities
	5	Clinical practice guideline–based on observational studies	723	2b	C	Polysomnography is recommended in children without specific comorbidities if uncertain need for surgery or discordance between history and examination
Postoperative hemorrhage	40,41	Systematic review of two randomized controlled trials	254	1a	A	No differences in postoperative hemorrhage rates are seen between TT techniques
	44,47,49	Retrospective case series with chart review	5812	4	C	TT might be associated with a lower risk of postoperative bleeding
Postoperative pain	19–22	Prospective randomized controlled trials	362	1b	B	No differences in postoperative pain rates are seen between TT techniques
	23,25,26,28,45,46,48	Prospective randomized controlled trials	842	1b	B	TT is not associated with a lower rate of postoperative pain

CRITICAL POINTS

- Although a large amount of literature is available and clinical guidelines exist, certain gaps in knowledge remain about perioperative management for tonsillectomy in children.
- Large, multicenter, prospective, randomized, controlled trials are needed on the effect of tonsillectomy on recurrent throat infections and SDB. Outcome measures should focus on not only recurrence of disease but also quality of life and school performance as indicators of well-being. Although a randomized controlled trial has shown reduction of throat infections after tonsillectomy in severely affected children, this effect in not seen in milder cases or for a postoperative period for more than 2 years.[8,9] Because the effect of tonsillectomy on throat infections was shown in a single study conducted in 1984, additional, newer, randomized, controlled trials may be needed to confirm these findings.
- Regarding SDB as an indication for surgery, certain topics must be addressed in more detail. No consensus exists on indications for a preoperative polysomnography in children without comorbidities. Currently, physicians are recommended to advocate for polysomnography in patients with SDB without comorbidities if the need for surgery is uncertain or in the presence of discordance between symptoms and physical examination. Future studies on polysomnography for SDB might be able to specify these rather wide criteria.
- Because some children may lack access to a sleep laboratory or have difficulty sleeping in a foreign environment, studies are need to evaluate PM. PM studies should focus on which parameters should be measured to replicate laboratory findings and accurately predict which children are at risk for postoperative complications.
- To the same extent, indications for postoperative polysomnography for SDB after tonsillectomy must be specified and studied further.
- With obesity rates increasing worldwide, a subject of growing concern is the management of obese children with SDB. A previous meta-analysis of four studies showed success rates of 10% to 20% for tonsillectomy for SDB in obese children,[7] whereas the resolution reported in normal-weight children is around 70% to 80%.[51] This discrepancy warrants future investigation of the extent to which obesity plays a role in failure to respond after tonsillectomy for SDB, and determination of the exact role of tonsillectomy in obese children.
- Currently, guidelines do not recommend specific tonsillectomy techniques. Although a large body of literature discusses various TT techniques that differ mainly in the instruments used, no substantial evidence exists for a general benefit of one instrument over another. The development of IT, which represents a different surgical strategy rather than a different instrumental technique, may be a field of further study that could eventually lead to new recommendations. Several studies have established benefits of IT over TT with respect to postoperative recovery and pain.[23,25,26,28,45,46,48] The finding of significantly lower postoperative bleeding rates for IT in retrospective case series[44,47,49] warrants further investigation and confirmation in prospective trials, but might hold the promise of future recommendations for surgical technique. Specific studies are needed on postoperative management after IT in patients in the younger age group (age<3 years) to confirm previous findings.[38] If positive, these studies may influence recommendations on inpatient versus outpatient surgery.

REFERENCES

1. Cullen KA, Hall MJ, Golosinsky A. Ambulatory surgery in the United States. Natl Health Stat Rep 2009;11:1–28.
2. Baugh R, Archer S, Mitchell R, et al. Clinical practice guideline: tonsillectomy in children. Otolaryngol Head Neck Surg 2011;144(Suppl):S1–30.
3. Johnson L, Elluru R, Myer C. Complications of adenotonsillectomy. Laryngoscope 2002;112:35–6.
4. Erickson B, Larson D, Stauver J. Changes in incidence and indications of tonsillectomy and adenotonsillectomy, 1970-2005. Otolaryngol Head Neck Surg 2009;140(6):894–901.
5. Roland P, Rosenfeld R, Brooks L, et al. Clinical practice guideline: polysomnography for sleep-disordered breathing prior to tonsillectomy in children. Otolaryngol Head Neck Surg 2011;145(Suppl):S1–15.
6. Friedman M, Wilson M, Lin CH, et al. Updated systematic review of tonsillectomy and adenoidectomy in the treatment of obstructive sleep apnea/hypopnea syndrome: a meta-analysis. Otolaryngol Head Neck Surg 2009;140(6):800–8.
7. Costa DJ, Mitchell R. Adenotonsillectomy for obstructive sleep apnea in obese children: a meta-analysis. Otolaryngol Head Neck Surg 2009;140(4):455–60.
8. Paradise JL, Bluestone CD, Bachmann RZ, et al. Efficacy of tonsillectomy for recurrent throat infection in severely affected children: results of parallel randomized and nonrandomized clinical trials. N Engl J Med 1984;310(11):674–83.
9. Paradise J, Bluestone CD, Colborn DK, et al. Tonsillectomy and adenotonsillectomy for recurrent throat infection in moderately affected children. Pediatrics 2002;110(1):7–15.
10. Morawska A, Lyszczarz J, Skladzien J. An analysis of orthodontic indications for surgical treatment of Waldeyer ring hyperplasia in pediatric patients of the otolaryngology and stomatology department of the university hospital of Krakow. Otolaryngol Pol 2008;62(3):272–7.
11. Burton MJ, Glasziou PP. Tonsillectomy or adenotonsillectomy versus non-surgical treatment for chronic/recurrent acute tonsillitis. Cochrane Database Syst Rev 2009;(1):CD001802.
12. Tanyeri HT, Polat S. Temperature-controlled radiofrequency tonsil ablation for the treatment of halitosis. Eur Arch Otorhinolaryngol 2011;268(2):267–72.
13. Brodsky L. Modern assessment of tonsils and adenoids. Pediatr Clin North Am 1989;36(6):1551–69.
14. Howard N, Brietzke S. Pediatric tonsil size: objective vs subjective measurements correlated to overnight polysomnogram. Otolaryngol Head Neck Surg 2009;140(5):675–81.
15. Arens R, McDonough J, Corbin A, et al. Upper airway size analysis by magnetic resonance imaging of children with obstructive sleep apnea syndrome. Am J Respir Crit Care Med 2003;167(1):65–70.
16. Brietzke SE, Katz ES, Robertson DW. Can history and physical examination reliably diagnose pediatric obstructive sleep apnea/hypopnea syndrome? A systematic review of the literature. Otolaryngol Head Neck Surg 2004;131(6):827–32.
17. Subcommittee on Obstructive Sleep Apnea Syndrome, American Academy of Pediatrics. Clinical practice guideline: diagnosis and management of childhood obstructive sleep apnea syndrome. Pediatrics 2002;109(4):704–12.
18. Vangelis AG, Salazar-Salvia MS, Jervis PN, et al. Modern technology-assisted vs conventional tonsillectomy: a meta-analysis of randomized controlled trials. Arch Otolaryngol Head Neck Surg 2011;137(6):558–70.

19. Parsons SP, Cordes SR, Comer B. Comparison of posttonsillectomy pain using the ultrasonic scalpel, coblator, and electrocautery. Otolaryngol Head Neck Surg 2006;134(1):106–13.

20. Stoker KE, Don DM, Kang DR, et al. Pediatric total tonsillectomy using coblation compared to conventional electrosurgery: a prospective, controlled single-blind study. Otolaryngol Head Neck Surg 2004;130(6):666–75.

21. Bäck L, Paloheimo M, Ylikoski J. Traditional tonsillectomy compared with bipolar radiofrequency thermal ablation tonsillectomy in adults: a pilot study. Arch Otolaryngol Head Neck Surg 2001;127(9):1106–12.

22. Philpott CM, Wild DC, Mehta D, et al. A double-blinded randomized controlled trial of coblation versus conventional dissection tonsillectomy on postoperative symptoms. Clin Otolaryngol 2005;30(2):143–8.

23. Wilson YL, Merer DM, Moscatleoo AL. Comparison of three common tonsillectomy techniques: a prospective randomized, double blinded clinical study. Laryngoscope 2009;119(1):162–70.

24. Ericsson E, Graf J, Hultcrantz E. Pediatric tonsillotomy with radiofrequency technique: long term follow-up. Laryngoscope 2006;116(10):1851–7.

25. Bitar MA, Rameh C. Microdebrider-assisted partial tonsillectomy: short- and long-term outcomes. Eur Arch Otorhinolaryngol 2008;265(4):459–63.

26. Derkay CS, Darrow DH, Welch C, et al. Post-tonsillectomy morbidity and quality of life in pediatric patients with obstructive tonsils and adenoid: microdebrider vs electrocautery. Otolaryngol Head Neck Surg 2006;134(1):114–20.

27. Chang KW. Randomized controlled trial of coblation versus electrocautery tonsillectomy. Otolaryngol Head Neck Surg 2005;132(2):273–80.

28. Chan KH, Friedman NR, Allen GC, et al. Randomized, controlled, multisite study of intracapsular tonsillectomy using low-temperature plasma excision. Arch Otolaryngol Head Neck Surg 2004;130(11):1303–7.

29. Schmidt R, Herzog A, Cook S, et al. Powered intracapsular tonsillectomy in the management of recurrent tonsillitis. Otolaryngol Head Neck Surg 2007;137(2):338–40.

30. Haberman RS, Shattuck TG, Dion NM. Is outpatient suction cautery tonsillectomy safe in a community hospital setting? Laryngoscope 1990;100(5):511–5.

31. Helmus C, Grin M, Westfall R. Same-day-stay adenotonsillectomy. Laryngoscope 1990;100(6):593–6.

32. McColley SA, April MM, Carroll JL, et al. Respiratory compromise after adenotonsillectomy in children with obstructive sleep apnea. Arch Otolaryngol Head Neck Surg 1992;118(9):940–3.

33. Nixon GM, Kermack AS, McGregor CD, et al. Sleep and breathing on the first night after adenotonsillectomy for obstructive sleep apnea. Pediatr Pulmonol 2005;39(4):332–8.

34. Nixon GM, Kermack AS, Davis GM, et al. Planning adenotonsillectomy in children with obstructive sleep apnea: the role of overnight oximetry. Pediatrics 2004;113(1 Pt 1):e19–25.

35. Tom LW, DeDio RM, Cohen DE, et al. Is outpatient tonsillectomy appropriate for young children? Laryngoscope 1992;102(3):277–80.

36. Rothschild MA, Catalano P, Biller HF. Ambulatory pediatric tonsillectomy and the identification of high-risk subgroups. Otolaryngol Head Neck Surg 1994;110(2):203–10.

37. Mitchell RB, Pereira KD, Friedman NR, et al. Outpatient adenotonsillectomy: is it safe in children younger than 3 years? Arch Otolaryngol Head Neck Surg 1997;123(7):681–3.

38. Bent JP, April MM, Ward RF, et al. Ambulatory powered intracapsular tonsillectomy and adenoidectomy in children younger than 3 years. Arch Otolaryngol Head Neck Surg 2004;130(10):1197–200.
39. Windfuhr JP, Chen YS, Remmert S. Hemorrhage following tonsillectomy and adenoidectomy in 15,218 patients. Otolaryngol Head Neck Surg 2006;132(2):281–6.
40. Pinder DK, Hilton MP. Dissection versus diathermy for tonsillectomy. Cochrane Database Syst Rev 2001;(4):CD002211.
41. Burton MJ, Doree C. Coblation versus other surgical techniques for tonsillectomy. Cochrane Database Syst Rev 2007;(3):CD004619.
42. Neumann C, Street I, Lowe D, et al. Harmonic scalpel tonsillectomy: a systematic review of evidence for postoperative hemorrhage. Otolaryngol Head Neck Surg 2007;137(3):378–84.
43. Leinbach RF, Markwell SJ, Colliver JA, et al. Hot versus cold tonsillectomy: a systematic review of the literature. Otolaryngol Head Neck Surg 2003;129(4):360–4.
44. Solares CA, Koempel JA, Hirose K, et al. Safety and efficacy of powered intracapsular tonsillectomy in children: a multi-center retrospective case series. In J Pediatr Otolaryngol 2005;69(1):21–6.
45. Hultcrantz E, Ericsson E. Pediatric tonsillotomy with the radiofrequency technique: less morbidity and pain. Laryngoscope 2004;114(5):871–7.
46. Korkmaz O, Bekas D, Cobanoglu B, et al. Partial tonsillectomy in children with obstructive tonsillar hypertrophy. Int J Pediatr Otorhinolaryngol 2008;72(7):1007–12.
47. Gallagher TQ, Wilcox L, McGuire E, et al. Analyzing factors associated with major complications after adenotonsillectomy in 4776 patients: comparing three tonsillectomy techniques. Otolaryngol Head Neck Surg 2010;142(6):886–92.
48. Chang KW. Intracapsular versus subcapsular coblation tonsillectomy. Otolaryngol Head Neck Surg 2008;138(2):153–7.
49. Schmidt R, Herzog A, Cook S, et al. Complications of tonsillectomy: a comparison of techniques. Arch Otolaryngol Head Neck Surg 2007;133(9):925–8.
50. Aurora RN, Zak RS, Karippot A, et al. Practice parameters for the respiratory indications for polysomnography in children. Sleep 2011;34(3):379–87.
51. Mitchell RB. Adenotonsillectomy for obstructive sleep apnea in children: outcome evaluated by pre-and postoperative polysomnography. Laryngoscope 2007;117(10):1844–54.

Evidence-Based Practice
Evaluation and Management of Unilateral Vocal Fold Paralysis

Stephanie Misono, MD, MPH[a],*, Albert L. Merati, MD[b]

KEYWORDS

- Evidence-based otolaryngology • Vocal cord paralysis • Larynx • Voice therapy
- Unilateral vocal fold paralysis

KEY POINTS

The following points list the level of evidence as based on Oxford Center for Evidence-Based Medicine.

- Unilateral vocal fold paralysis (UVFP) has a broad range of causes, including postsurgical, idiopathic, and neoplasm-related (evidence grade C).
- Work-up for UVFP should include computed tomography imaging, but not serology. Electromyography is useful for predicting poor prognosis (evidence grade C).
- Voice therapy can be beneficial, but is not sufficient for many patients with UVFP. In the short term, injection medialization can achieve comparable clinical results with medialization thyroplasty. Thyroplasty and reinnervation also achieve comparable voice outcomes (evidence grade B).

Abbreviations: UNILATERAL VOCAL FOLD PARALYSIS	
CT	Computed tomography
CXR	Chest x-ray/radiograph
LEMG	Laryngeal electromyography
UVFP	Unilateral vocal fold paralysis

OVERVIEW

Unilateral vocal fold paralysis (UVFP) continues to command attention as a fundamental clinical problem in otolaryngology. Its impact on voice, swallowing, and even airway function is notable. Patients and their physicians have many helpful diagnostic

The authors have no financial disclosures.
[a] Department of Otolaryngology/Head and Neck Surgery, University of Minnesota, 420 Delaware Street Southeast, MMC 396, Minneapolis, MN 55455, USA; [b] Department of Otolaryngology/Head and Neck Surgery, University of Washington, 1959 Northeast Pacific Street, Box 356515, Seattle, WA 98195, USA
* Corresponding author.
E-mail address: smisono@umn.edu

and therapeutic options for treatment, but at times this clinical decision making must occur without the luxury of scientifically established principles and practices. This article provides an evidence-based overview of (1) the causes and symptoms, (2) evaluation, and (3) management of UVFP. Publications addressing aspects of this topic number in the thousands, and therefore selected articles are presented to provide a sense of how the evidence has been developed and assessed. The discussion focuses primarily on UVFP rather than on the broader topic of unilateral vocal fold immobility. For each topic, the Oxford Center for Evidence-Based Medicine levels of evidence are listed.

Causes of UVFP (Evidence Level 3–4)

The list of potential causes of UVFP is broad, and includes:

- Iatrogenic
- Traumatic
- Neoplasms and thoracic diseases
- Systemic

Iatrogenic

Iatrogenic injury is commonly related to retraction and/or dissection along the route of the recurrent laryngeal nerve or even the vagus itself. Procedures associated with risk of postoperative vocal fold paralysis include thyroidectomy (0.8%–2.3% rate of permanent UVFP),[1–3] anterior cervical spine surgery (less than 1% risk of permanent UVFP per recent data),[4–7] esophagectomy (~11% risk),[7] cardiac/aortic surgery (~2% risk),[8] mediastinoscopy (0.2%–6% risk),[9,10] and carotid endarterectomy (~4% risk).[11,12]

Interpretation of the risks of UVFP associated with surgical procedures can be confusing because of the difficulty of determining the contribution of underlying disorders to the postoperative outcome. Without systematic preoperative and postoperative assessment of laryngeal function, which may not be clinically feasible, precise risk of UVFP associated with a given surgical procedure can be difficult to estimate. The picture is further clouded by the association of endotracheal intubation[13] or laryngeal mask airway[14] with UVFP, although some work has shown that the risk of iatrogenic UVFP related to retraction may be decreased by ongoing monitoring and adjustment of endotracheal tube pressure, particularly when retractors are placed or repositioned.[7]

Traumatic

Traumatic causes associated with UVFP include high vagal nerve injury caused by direct trauma, although vagal nerve injuries more commonly result from surgical removal of masses involving the vagus itself.[15] Arytenoid dislocation has been proposed as a cause of unilateral vocal fold immobility but this topic remains controversial; a recent review suggests that the diagnosis cannot be made by laryngoscopy alone and that there is insufficient evidence in the literature to characterize arytenoid dislocation as a unique entity.[16]

Neoplasms and thoracic diseases

Tumors and thoracic problems have also been implicated in the pathophysiology of UVFP, including lung cancer, thoracic aortic aneurysm, metastases, pulmonary/mediastinal tuberculosis, esophageal cancer,[11] patent ductus arteriosus,[12] and laryngeal chondrosarcoma.[17] Direct infiltration of the recurrent laryngeal nerve can also occur with thyroid carcinomas in addition to lung carcinomas as mentioned earlier.[18] UVFP has also been reported after iodine-131 treatment of thyrotoxicosis[19,20] or radiation of other types to the head and neck[21] or upper chest.[22,23] Tumors in the central nervous system can also cause UVFP, but typically have a constellation of associated symptoms.

Systemic

Systemic causes can be divided into a variety of categories. Infectious causes include West Nile,[24] varicella[25] and herpes,[26] Lyme,[27] and syphilis,[28] while inflammatory processes can include sarcoidosis,[29] lupus,[30] amyloidosis, polyarteritis nodosa, and silicosis. Neurologic diagnoses associated with vocal fold paralysis include myasthenia gravis,[31] severe degenerative spine disease,[32] multiple sclerosis,[33] amyotrophic lateral sclerosis,[34] Guillain-Barré (although typically bilateral),[35] Parkinson (also more commonly described as bilateral),[36] Charcot-Marie-Tooth, and familial hypokalemic periodic paralysis. Diabetes[37] or malnutrition, such as B12 deficiency,[38] can contribute, as can medications such as vinca alkaloids.[39] Idiopathic UVFP is a diagnosis of exclusion and, in those cases, the pathogenesis remains poorly understood.

Evolving Distribution of Causes (Levels 3–4)

Both in the United States and elsewhere, numerous studies have focused on the relative distribution of causes for UVFP. Neoplasm, trauma, and surgery were the most consistently cited causes in the 1970s, but the distribution has evolved over time.[40–42] In 1998, a retrospective review by Ramadan and colleagues[43] examined causes in 98 patients with UVFP; they were categorized as neoplastic in 32%, surgical in 30%, idiopathic in 16%, traumatic in 11%, central in 8%, and infectious in 3%. Several years later, a large comparative retrospective analysis spanning a 20-year period was presented by Rosenthal and colleagues,[44] comprising 827 patients who were seen with vocal fold immobility. In the first decade, spanning 1985 to 1995, the most common cause was malignancy (mostly lung). By contrast, in the second decade, 1996 to 2005, the most common cause was nonthyroid surgery (including anterior cervical spine, carotid). Consistent with these findings, a 1-year retrospective study published in 2006 reported a greater proportion of anterior cervical spine surgery than thyroid, thoracic, or cranial procedures among patients with iatrogenic vocal fold motion impairment.[6]

Thus, although the distribution of causes has evolved over time and may vary depending on geographic location,[45–47] commonly reported causes include neoplasms, particularly lung and thyroid neoplasms, and postsurgical causes (commonly spine surgery, carotid surgery, and thyroidectomy), with a persistent minority remaining idiopathic after thorough evaluation.

Natural History of Idiopathic UVFP (Level 4)

Observational studies have provided some insight into the natural history of UVFP. A retrospective review of 633 patients with vocal fold paralysis diagnosed between 1940 and 1949 included 181 of unknown cause. Of those, 31 had respiratory infection before onset of symptoms, and 29 had incidental findings such as goiter or pharyngoesophageal diverticulum, but most had no apparent predisposing factors. Long-term survival data suggested that patients with truly idiopathic UVFP seemed to have normal life spans, with 33% chance of vocal improvement over time.[48] More recently, Sulica[49] performed a review of the literature and identified 20 articles reporting 717 cases of idiopathic vocal fold paralysis. He reported that idiopathic vocal fold paralysis comprises 24% ± 10% of UVFP. When findings from all of the studies were summarized, complete recovery of motion was observed in 36% ± 22% and some recovery (complete and partial) in 39% ± 20%. Complete recovery of voice was reported in 52% ± 17%, and some recovery in 61% ± 22%. Most recovered in less than a year, but a small minority (5/717) described recovery after more than a year. As noted in the review, the variable recovery rates reported in different studies likely relates to heterogeneity of timeframe as well as criteria for defining recovery,[49] but most patients with idiopathic UVFP showed some vocal improvement, typically in less than a year.

Symptoms (Levels 3–4)

Although evaluation of UVFP is frequently focused on voice complaints (discussed later), dysphagia and other complaints appear fairly common. In a survey of 63 patients with UVFP secondary to a variety of causes, all patients with UVFP reported voice problems, 60% reported swallowing problems, and 75% reported subjective dyspnea.[50] In patients with dysphagia and UVFP who underwent flexible endoscopic evaluation of swallowing studies, liquid bolus retention and penetration were associated with aspiration in nearly half,[51] and the pharyngeal residues were noted at the base of tongue, valleculae, and piriform sinuses.[52] These findings may suggest that difficulty with swallowing in patients with UVFP is not solely explained by the vocal fold problem and may reflect associated problems, possibly secondary to the underlying cause of the UVFP.[52]

Quality of Life at Presentation (Levels 3–4)

It is intuitive that UVFP would have a considerable effect on quality of life given the findings described earlier, and validated scales have shown this impact. In a study at Vanderbilt University, patients with UVFP prospectively completed The Medical Outcomes Study Short Form 36-Item Health Survey (SF-36),[53] Voice Handicap Index (VHI),[54] and Voice Outcome Survey (VOS)[55] at presentation and at first postoperative visit after thyroplasty with or without arytenoid adduction. The SF-36 is a general health status measure, the VHI is a voice-specific handicap measure, and the VOS is a survey designed to assess vocal quality and life impact of voice-related problems specifically in patients with UVFP. At presentation, patients with UVFP scored significantly lower (worse) than normal on all domains of the SF-36 and on the VOS. After surgery, acoustic and aerodynamic measures of voice were improved. All domains of the SF-36 were observed to have a trend toward increased scores, with some domains showing a statistically significant increase. The VHI and its subscales, as well as the VOS, had significant improvement.[56] Several other measures of voice-related patient-reported quality of life have been used, including the Voice-Related Quality of Life (VRQOL)[57] and a variety of study-specific scales. These and other studies[58] underscore the significant impact of UVFP on both voice-related and overall health-related quality of life.

EVIDENCE-BASED CLINICAL ASSESSMENT
Examination for UVFP (Levels 3–5)

Examination of the patient who presents with suspected UVFP may include several components, including:

- Auditory-perceptual evaluation of voice
- Acoustic/aerodynamic measurements
- Intensity measures
- Laryngoscopy

Auditory-perceptual evaluation

Auditory-perceptual evaluation using the GRBAS (grade, roughness, breathiness, asthenia, strain) scale shows that patients with UVFP are rated significantly worse than normal.[59] More recently, the Consensus Auditory Perceptual Evaluation of Voice (CAPE-V) was developed for voice disorders in general. Little information is available in the literature about CAPE-V evaluation of UVFP, but work in postthyroidectomy patients at Walter Reed Hospital suggest that overall severity, habitual loudness, habitual pitch, and roughness are parameters that may be affected.[60] The challenges with auditory-perceptual evaluation of voice are well documented and include issues of interrater and intrarater reliability[61,62] as well as the impact of listener experience[63] and knowledge of the patient's history and/or diagnosis.[64] In addition, patients' perceptual self-ratings seemed to be distinct from those of trained listeners.[65] Patient ratings of the impact of vocal problems on quality of life do not correlate well with auditory-perceptual judgments.[66] Nonetheless, these judgments do allow raters to follow voice changes over time.

Acoustic and aerodynamic evaluation

Acoustic and aerodynamic evaluation in UVFP shows worse jitter, shimmer, noise/harmonic ratio, and maximum phonation time compared with normal voice.[59] As noted by Behrman,[67] acoustic and aerodynamic measures, although sometimes thought to be objective, are not truly so, because of the need for behavioral investment on the part of both patient and clinician to obtain representative phonatory samples and the challenge of performing some of these measurements when vocal fold vibration is irregular.[67] The relevance and validity of measures such as maximum phonation time and s/z ratio is also questioned because, in some cases, suboptimal techniques such as excessive supraglottic recruitment can lead to apparently improved maximum vocal performance measures. Nonetheless, these measures are frequently reported. Development of nonlinear, random time-series analysis may provide further information, but is in its early stages.[68] Another potentially promising technique is spectral moment analysis.[69] Reduction of cepstral peak prominence has been observed in patients with UVFP compared with controls, but it is unclear whether this is diagnostic.[70]

Intensity

Intensity has been used occasionally as a measure of vocal function, particularly habitual speaking intensity (loudness) and/or maximum physiologic dynamic range; these measures may be more closely related to the patient's assessment of vocal impact of vocal fold paralysis.[67]

Laryngoscopy

Laryngoscopy is an essential part of the evaluation of UVFP. The most common laryngoscopic findings beyond vocal fold motion impairment include bowing, incomplete glottal closure, and phase asymmetry on videostroboscopy.[59] The position of the vocal fold (eg, paramedian vs lateral) does not necessarily clarify the location of the lesion along the neurologic pathway from brain to motion of vocal fold.[71] However, the paralyzed side does tend to be shortened and arytenoid is commonly anteriorly rotated.[71] Passive gliding motion of arytenoid is seen in 91% patients with UVFP examined by three-dimensional (3D) computed tomography (CT), and caudal displacement in 100%.[72] Some have suggested that the position and shape of the false vocal fold may be informative, but this is controversial.[73] The specific value of stroboscopy compared with routine flexible fiberoptic laryngoscopy has also been debated, and its use is limited by challenges in capturing an adequate signal in profoundly dysphonic patients.[74]

Imaging for UVFP (Levels 3–5)

A variety of imaging techniques have been used in the work-up of patients with suspected UVFP. In a survey of members of the American Broncho-Esophagological Association, respondents indicated[75] that: Chest radiography (CXR) and/or neck/chest CT is always or often necessary (69%–72%). Magnetic resonance imaging (MRI) was thought to be always or often necessary by 39%, sometimes by 51%.

CXR and CT

An area of particular interest is the comparison of CXR versus neck/chest CT (typically with contrast) for evaluation of possible causes of UVFP given the considerable differences in cost and exposure to radiation. CXR can detect important diagnoses such as goiter and pulmonary fibrosis,[48] but may miss findings detected by CT,[76] particularly those in the left aortopulmonary window.[77] It has also been suggested that MRI is more sensitive, but carries a higher rate of false-positives.[78]

Because of the false-negative rate seen on CXR, several algorithms have been proposed for imaging used as part of the work-up of UVFP. Altman and Benninger[79] described starting with CXR and proceeding with CT or MRI if the CXR is negative. The CT is performed from skull base to thoracic inlet for right UVFP, and skull base to aortic triangle for left UVFP. In contrast, El Badawey and colleagues[45] described primary use of CT, without routine use of CXR.

Liu and colleagues[78] described stratification of patients with newly diagnosed UVFP using clinical findings (such as a history of malignancy) to divide into high-suspicion and low-suspicion groups. They then examined costs associated with imaging for each group. The high-suspicion group work-up (which included MR and/or CT) cost $2304 per true-positive, whereas the low-suspicion group cost $10,849 per true-positive case.[78] An implication of these findings is that imaging could be deferred for the low-suspicion group, but the associated risks and costs of delayed diagnosis need to be evaluated thoroughly before making such a recommendation.

Ultrasound

The use of ultrasound has attracted more attention in recent years[47]; neck ultrasonography identified subclinical tumors in 30% of 53 patients with UVFP, including papillary thyroid carcinoma and metastatic cervical lymph nodes from lung and other cancers.[80] Some describe using ultrasound if physical examination suggests low right recurrent laryngeal nerve impairment.[81]

Positron emission tomography

Although positron emission tomography (PET) scanning is not routinely used in the diagnosis of UVFP, it is important to be aware of the potential for misleading results on PET that are related to the presence of UVFP. Several studies have shown that, when UVFP is present, the contralateral normal side can have high fluorodeoxyglucose uptake thought to be secondary to attempted compensatory motion, potentially raising misleading concern for malignancy.[82,83] These findings have most commonly been described in patients with primary lung malignancies who had secondary unilateral recurrent laryngeal nerve paralysis. Other potentially misleading findings arise from the treatment of UVFP; granulomas that arise from the use of Teflon (polytetrafluoroethylene, DuPont, Wilmington, DE) for injection medialization can lead to false-positive findings on PET,[84] as can an elastomer suspension implant (trade name Vox, Uroplasty Inc., Minnetonka, MN).[85]

Summary of evidence on recommended imaging

The ideal algorithm for imaging in the work-up of UVFP remains controversial. Evidence in the literature is inadequate to make a blanket recommendation, but numerous studies have reported the use of imaging to identify significant abnormalities in patients who present with idiopathic vocal fold paralysis, and cross-sectional imaging is likely indicated. It can be difficult to directly synthesize across studies given different recruitment and/or inclusion criteria. Prospective controlled studies are necessary for further evaluation. Other factors to consider include cost and exposure to radiation.[86]

Serology in UVFP (Levels 3–5)

Use of serology in the evaluation of patients with UVFP has been described in a variety of studies. A survey of American Broncho-Esophagological Association members indicated that 54% of respondents indicated that serum tests could be considered as part of a work-up, but most (80%) of these indicated that the tests were appropriate only occasionally or rarely. The most commonly mentioned tests were rheumatoid factor (38%), Lyme titer (36%), erythrocyte sedimentation rate (34%), and antinuclear antibody (ANA) (33%).[75] Review of the literature at that time showed mostly case reports, with 1 case-control study on diabetes[37,75]; sarcoidosis and ANA were also frequently addressed but there remains no population-based information. There remains no definite evidence to support routine serology in patients with UVFP who do not have signs/symptoms of underlying disease, and practitioners are likely best served by ordering serology only if they have a clinical index of suspicion for particular associated diseases.

Laryngeal Electromyography (Levels 2–5)

The inclusion of laryngeal electromyography (LEMG) in the evaluation of patients with UVFP has garnered attention as a technique that could evaluate the current neurologic status of the affected vocal fold and perhaps provide prognostic information. Although the increasing popularity of injection medialization has perhaps tempered the impact of LEMG because immediate and temporary intervention is now available, interest in electromyography (EMG) continues. In a 2005 survey of members of the American Broncho-Esophagological Association, 75% of respondents used EMG to evaluate UVFP. These evaluations were typically performed in an unblinded fashion (85%); 66% of respondents thought that having clinical information was helpful. Congruent results were generally reported, with some variability.[87]

In 2009, the Neurolaryngology Study Group of the American Academy of Otolaryngology/Head and Neck Surgery convened a multidisciplinary panel to develop recommendations based on available evidence combined with expert opinion in areas in which evidence was not yet available. They summarized data that may suggest usefulness of EMG, but concluded that EMG was primarily a qualitative, not quantitative, examination. The study group advocated caution regarding the use of EMG data for early management of UVFP, and encouraged consideration of serial examinations. General recommendations included the need for prospective and blinded studies as well as standardized methods and interpretations.[88] A 2012 meta-analysis by Rickert and colleagues[89] examined the usefulness of LEMG for prognosis in vocal fold palsy using laryngoscopy as the gold standard; their analysis showed that, among patients with abnormal findings such as fibrillations, positive sharp waves, and absent or reduced voluntary motor unit potentials, 91% had no recovery of vocal fold mobility, although the length of follow-up was variable across the included studies.[89] Other proposed methods for LEMG interpretation include interference pattern analysis, which allows description of motor unit recruitment[90] in patients with UVFP, and the use of the ratio of mean peak-to-peak amplitude comparing motor unit amplitude on sniff versus sustained phonation for evaluation of synkinesis and associated poor prognosis for recovery.[91]

The current evidence indicates that LEMG with negative prognostic factors is likely to predict a poor functional outcome, but the optimal timing of LEMG in relation to symptom onset remains unclear. Prospective blinded studies are needed to confirm these and other potential ways to use LEMG in a quantitative, objective, and reproducible fashion.

EVIDENCE-BASED MEDICAL MANAGEMENT AND SURGICAL TECHNIQUE
Speech Pathology

Voice therapy (Level 4)
Several studies have described the use of voice therapy in the management of UVFP, although there is an opportunity in the literature for further examination of this issue. Although swallowing therapy is outside the scope of this article, techniques may include chin tuck, neck extension, head turn, supraglottic and supersupraglottic swallow, and/or dietary modification. Some patients also benefit from oral motor exercises, vocal adduction exercises, Valsalva swallow, and Mendelsohn maneuvers.[92]

Voice therapy in UVFP is typically directed at abdominal breathing and humming/resonant voice to improve closure of the glottis, encourage abdominal breath support, and improve vocal fold function while avoiding supraglottic hyperfunction.

Depending on the study, significant numbers of patients with UVFP who opted for voice therapy reported vocal improvement subjectively or as measured by glottal closure, acoustic measurements, pitch range, and/or patient-reported voice handicap.[93,94] Interpretation of the impact of voice therapy in UVFP may be obscured by returning neurologic function,[95] and it is unknown whether there is a relationship between voice therapy and neurologic recovery.

Other studies have also suggested the usefulness of voice therapy in the management of UVFP,[96,97] but there is often no comparison group, making it difficult to assess whether voice therapy affected the likelihood of these improvements. Randomized controlled studies may be difficult to perform in this area because patients who desire surgery may not be receptive to randomization into voice therapy, and vice versa, but controlled studies may be possible using alternate study designs. An additional challenge to studying this topic is the variability of therapy techniques across institutions or across individual therapists.

Surgical Techniques for UVFP

Medialization
One of the mainstays of surgical treatment of UVFP is the concept of medialization, in which the paralyzed vocal fold is displaced toward the midline to facilitate glottal closure. The ideal timing for medialization remains unclear. Some have postulated that the immobile cricoarytenoid joint may become fixed over time,[98] whereas other studies suggest that joint mobility may remain intact even many years after onset of paralysis.[99,100] Other studies examine voice and other functional outcomes after early medialization versus late medialization, and these are discussed later.

Injection medialization (levels 1–4) Injection medialization of the vocal fold was first performed in 1911 by Brunings via peroral injection using paraffin. This technique lost popularity until the development of other injectables that were thought to be less reactogenic. A recent retrospective review from multiple institutions summarized characteristics and complications of 460 injections for augmentation of the vocal folds of which 54% were performed for vocal fold paralysis. There was an even split between awake injections performed in clinic versus those performed under general anesthesia. Most awake injections (47%) were performed via transcricothyroid approach. Also frequent were: Perioral: 23% and Transthyrohyoid: 21%.

Reported technical success rates were 97% or greater and complication rates were 3% or less, with no difference between awake and asleep techniques. Use of injection augmentation in awake patients is increasing; over the 5-year period from 2003 to 2008, the rate increased from 11% to 43%.[101] The goal of injection medialization is to reposition the vocal fold medially, allowing contact between the affected side and the normal side (**Fig. 1**). Recent data suggest that injection medialization causes passive medial rotation and translation of the arytenoid cartilage.[102]

Injection medialization materials A variety of materials is now available for use in injection medialization. The literature was recently summarized by Paniello,[103] who examined findings from 42 articles describing up to 30 patients each with follow-up time up to 1 year, describing injection medialization and voice outcomes as reflected by a variety of measures.

- All studies showed vocal improvement after injection medialization.
- There were 2 level I studies, both by Hertegard and colleagues,[104,105] describing the use of hyaluronan versus collagen for injection; their findings suggested better vibratory function and less resorption of hyaluron over time.
- The remainder of the studies described injection with fat, collagen, acellular dermis, fascia, Teflon, silicone, and other materials.
- The largest proportion of articles described the use of fat injection.
- Most did not compare different types of injectables, and longer clinical follow-up was not available.[103]

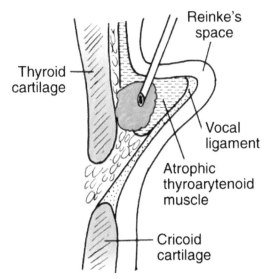

Fig. 1. A hemicoronal section through the larynx, showing the placement of an injectable material to medialize the affected vocal fold. (*From* Fakhry C, Flint PW, Cummings CW. Medialization thyroplasty. In: Cummings otolaryngology. 5th edition. Philadelphia: Mosby Elsevier; 2010; with permission.)

The multi-institutional retrospective review by Sulica and colleagues[101] gave a sense of current practice patterns:

Used most commonly for awake injections:
- Methylcellulose: 35%
- Bovine collagen: 28%
- Calcium hydroxylapatite: 26%

Used most commonly in the operating room:
- Calcium hydroxylapatite: 36%
- Methylcellulose: 35%

Though Teflon was previously popular because of its long duration and because it is easy to inject, Teflon injection is associated with giant cell granulomas that persist decades after injection[106] and are challenging to address surgically.[107] Some problems may have been related to technique,[108,109] and some investigators describe vocal rehabilitation with multiple surgical procedures, but the potential disadvantages render Teflon difficult to support except in rare cases, particularly when other alternatives exist.

Individual surgeon preferences for use of a given injectable may also depend on characteristics of each material, including duration, ease of use, cost, and rheologic properties. Several of the commonly used injectable materials are summarized in **Table 1**.

Although there is an estimated duration of effect quoted for each injectable, the literature reveals a wide range of reported durations. For example, several studies described an effect of greater than 1 year in patients with UVFP who underwent injections with micronized dermis.[115,116] The assessment of duration of effect for injection medialization may be complex because of the possibility of partial improvement in neurologic function, which may improve the tone of the paralyzed vocal fold without restoring motion.

Numerous injectables are in active use, which suggests that no single injectable is definitively superior to the others, and nuanced decision making with respect to selection of injectable may be appropriate. Further investigation, perhaps with more randomized head-to-head comparisons, may clarify the potential usefulness of different substances.

Complications of injection medialization As described earlier, complications are rare. Reported risks include prolonged stridor, need for intubation, and postinjection dysphonia[121] secondary to subepithelial injection and/or overinjection.[101] Particular caution is important to avoid superficial injection, because injectate can persist for years.[122] Rare risks include intralaryngeal migration of injectate[123] and abscess at the site of injection.[124]

Timing of injection medialization Timing of injection medialization may affect long-term outcomes. In all comers, overall need for permanent medialization (eg, medialization thyroplasty) is approximately 20% to 30% after injection.[116,125] Early medialization (1–4 days) after the onset of UVFP after thoracic surgery has been associated with significantly fewer cases of pneumonia and a shorter length of stay compared with late medialization (greater than 5 days after onset).[126] There are now data to suggest that early injection medialization may be associated with a lower rate of eventual need for permanent medialization thyroplasty.[127,128] Taken together, these data suggest that early injection medialization may be helpful, and that early

Table 1
Examples of vocal fold injection materials

Material	Sample Trade Names	Length of Effect	Amount Injected	Needle Gauge	FDA Approval	Comments	Estimated Cost
Autologous fascia	NA	? months to year	Overinject	18–22	NA	Requires harvest	NA
Autologous fat	NA	? y; variable	Overinject	18–22	NA	Requires harvest	NA
Cadaveric micronized dermis	Cymetra (LifeCell, Branchburg, NJ)	2–4 mo; some >1 y	Overinject	18–25	Yes	Requires preparation	$400
Calcium hydroxylapatite	Radiesse Voice (Merz Aesthetics, San Mateo, CA)	>1 y	Slightly overinject	25	Yes	Place lateral to ligament; poor rheologic properties	$260
Carboxymethylcellulose	Radiesse Voice Gel (Merz Aesthetics)	2–3 mo	Slightly overinject	27	Yes	—	$220
Hyaluronic acid gels	Restylane, Perlane (Medicis Aesthetics, Scottsdale, AZ)	6–9 mo	Slightly overinject	27	No	Good compliance, rheologic properties	?230
Porcine gelatin	Gelfoam (Pfizer, New York, NY)	4–8 wk	Overinject	18	No	Requires preparation	?$60

Several collagen preparations, including Zyplast, Cosmoplast, and Cosmoderm, and the hyaluronic acid preparations Hylaform and Hylaform Plus (Allergan, Irvine CA), have been discontinued in recent years. Information presented in this table was acquired from multiple sources, including relevant articles in the literature[110–120] and vendor/manufacturer information. FDA, US Food and Drug Administration; NA, not applicable. "?" indicates that the effect/cost shown is speculative.

positioning of the vocal fold may affect long-term outcomes, but further studies are necessary to develop refined recommendations for patients with newly diagnosed UVFP.

Medialization thyroplasty (levels 2–4) A more long-lasting approach to medialization of the paralyzed true vocal fold was originally described by Payr[129] in 1915, who used a cartilage flap pressed inward from a thyroid cartilage window to reposition the paralyzed vocal fold. This technique was later modified by Isshiki,[130,131] who described use of mobilized thyroid cartilage inserted through the window, and further adapted it with the use of alloplastic material. As with injection medialization, early medialization thyroplasty has been associated with fewer diagnoses of pneumonia and shorter lengths of stay after thoracic surgeries, as mentioned earlier.[126] The procedure has commonly necessitated overnight observation, but some have moved toward risk stratification,[132] suggesting that, in patients with low risk factors for complications, day surgery could be considered.[133]

Thyroplasty materials As with injection medialization, a variety of implant types is available, although the current literature most commonly presents data for patients undergoing medialization with a carved Silastic (polymeric silicone, Dow Corning, Midland, MI) implant (**Fig. 2**). In a 2008 comprehensive evidence-based review by Paniello, 52 articles describing the impact of open implant medialization on subjective and objective voice outcomes were summarized:

- There was no level 1 evidence.
- There was some level 2 evidence for Silastic, Montgomery (Boston Medical Products, Westborough, MA), GORE-TEX (W.L. Gore and Associates, Elkton, MD), and other types of implants.
- Most reported improvement in voice outcomes using auditory-perceptual and aerodynamic/acoustic measures.[103]

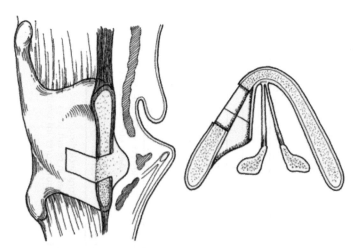

Fig. 2. A polymer implant used in a medialization thyroplasty to permanently medially displace the vocal fold. This procedure allows adjustment of the position of the vocal fold in 3 dimensions. On the left is an oblique coronal view, on the right is an axial view. (*From* Fried MP, editor. The larynx. 2nd edition. St Louis (MO): Elsevier; 1996. p. 213; with permission.)

More recently, some direct comparisons between titanium implants and other materials have been published, with some suggestion that titanium may be superior[134,135] for restoration of voice quality, but additional work is necessary before a definitive conclusion is possible.

Thyroplasty procedure Although the details of the procedure may be surgeon specific, intraoperative measurement of maximum phonation time may be useful in predicting postoperative outcomes. Although the maximum phonation time is typically lower when supine, and may be lower under sedation, the relative improvement in maximum phonation time at the time of medialization is thought to be informative.[136]

Adjunct procedures at the time of medialization thyroplasty may include arytenoid adduction,[137] arytenopexy,[138] or even cricothyroid approximation.[139] Arytenoid adduction does not necessarily change the laryngoscopic appearance in a predictable way.[140] Some data suggest that arytenopexy may also lead to improved phonatory results[141]; a cadaver study suggests improved harmonic profile with arytenopexy compared with arytenoid adduction.[142] To our knowledge, there are no studies that directly compare results of the 2 techniques in vivo.

Thyroplasty complications For medialization thyroplasty, there is an 8% estimated rate of complications requiring medical or surgical intervention,[143] including:

- Edema
- Wound complications
- Extrusion
- Need for tracheotomy

Higher complication risks have been observed in patients on anticoagulation, with atrophic/absent tissue, and/or undergoing revision surgery.[133]

Rare reported complications include creation of a window in cricoid cartilage, leading to airway obstruction when the implant was placed,[144] as well as implant extrusion in 2.1% and implant malpositioning in 1.3%.[103]

Common indications for revision surgery include:[145]

- Arytenoid rotation with persistent posterior glottic gap
- Implant malposition
- Implant extrusion

Airway complications are more commonly reported after arytenoid adduction than after medialization laryngoplasty.[146] Although medialization is often described as reversible because the implant may be removed, placement of the implant has been associated with permanent changes in joint mobility and/or fibrosis in an experimental animal model.[147]

Thyroplasty outcomes Medialization thyroplasty has a very good overall and long-term effect. Although some have raised the question of late-onset vocal fold atrophy and whether that renders implant medialization less effective over time,[145] most investigators show excellent persistence of vocal improvement at 3 months after surgery, with stable or greater improvement at the 1-year time point.[148–152] Longer-term data are scant, but Leder and Sasaki[149] showed long-term improvement in maximum phonation time and other characteristics that persisted more than 3 years after medialization thyroplasty. Despite possible variability in the first several months after medialization, the overall vocal improvement seems robust and long lasting.

Although medialization thyroplasty is effective, there may be room for improvement. Gray and colleagues[153] assessed vocal function in 15 patients 1 year after type I thyroplasty with cartilage, Silastic, or GORE-TEX, and variable causes of vocal fold paralysis:

- Some voice characteristics (pitch, intonation, loudness) were not statistically different from normal.
- Other voice characteristics (strain, breathiness, hoarseness, harshness, unsteadiness) were different.
- When patients were surveyed:
  - 92% reported that surgery helped with their voices
  - 73% were generally or extremely satisfied
  - 87% thought that their voices were still abnormal
  - 25% had adjusted their employment to accommodate their voices

This information is important to keep in mind when counseling patients regarding postoperative expectations.

Comparing injection medialization versus medialization thyroplasty: level 3
Voice Several studies have compared results of injection medialization and medialization thyroplasty. Many have not showed a meaningful difference between the 2 techniques,[154–156] but several reported a trend toward greater improvement after medialization thyroplasty in the long term.[157–159] As noted by Paniello in systematic review of a subset of these articles, a challenge to the interpretation of these data is the variable length of follow-up time and small sample sizes. Studies with longer follow-up time tended to favor results of medialization thyroplasty.[103] Different injection materials across studies and, in some cases, incomplete data render overall comparisons difficult to make. In addition, randomization to injection medialization versus medialization thyroplasty may not be acceptable to patients. The available data suggest that, in the short term, injection medialization and medialization thyroplasty are likely comparable with respect to voice outcomes but that, in the long term, medialization thyroplasty may provide better voice results. More investigation is needed to clarify and compare long-term outcomes.

Swallowing Few studies have compared the impact of injection medialization to that of medialization thyroplasty on swallowing, but no significant difference has been detected in the improvement of swallowing between patients who underwent injection medialization versus those who underwent medialization thyroplasty.[160,161]

Medialization thyroplasty versus medialization thyroplasty with arytenoid adduction (levels 3–4)
Another debated topic is the consideration of arytenoid adduction when medialization thyroplasty is performed. In excised canine larynges, studies suggested differences between injection, thyroplasty, and thyroplasty with arytenoid adduction; injection reduced mucosal wave amplitude, but medialization thyroplasty with or without arytenoid adduction increased amplitude. Overall, medialization with arytenoid adduction resulted in the greatest improvement in phonatory measurements including phonation threshold flow, phonation threshold power, and signal/noise ratio.[162]

A small number of studies have undertaken this comparison in patients, with some showing no difference between the 2 groups[143] and others showing greater improvement or a trend in that direction after medialization thyroplasty with arytenoid adduction.[143,163–165] Formal summary evaluation of these studies is difficult because of heterogeneous patient groups, implant types, and measurement of preoperative and postoperative outcomes. There is little evidence on whether these techniques have a differential impact on swallowing.

Laryngeal reinnervation (levels 1–4) Another approach to the management of UVFP has been laryngeal reinnervation, which takes advantage of the presence of other functioning nerves in the anatomic vicinity to improve tone and/or mobility of the paralyzed side.[166] Options for laryngeal reinnervation include ansa,[98] phrenic,[98] hypoglossal,[167] and nerve-muscle pedicles (**Fig. 3**).[168–170] Approaches have included selective innervation of different muscles in the same setting (eg, adductor and abductor)[98] or targeted reinnervation of a selected muscle (eg, lateral cricoarytenoid or thyroarytenoid).[170] Some studies have described the use of various laryngeal reinnervation techniques in combination with arytenoid adduction.[171–173]

In a systematic review of the literature, Paniello identified 11 studies, levels 3 to 4, with either a trend toward or statistically significant improvement of voice parameters as assessed by auditory-perceptual evaluation, acoustic/aerodynamic measures, and/or laryngoscopy or stroboscopy. The complication rate was low, with 1 delayed tracheostomy tube placement reported (2%).[103] As he noted, there is great clinical variability

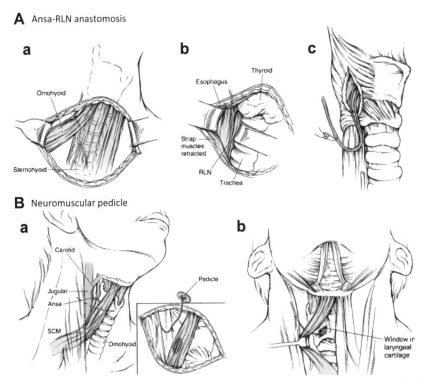

Fig. 3. Reinnervation techniques. Different methods for laryngeal reinnervation, including (*A*) direct ansa–recurrent laryngeal nerve (RLN) anastomoses: (*Aa*) identification of ansa cervicalis branch to sternohyoid muscle, (*Ab*) identification of recurrent laryngeal nerve, (*Ac*) anastomosis of the 2 nerves, and (*B*) use of neuromuscular pedicle: (*Ba*) neuromuscular pedicle harvest using ansa cervicalis branch to omohyoid muscle, (*Bb*) neuromuscular pedicle placement into lateral cricoarytenoid muscle via laryngeal cartilage window. SCM, sternocleidomastoid muscle. (*From* Cummings otolaryngology. 5th edition. Mosby: Elsevier. Fig. 68-2 and 68-1; with permission.)

in the evidence currently in the literature; depending on the study, there are different reinnervation techniques, possible concomitant procedures, different timing of reinnervation, patient ages, and length of follow-up.[103] A varying degree of synkinesis from misdirected reinnervation of laryngeal abductors and/or adductors can also complicate the picture,[91,174–176] as can the use of voice therapy.

Medialization thyroplasty versus laryngeal reinnervation (levels 1–3)

Tucker[177] compared nerve-muscle pedicle with medialization thyroplasty versus medialization thyroplasty alone; expert listeners rated voice outcomes better after combined reinnervation and medialization thyroplasty. This study was not randomized, but helped to lay the groundwork for a major trial.

Paniello and colleagues[178] performed a multicenter randomized clinical trial comparing medialization thyroplasty versus reinnervation using the ansa cervicalis nerve. The trial included 24 patients, 12 in each arm. Preoperative and postoperative voice was evaluated using perceptual rating by untrained listeners, blinded speech pathologists' GRBAS ratings, the VRQOL scale, and, secondarily, maximum phonation time, cepstral analysis, and EMG. At 12 months after surgery:

- Both groups had significant improvement in perceptual ratings, GRBAS, and VRQOL, and no significant difference between the groups; however, more detailed analysis revealed that patient age seemed to be an important variable.
- Patients less than 52 years old who underwent reinnervation had better postoperative auditory-perceptual ratings than those in the same age group who underwent medialization.
- Patients less than 52 years old who underwent reinnervation had better voice results than those more than 52 years old who underwent reinnervation.
- Among those more than 52 years old, voice results were better after medialization thyroplasty than after reinnervation.
- As in prior studies of surgical intervention for UVFP, most of the voice results did not reach normal as measured by GRBAS and VRQOL. However, cepstral analysis showed better voicing in the reinnervated group, and reinnervated patients less than 52 years old approached normal values.
- At the conclusion of study, several additional surgeries were planned for study patients, including injection augmentation in 2 of the medialization patients and thyroplasties in 2 of the reinnervated patients, suggesting that some patients may benefit from multiple procedures.

In addition to a new nuanced picture of tailored surgical approaches for patients of different ages who present with UVFP, this trial provided some valuable insights into the challenges of performing this type of study. The investigators described difficulty with both accrual and randomization, noting that both patients and surgeons had difficulty accepting randomization. Nonetheless, it stands as an inspiring example of a well-conducted study that addressed a focused and meaningful clinical question.

WHAT DOES THE EVIDENCE TELL US?

- Presentation (evidence grade C). A wide variety of causes can lead to UVFP; the distribution of these causes has evolved over time. Post-surgical, idiopathic, and neoplasm-related UVFP remain common.
- Evaluation (evidence grade C). In the work-up of UVFP, imaging may be reasonable (CXR is not sufficient, CT is more informative, ultrasound may be useful), but the routine use of serology is not well supported. LEMG with fibrillations, positive

sharp waves, and/or absent or reduced voluntary motor unit potentials predicts a lack of functionally meaningful recovery, but the ideal timing of LEMG after symptom onset remains to be defined.

- Management (evidence grade B). Data on voice therapy suggest a positive impact, but further studies are needed. Injection medialization is widely used, and a variety of injectables may be considered. Current evidence suggests that initial voice outcomes after injection medialization are similar to those after medialization thyroplasty, but long-term results may favor the latter. Laryngeal reinnervation has been shown to have comparable vocal impact with that of medialization thyroplasty, and surgical decision making should take patient age into account. Some patients may benefit from multiple procedures.
- There is a need for ongoing systematic reviews of the literature and more randomized controlled trials.

Critical Points

- UVFP has a broad range of causes, including postsurgical, idiopathic, and neoplasm-related causes (evidence grade C).
- Work-up should include cross-sectional imaging, but not serology. EMG is useful for predicting poor prognosis (evidence grade C).
- Voice therapy can be beneficial, but is not sufficient for many patients with UVFP. In the short term, injection medialization can achieve comparable clinical results with medialization thyroplasty. Thyroplasty and reinnervation also achieve comparable voice outcomes (evidence grade B).

REFERENCES

1. Bhattacharyya N, Fried MP. Assessment of the morbidity and complications of total thyroidectomy. Arch Otolaryngol Head Neck Surg 2002;128(4):389–92.
2. Jeannon JP, Orabi AA, Bruch GA, et al. Diagnosis of recurrent laryngeal nerve palsy after thyroidectomy: a systematic review. Int J Clin Pract 2009;63(4):624–9.
3. Lee KE, Koo do H, Kim SJ, et al. Outcomes of 109 patients with papillary thyroid carcinoma who underwent robotic total thyroidectomy with central node dissection via the bilateral axillo-breast approach. Surgery 2010;148(6):1207–13.
4. Netterville JL, Koriwchak MJ, Winkle M, et al. Vocal fold paralysis following the anterior approach to the cervical spine. Ann Otol Rhinol Laryngol 1996;105(2):85–91.
5. Heeneman H. Vocal cord paralysis following approaches to the anterior cervical spine. Laryngoscope 1973;83(1):17–21.
6. Merati AL, Shemirani N, Smith TL, et al. Changing trends in the nature of vocal fold motion impairment. Am J Otolaryngol 2006;27(2):106–8.
7. Kriskovich MD, Apfelbaum RI, Haller JR. Vocal fold paralysis after anterior cervical spine surgery: incidence, mechanism, and prevention of injury. Laryngoscope 2000;110(9):1467–73.
8. Itagaki T, Kikura M, Sato S. Incidence and risk factors of postoperative vocal cord paralysis in 987 patients after cardiovascular surgery. Ann Thorac Surg 2007;83(6):2147–52.
9. Widstrom A. Palsy of the recurrent nerve following mediastinoscopy. Chest 1975;67(3):365–6.
10. Roberts JR, Wadsworth J. Recurrent laryngeal nerve monitoring during mediastinoscopy: predictors of injury. Ann Thorac Surg 2007;83(2):388–91 [discussion: 391–2].

11. Bando H, Nishio T, Bamba H, et al. Vocal fold paralysis as a sign of chest diseases: a 15-year retrospective study. World J Surg 2006;30(3):293–8.

12. Hardy JD, Webb WR, Timmis H, et al. Patent ductus arteriosus: operative treatment of 100 consecutive patients with isolated lesions without mortality. Ann Surg 1966;164(5):877–82.

13. Kikura M, Suzuki K, Itagaki T, et al. Age and comorbidity as risk factors for vocal cord paralysis associated with tracheal intubation. Br J Anaesth 2007;98(4): 524–30.

14. Lowinger D, Benjamin B, Gadd L. Recurrent laryngeal nerve injury caused by a laryngeal mask airway. Anaesth Intensive Care 1999;27(2):202–5.

15. Fang TJ, Tam YY, Courey MS, et al. Unilateral high vagal paralysis: relationship of the severity of swallowing disturbance and types of injuries. Laryngoscope 2011;121(2):245–9.

16. Norris BK, Schweinfurth JM. Arytenoid dislocation: an analysis of the contemporary literature. Laryngoscope 2011;121(1):142–6.

17. Leonetti JP, Collins SL, Jablokow V, et al. Laryngeal chondrosarcoma as a late-appearing cause of "idiopathic" vocal cord paralysis. Otolaryngol Head Neck Surg 1987;97(4):391–5.

18. McCaffrey TV, Lipton RJ. Thyroid carcinoma invading the upper aerodigestive system. Laryngoscope 1990;100(8):824–30.

19. Coover LR. Permanent iatrogenic vocal cord paralysis after I-131 therapy: a case report and literature review. Clin Nucl Med 2000;25(7):508–10.

20. Snyder S. Vocal cord paralysis after radioiodine therapy. J Nucl Med 1978;19(8): 975–6.

21. Stern Y, Marshak G, Shpitzer T, et al. Vocal cord palsy: possible late complication of radiotherapy for head and neck cancer. Ann Otol Rhinol Laryngol 1995; 104(4 Pt 1):294–6.

22. Lau DP, Lo YL, Wee J, et al. Vocal fold paralysis following radiotherapy for nasopharyngeal carcinoma: laryngeal electromyography findings. J Voice 2003;17(1):82–7.

23. Westbrook KC, Ballantyne AJ, Eckles NE, et al. Breast cancer and vocal cord paralysis. South Med J 1974;67(7):805–7.

24. Steele NP, Myssiorek D. West Nile virus induced vocal fold paralysis. Laryngoscope 2006;116(3):494–6.

25. Chitose SI, Umeno H, Hamakawa S, et al. Unilateral associated laryngeal paralysis due to varicella-zoster virus: virus antibody testing and videofluoroscopic findings. J Laryngol Otol 2008;122(2):170–6.

26. Magnussen CR, Patanella HP. Herpes simplex virus and recurrent laryngeal nerve paralysis. Report of a case and review of the literature. Arch Intern Med 1979;139(12):1423–4.

27. Schroeter V, Belz GG, Blenk H. Paralysis of recurrent laryngeal nerve in Lyme disease. Lancet 1988;2(8622):1245.

28. Rabkin R. Paralysis of the larynx due to central nervous system syphilis. Eye Ear Nose Throat Mon 1963;42:53.

29. Chijimatsu Y, Tajima J, Washizaki M, et al. Hoarseness as an initial manifestation of sarcoidosis. Chest 1980;78(5):779–81.

30. Kraus A, Guerra-Bautista G. Laryngeal involvement as a presenting symptom of systemic lupus erythematosus. Ann Rheum Dis 1990;49(6):421.

31. Carpenter RJ 3rd, McDonald TJ, Howard FM Jr. The otolaryngologic presentation of myasthenia gravis. Laryngoscope 1979;89(6 Pt 1):922–8.

32. Yoskovitch A, Kantor S. Cervical osteophytes presenting as unilateral vocal fold paralysis and dysphagia. J Laryngol Otol 2001;115(5):422–4.

33. Rontal E, Rontal M, Wald J, et al. Botulinum toxin injection in the treatment of vocal fold paralysis associated with multiple sclerosis: a case report. J Voice 1999;13(2):274–9.
34. Polkey MI, Lyall RA, Green M, et al. Expiratory muscle function in amyotrophic lateral sclerosis. Am J Respir Crit Care Med 1998;158(3):734–41.
35. Holinger LD, Holinger PC, Holinger PH. Etiology of bilateral abductor vocal cord paralysis: a review of 389 cases. Ann Otol Rhinol Laryngol 1976;85(4 Pt 1): 428–36.
36. Plasse HM, Lieberman AN. Bilateral vocal cord paralysis in Parkinson's disease. Arch Otolaryngol 1981;107(4):252–3.
37. Schechter GL, Kostianovsky M. Vocal cord paralysis in diabetes mellitus. Trans Am Acad Ophthalmol Otolaryngol 1972;76(3):729–40.
38. Ahn TB, Cho JW, Jeon BS. Unusual neurological presentations of vitamin B(12) deficiency. Eur J Neurol 2004;11(5):339–41.
39. Burns BV, Shotton JC. Vocal fold palsy following vinca alkaloid treatment. J Laryngol Otol 1998;112(5):485–7.
40. Titche LL. Causes of recurrent laryngeal nerve paralysis. Arch Otolaryngol 1976; 102(5):259–61.
41. Parnell FW, Brandenburg JH. Vocal cord paralysis. A review of 100 cases. Laryngoscope 1970;80(7):1036–45.
42. Maisel RH, Ogura JH. Evaluation and treatment of vocal cord paralysis. Laryngoscope 1974;84(2):302–16.
43. Ramadan HH, Wax MK, Avery S. Outcome and changing cause of unilateral vocal cord paralysis. Otolaryngol Head Neck Surg 1998;118(2):199–202.
44. Rosenthal LH, Benninger MS, Deeb RH. Vocal fold immobility: a longitudinal analysis of etiology over 20 years. Laryngoscope 2007;117(10):1864–70.
45. El Badawey MR, Punekar S, Zammit-Maempel I. Prospective study to assess vocal cord palsy investigations. Otolaryngol Head Neck Surg 2008;138(6): 788–90.
46. Chen HC, Jen YM, Wang CH, et al. Etiology of vocal cord paralysis. ORL J Otorhinolaryngol Relat Spec 2007;69(3):167–71.
47. Furukawa M, Furukawa MK, Ooishi K. Statistical analysis of malignant tumors detected as the cause of vocal cord paralysis. ORL J Otorhinolaryngol Relat Spec 1994;56(3):161–5.
48. Huppler EG, Schmidt HW, Devine KD, et al. Ultimate outcome of patients with vocal-cord paralysis of undetermined cause. Am Rev Tuberc 1956;73(1): 52–60.
49. Sulica L. The natural history of idiopathic unilateral vocal fold paralysis: evidence and problems. Laryngoscope 2008;118(7):1303–7.
50. Brunner E, Friedrich G, Kiesler K, et al. Subjective breathing impairment in unilateral vocal fold paralysis. Folia Phoniatr Logop 2011;63:142–6.
51. Leder SB, Ross DA. Incidence of vocal fold immobility in patients with dysphagia. Dysphagia 2005;20(2):163–7 [discussion: 168–9].
52. Bhattacharyya N, Kotz T, Shapiro J. The effect of bolus consistency on dysphagia in unilateral vocal cord paralysis. Otolaryngol Head Neck Surg 2003;129(6):632–6.
53. McHorney CA, Ware JE Jr, Raczek AE. The MOS 36-Item Short-Form Health Survey (SF-36): II. Psychometric and clinical tests of validity in measuring physical and mental health constructs. Med Care 1993;31(3):247–63.
54. Jacobson BH, Johnson A, Grywalski C, et al. The Voice Handicap Index (VHI): development and validation. Am J Speech Lang Pathol 1997;6(3):66–70.

55. Gliklich RE, Glovsky RM, Montgomery WW. Validation of a voice outcome survey for unilateral vocal cord paralysis. Otolaryngol Head Neck Surg 1999;120(2): 153–8.

56. Spector BC, Netterville JL, Billante C, et al. Quality-of-life assessment in patients with unilateral vocal cord paralysis. Otolaryngol Head Neck Surg 2001;125(3): 176–82.

57. Hogikyan ND, Wodchis WP, Terrell JE, et al. Voice-related quality of life (V-RQOL) following type I thyroplasty for unilateral vocal fold paralysis. J Voice 2000;14(3):378–86.

58. Billante CR, Spector B, Hudson M, et al. Voice outcome following thyroplasty in patients with cancer-related vocal fold paralysis. Auris Nasus Larynx 2001; 28(4):315–21.

59. Wang W, Chen D, Chen S, et al. Laryngeal reinnervation using ansa cervicalis for thyroid surgery-related unilateral vocal fold paralysis: a long-term outcome analysis of 237 cases. PLoS One 2011;6(4):e19128.

60. Stojadinovic A, Henry LR, Howard RS, et al. Prospective trial of voice outcomes after thyroidectomy: evaluation of patient-reported and clinician-determined voice assessments in identifying postthyroidectomy dysphonia. Surgery 2008; 143(6):732–42.

61. Kreiman J, Gerratt BR, Ito M. When and why listeners disagree in voice quality assessment tasks. J Acoust Soc Am 2007;122(4):2354–64.

62. Kreiman J, Gerratt BR. Sources of listener disagreement in voice quality assessment. J Acoust Soc Am 2000;108(4):1867–76.

63. Kreiman J, Gerratt BR, Precoda K. Listener experience and perception of voice quality. J Speech Hear Res 1990;33(1):103–15.

64. Eadie T, Sroka A, Wright DR, et al. Does knowledge of medical diagnosis bias auditory-perceptual judgments of dysphonia? J Voice 2011;25(4):420–9.

65. Eadie TL, Kapsner M, Rosenzweig J, et al. The role of experience on judgments of dysphonia. J Voice 2010;24(5):564–73.

66. Karnell MP, Melton SD, Childes JM, et al. Reliability of clinician-based (GRBAS and CAPE-V) and patient-based (V-RQOL and IPVI) documentation of voice disorders. J Voice 2007;21(5):576–90.

67. Behrman A. Evidence-based treatment of paralytic dysphonia: making sense of outcomes and efficacy data. Otolaryngol Clin North Am 2004;37(1):75–104, vi.

68. Little MA, Costello DA, Harries ML. Objective dysphonia quantification in vocal fold paralysis: comparing nonlinear with classical measures. J Voice 2011;25(1): 21–31.

69. Colton RH, Paseman A, Kelley RT, et al. Spectral moment analysis of unilateral vocal fold paralysis. J Voice 2011;25(3):330–6.

70. Balasubramanium RK, Bhat JS, Fahim S 3rd, et al. Cepstral analysis of voice in unilateral adductor vocal fold palsy. J Voice 2011;25(3):326–9.

71. Woodson GE. Configuration of the glottis in laryngeal paralysis. I: Clinical study. Laryngoscope 1993;103(11 Pt 1):1227–34.

72. Hiramatsu H, Tokashiki R, Nakamura M, et al. Characterization of arytenoid vertical displacement in unilateral vocal fold paralysis by three-dimensional computed tomography. Eur Arch Otorhinolaryngol 2009;266(1):97–104.

73. Steffen N, Vieira VP, Yazaki RK, et al. Modifications of vestibular fold shape from respiration to phonation in unilateral vocal fold paralysis. J Voice 2011;25(1): 111–3.

74. Harries ML, Morrison M. The role of stroboscopy in the management of a patient with a unilateral vocal fold paralysis. J Laryngol Otol 1996;110(2):141–3.

75. Merati AL, Halum SL, Smith TL. Diagnostic testing for vocal fold paralysis: survey of practice and evidence-based medicine review. Laryngoscope 2006; 116(9):1539–52.
76. Song SW, Jun BC, Cho KJ, et al. CT evaluation of vocal cord paralysis due to thoracic diseases: a 10-year retrospective study. Yonsei Med J 2011;52(5):831–7.
77. Glazer HS, Aronberg DJ, Lee JK, et al. Extralaryngeal causes of vocal cord paralysis: CT evaluation. AJR Am J Roentgenol 1983;141(3):527–31.
78. Liu AY, Yousem DM, Chalian AA, et al. Economic consequences of diagnostic imaging for vocal cord paralysis. Acad Radiol 2001;8(2):137–48.
79. Altman JS, Benninger MS. The evaluation of unilateral vocal fold immobility: is chest X-ray enough? J Voice 1997;11(3):364–7.
80. Wang CP, Chen TC, Lou PJ, et al. Neck ultrasonography for the evaluation of the etiology of adult unilateral vocal fold paralysis. Head Neck 2012;34(5):643–8.
81. Robinson S, Pitkaranta A. Radiology findings in adult patients with vocal fold paralysis. Clinical Radiology 2006;61(10):863–7.
82. Heller MT, Meltzer CC, Fukui MB, et al. Superphysiologic FDG uptake in the non-paralyzed vocal cord. Resolution of a false-positive PET result with combined PET-CT imaging. Clin Positron Imaging 2000;3(5):207–11.
83. Kamel EM, Goerres GW, Burger C, et al. Recurrent laryngeal nerve palsy in patients with lung cancer: detection with PET-CT image fusion – report of six cases. Radiology 2002;224(1):153–6.
84. Yeretsian RA, Blodgett TM, Branstetter BF 4th, et al. Teflon-induced granuloma: a false-positive finding with PET resolved with combined PET and CT. AJNR Am J Neuroradiol 2003;24(6):1164–6.
85. Tessonnier L, Fakhry N, Taieb D, et al. False-positive finding on FDG-PET/CT after injectable elastomere implant (Vox implant) for vocal cord paralysis. Otolaryngol Head Neck Surg 2008;139(5):738–9.
86. Hall EJ, Brenner DJ. Cancer risks from diagnostic radiology. Br J Radiol 2008; 81(965):362–78.
87. Halum SL, Patel N, Smith TL, et al. Laryngeal electromyography for adult unilateral vocal fold immobility: a survey of the American Broncho-Esophagological Association. Ann Otol Rhinol Laryngol 2005;114(6):425–8.
88. Blitzer A, Crumley RL, Dailey SH, et al. Recommendations of the Neurolaryngology Study Group on laryngeal electromyography. Otolaryngol Head Neck Surg 2009;140(6):782–93.
89. Rickert SM, Childs LF, Carey BT, et al. Laryngeal electromyography for prognosis of vocal fold palsy: a meta-analysis. Laryngoscope 2012;122(1):158–61.
90. Statham MM, Rosen CA, Nandedkar SD, et al. Quantitative laryngeal electromyography: turns and amplitude analysis. Laryngoscope 2010;120(10):2036–41.
91. Statham MM, Rosen CA, Smith LJ, et al. Electromyographic laryngeal synkinesis alters prognosis in vocal fold paralysis. Laryngoscope 2010;120(2):285–90.
92. Peterson KL, Fenn J. Treatment of dysphagia and dysphonia following skull base surgery. Otolaryngol Clin North Am 2005;38(4):809–17, xi.
93. D'Alatri L, Galla S, Rigante M, et al. Role of early voice therapy in patients affected by unilateral vocal fold paralysis. J Laryngol Otol 2008;122(9):936–41.
94. Heuer RJ, Thayer Sataloff R, Emerich K, et al. Unilateral recurrent laryngeal nerve paralysis: the importance of "preoperative" voice therapy. J Voice 1997; 11(1):88–94.
95. Mattioli F, Bergamini G, Alicandri-Ciufelli M, et al. The role of early voice therapy in the incidence of motility recovery in unilateral vocal fold paralysis. Logoped Phoniatr Vocol 2011;36(1):40–7.

96. Kelchner LN, Stemple JC, Gerdeman E, et al. Etiology, pathophysiology, treatment choices, and voice results for unilateral adductor vocal fold paralysis: a 3-year retrospective. J Voice 1999;13(4):592–601.
97. Schindler A, Bottero A, Capaccio P, et al. Vocal improvement after voice therapy in unilateral vocal fold paralysis. J Voice 2008;22(1):113–8.
98. Crumley RL. Selective reinnervation of vocal cord adductors in unilateral vocal cord paralysis. Ann Otol Rhinol Laryngol 1984;93(4 Pt 1):351–6.
99. Gacek M, Gacek RR. Cricoarytenoid joint mobility after chronic vocal cord paralysis. Laryngoscope 1996;106(12 Pt 1):1528–30.
100. Colman MF, Schwartz I. The effect of vocal cord paralysis on the cricoarytenoid joint. Otolaryngol Head Neck Surg 1981;89(3 Pt 1):419–22.
101. Sulica L, Rosen CA, Postma GN, et al. Current practice in injection augmentation of the vocal folds: indications, treatment principles, techniques, and complications. Laryngoscope 2010;120(2):319–25.
102. Mau T, Weinheimer KT. Three-dimensional arytenoid movement induced by vocal fold injections. Laryngoscope 2010;120(8):1563–8.
103. Shin JL, Hartnick CJ, Randolph GW, editors. Evidence-based otolaryngology. New York: Springer; 2008.
104. Hertegard S, Hallen L, Laurent C, et al. Cross-linked hyaluronan used as augmentation substance for treatment of glottal insufficiency: safety aspects and vocal fold function. Laryngoscope 2002;112:2211–9.
105. Hertegard S, Hallen L, Laurent C, et al. Cross-linked hyaluronan versus collagen for injection treatment of glottal insufficiency: 2-year follow-up. Acta Otolaryngol 2004;124:1208–14.
106. Dedo HH, Carlsoo B. Histologic evaluation of Teflon granulomas of human vocal cords. A light and electron microscopic study. Acta Otolaryngol 1982;93(5–6): 475–84.
107. Ossoff RH, Koriwchak MJ, Netterville JL, et al. Difficulties in endoscopic removal of Teflon granulomas of the vocal fold. Ann Otol Rhinol Laryngol 1993;102(6): 405–12.
108. Nakayama M, Ford CN, Bless DM. Teflon vocal fold augmentation: failures and management in 28 cases. Otolaryngol Head Neck Surg 1993;109(3 Pt 1): 493–8.
109. Kasperbauer JL, Slavit DH, Maragos NE. Teflon granulomas and overinjection of Teflon: a therapeutic challenge for the otorhinolaryngologist. Ann Otol Rhinol Laryngol 1993;102(10):748–51.
110. Schramm VL, May M, Lavorato AS. Gelfoam paste injection for vocal cord paralysis: temporary rehabilitation of glottic incompetence. Laryngoscope 1978;88(8 Pt 1):1268–73.
111. O'Leary MA, Grillone GA. Injection laryngoplasty. Otolaryngol Clin North Am 2006;39(1):43–54.
112. Lau DP, Lee GA, Wong SM, et al. Injection laryngoplasty with hyaluronic acid for unilateral vocal cord paralysis. Randomized controlled trial comparing two different particle sizes. J Voice 2010;24(1):113–8.
113. Rosen CA, Gartner-Schmidt J, Casiano R, et al. Vocal fold augmentation with calcium hydroxylapatite: twelve-month report. Laryngoscope 2009;119(5): 1033–41.
114. Kwon TK, Rosen CA, Gartner-Schmidt J. Preliminary results of a new temporary vocal fold injection material. J Voice 2005;19(4):668–73.
115. Milstein CF, Akst LM, Hicks MD, et al. Long-term effects of micronized Alloderm injection for unilateral vocal fold paralysis. Laryngoscope 2005;115(9):1691–6.

116. Tan M, Woo P. Injection laryngoplasty with micronized dermis: a 10-year experience with 381 injections in 344 patients. Laryngoscope 2010;120(12):2460–6.

117. Mikaelian DO, Lowry LD, Sataloff RT. Lipoinjection for unilateral vocal cord paralysis. Laryngoscope 1991;101(5):465–8.

118. McCulloch TM, Andrews BT, Hoffman HT, et al. Long-term follow-up of fat injection laryngoplasty for unilateral vocal cord paralysis. Laryngoscope 2002; 112(7 Pt 1):1235–8.

119. Reijonen P, Tervonen H, Harinen K, et al. Long-term results of autologous fascia in unilateral vocal fold paralysis. Eur Arch Otorhinolaryngol 2009;266(8):1273–8.

120. Reijonen P, Lehikoinen-Soderlund S, Rihkanen H. Results of fascial augmentation in unilateral vocal fold paralysis. Ann Otol Rhinol Laryngol 2002;111(6): 523–9.

121. Anderson TD, Sataloff RT. Complications of collagen injection of the vocal fold: report of several unusual cases and review of the literature. J Voice 2004;18(3): 392–7.

122. Ford CN, Bless DM. Clinical experience with injectable collagen for vocal fold augmentation. Laryngoscope 1986;96(8):863–9.

123. Bock JM, Lee JH, Robinson RA, et al. Migration of Cymetra after vocal fold injection for laryngeal paralysis. Laryngoscope 2007;117(12):2251–4.

124. Zapanta PE, Bielamowicz SA. Laryngeal abscess after injection laryngoplasty with micronized AlloDerm. Laryngoscope 2004;114(9):1522–4.

125. Arviso LC, Johns MM 3rd, Mathison CC, et al. Long-term outcomes of injection laryngoplasty in patients with potentially recoverable vocal fold paralysis. Laryngoscope 2010;120(11):2237–40.

126. Bhattacharyya N, Batirel H, Swanson SJ. Improved outcomes with early vocal fold medialization for vocal fold paralysis after thoracic surgery. Auris Nasus Larynx 2003;30(1):71–5.

127. Friedman AD, Burns JA, Heaton JT, et al. Early versus late injection medialization for unilateral vocal cord paralysis. Laryngoscope 2010;120(10):2042–6.

128. Yung KC, Likhterov I, Courey MS. Effect of temporary vocal fold injection medialization on the rate of permanent medialization laryngoplasty in unilateral vocal fold paralysis patients. Laryngoscope 2011;121(10):2191–4.

129. Payr E. Plastik am Schildknorpel zur Behebung der Folgen einseitiger Stimmbanclahmung. Deutsche Medizinische Wochenschrift 1915;43:1265–70 [in German].

130. Isshiki N, Okamura H, Ishikawa T. Thyroplasty type I (lateral compression) for dysphonia due to vocal cord paralysis or atrophy. Acta Otolaryngol 1975; 80(5–6):465–73.

131. Isshiki N, Taira T, Kojima H, et al. Recent modifications in thyroplasty type I. Ann Otol Rhinol Laryngol 1989;98(10):777–9.

132. Zhao X, Roth K, Fung K. Type I thyroplasty: risk stratification approach to inpatient versus outpatient postoperative management. J Otolaryngol Head Neck Surg 2010;39(6):757–61.

133. Bray D, Young JP, Harries ML. Complications after type one thyroplasty: is daycase surgery feasible? J Laryngol Otol 2008;122(7):715–8.

134. van Ardenne N, Vanderwegen J, Van Nuffelen G, et al. Medialization thyroplasty: vocal outcome of silicone and titanium implant. Eur Arch Otorhinolaryngol 2011; 268(1):101–7.

135. Storck C, Fischer C, Cecon M, et al. Hydroxyapatite versus titanium implant: comparison of the functional outcome after vocal fold medialization in unilateral recurrent nerve paralysis. Head Neck 2010;32(12):1605–12.

136. Lundy DS, Casiano RR, Xue JW. Can maximum phonation time predict voice outcome after thyroplasty type I? Laryngoscope 2004;114(8):1447–54.
137. Isshiki N, Tanabe M, Sawada M. Arytenoid adduction for unilateral vocal cord paralysis. Arch Otolaryngol 1978;104(10):555–8.
138. Zeitels SM, Hochman I, Hillman RE. Adduction arytenopexy: a new procedure for paralytic dysphonia with implications for implant medialization. Ann Otol Rhinol Laryngol Suppl 1998;173:2–24.
139. Thakar A, Sikka K, Verma R, et al. Cricothyroid approximation for voice and swallowing rehabilitation of high vagal paralysis secondary to skull base neoplasms. Eur Arch Otorhinolaryngol 2011;268(11):1611–6.
140. Li AJ, Johns MM, Jackson-Menaldi C, et al. Glottic closure patterns: type I thyroplasty versus type I thyroplasty with arytenoid adduction. J Voice 2011;25(3): 259–64.
141. Franco RA, Andrus JG. Aerodynamic and acoustic characteristics of voice before and after adduction arytenopexy and medialization laryngoplasty with GORE-TEX in patients with unilateral vocal fold immobility. J Voice 2009;23(2): 261–7.
142. McNamar J, Montequin DW, Welham NV, et al. Aerodynamic, acoustic, and vibratory comparison of arytenoid adduction and adduction arytenopexy. Laryngoscope 2008;118(3):552–8.
143. Abraham MT, Gonen M, Kraus DH. Complications of type I thyroplasty and arytenoid adduction. Laryngoscope 2001;111(8):1322–9.
144. Senkal HA, Yilmaz T. Type I thyroplasty revision 1 year after a window was mistakenly created on the cricoid cartilage. Ear Nose Throat J 2010;89(5):E14–6.
145. Woo P, Pearl AW, Hsiung MW, et al. Failed medialization laryngoplasty: management by revision surgery. Otolaryngol Head Neck Surg 2001;124(6):615–21.
146. Rosen CA. Complications of phonosurgery: results of a national survey. Laryngoscope 1998;108(11 Pt 1):1697–703.
147. Paniello RC, Dahm JD. Reversibility of medialization laryngoplasty. An experimental study. Ann Otol Rhinol Laryngol 1997;106(11):902–8.
148. Sasaki CT, Leder SB, Petcu L, et al. Longitudinal voice quality changes following Isshiki thyroplasty type I: the Yale experience. Laryngoscope 1990;100(8): 849–52.
149. Leder SB, Sasaki CT. Long-term changes in vocal quality following Isshiki thyroplasty type I. Laryngoscope 1994;104(3 Pt 1):275–7.
150. Netterville JL, Stone RE, Luken ES, et al. Silastic medialization and arytenoid adduction: the Vanderbilt experience. A review of 116 phonosurgical procedures. Ann Otol Rhinol Laryngol 1993;102(6):413–24.
151. Billante CR, Clary J, Childs P, et al. Voice gains following thyroplasty may improve over time. Clin Otolaryngol Allied Sci 2002;27(2):89–94.
152. Lundy DS, Casiano RR, Xue JW, et al. Thyroplasty type I: short- versus long-term results. Otolaryngol Head Neck Surg 2000;122(4):533–6.
153. Gray SD, Barkmeier J, Jones D, et al. Vocal evaluation of thyroplastic surgery in the treatment of unilateral vocal fold paralysis. Laryngoscope 1992;102(4): 415–21.
154. Dejonckere PH. Teflon injection and thyroplasty: objective and subjective outcomes. Rev Laryngol Otol Rhinol (Bord) 1998;119(4):265–9.
155. Lundy DS, Casiano RR, McClinton ME, et al. Early results of transcutaneous injection laryngoplasty with micronized acellular dermis versus type-I thyroplasty for glottic incompetence dysphonia due to unilateral vocal fold paralysis. J Voice 2003;17(4):589–95.

156. Morgan JE, Zraick RI, Griffin AW, et al. Injection versus medialization laryngo-plasty for the treatment of unilateral vocal fold paralysis. Laryngoscope 2007; 117(11):2068–74.
157. Tsuzuki T, Fukuda H, Fujioka T, et al. Voice prognosis after liquid and solid sili-cone injection. Am J Otolaryngol 1991;12(3):165–9.
158. D'Antonio LL, Wigley TL, Zimmerman GJ. Quantitative measures of laryngeal function following Teflon injection or thyroplasty type I. Laryngoscope 1995; 105(3 Pt 1):256–62.
159. Vinson KN, Zraick RI, Ragland FJ. Injection versus medialization laryngoplasty for the treatment of unilateral vocal fold paralysis: follow-up at six months. Laryn-goscope 2010;120(9):1802–7.
160. Bhattacharyya N, Kotz T, Shapiro J. Dysphagia and aspiration with unilateral vocal cord immobility: incidence, characterization, and response to surgical treatment. Ann Otol Rhinol Laryngol 2002;111(8):672–9.
161. Nayak VK, Bhattacharyya N, Kotz T, et al. Patterns of swallowing failure following medialization in unilateral vocal fold immobility. Laryngoscope 2002;112(10): 1840–4.
162. Hoffman MR, Witt RE, Chapin WJ, et al. Multiparameter comparison of injection laryngoplasty, medialization laryngoplasty, and arytenoid adduction in an ex-cised larynx model. Laryngoscope 2010;120(4):769–76.
163. McCulloch TM, Hoffman HT, Andrews BT, et al. Arytenoid adduction combined with Gore-Tex medialization thyroplasty. Laryngoscope 2000;110(8):1306–11.
164. Thompson DM, Maragos NE, Edwards BW. The study of vocal fold vibratory patterns in patients with unilateral vocal fold paralysis before and after type I thyroplasty with or without arytenoid adduction. Laryngoscope 1995;105(5 Pt 1): 481–6.
165. Mortensen M, Carroll L, Woo P. Arytenoid adduction with medialization laryngo-plasty versus injection or medialization laryngoplasty: the role of the arytenoido-pexy. Laryngoscope 2009;119(4):827–31.
166. Tucker HM. Reinnervation of the paralyzed larynx: a review. Head Neck Surg 1979;1(3):235–42.
167. Paniello RC, Lee P, Dahm JD. Hypoglossal nerve transfer for laryngeal reinner-vation: a preliminary study. Ann Otol Rhinol Laryngol 1999;108(3):239–44.
168. Tucker HM, Rusnov M. Laryngeal reinnervation for unilateral vocal cord paral-ysis: long-term results. Ann Otol Rhinol Laryngol 1981;90(5 Pt 1):457–9.
169. Tucker HM. Long-term results of nerve-muscle pedicle reinnervation for laryn-geal paralysis. Ann Otol Rhinol Laryngol 1989;98(9):674–6.
170. Goding GS Jr. Nerve-muscle pedicle reinnervation of the paralyzed vocal cord. Otolaryngol Clin North Am 1991;24(5):1239–52.
171. Hassan MM, Yumoto E, Baraka MA, et al. Arytenoid rotation and nerve-muscle pedicle transfer in paralytic dysphonia. Laryngoscope 2011;121(5):1018–22.
172. Yumoto E, Sanuki T, Toya Y, et al. Nerve-muscle pedicle flap implantation combined with arytenoid adduction. Arch Otolaryngol Head Neck Surg 2010; 136(10):965–9.
173. Chhetri DK, Gerratt BR, Kreiman J, et al. Combined arytenoid adduction and laryngeal reinnervation in the treatment of vocal fold paralysis. Laryngoscope 1999;109(12):1928–36.
174. Woo P, Mangaro M. Aberrant recurrent laryngeal nerve reinnervation as a cause of stridor and laryngospasm. Ann Otol Rhinol Laryngol 2004;113(10):805–8.
175. Maronian NC, Robinson L, Waugh P, et al. A new electromyographic definition of laryngeal synkinesis. Ann Otol Rhinol Laryngol 2004;113(11):877–86.

176. Crumley RL. Laryngeal synkinesis revisited. Ann Otol Rhinol Laryngol 2000; 109(4):365–71.

177. Tucker HM. Long-term preservation of voice improvement following surgical medialization and reinnervation for unilateral vocal fold paralysis. J Voice 1999; 13(2):251–6.

178. Paniello RC, Edgar JD, Kallogjeri D, et al. Medialization versus reinnervation for unilateral vocal fold paralysis: a multicenter randomized clinical trial. Laryngoscope 2011;121(10):2172–9.

Otolaryngology Clinic of North America: Evidence-Based Practice

Management of Hoarseness/Dysphonia

Jaime I. Chang, MD[a], Scott E. Bevans, MD[b],
Seth R. Schwartz, MD, MPH[a],*

KEYWORDS

- Dysphonia • Hoarseness • Evidence-based otolaryngology • Laryngoscopy
- Laryngostroboscopy • Laryngeal imaging • Laryngeal electromyography

KEY POINTS

The following points list the level of evidence as based on Oxford Center for Evidence-Based Medicine. Additional critical points are provided and points here are expanded at the conclusion of this article.

- The otolaryngologist must rule out malignancy in patients with persistent dysphonia [Level 5].
- Angled rigid endoscopy, although not as well tolerated, enhances diagnostic yield [Level 4].
- Laryngeal electromyography offers diagnostic and prognostic information in vocal fold paralysis/paresis [Level 3a].
- Some benign causes of dysphonia respond to voice therapy [Level 3].
- Antibiotics are not useful for dysphonia, excepting specific bacterial infections of the airway [Level 1a].
- Targeted use of antireflux medications can be beneficial to control laryngeal inflammation and reflux symptoms [Level 1b-], but remains unproven as empiric therapy for isolated dysphonia.

OVERVIEW

Hoarseness is a common patient complaint and can be the main symptom for a wide range of medical problems. It can result from mild self-limited inflammation of the

All authors have nothing to disclose.
The opinions and assertions contained herein are the private views of the authors and should not be construed as official or reflecting the views of the Department of Defense or the Department of the Army.
[a] Otolaryngology-Head and Neck Surgery, Virginia Mason Medical Center, Seattle, WA, USA;
[b] Otolaryngology-Head and Neck Surgery, Madigan Healthcare System, Tacoma, WA, USA
* Corresponding author.
E-mail address: Seth.Schwartz@vmmc.org

Otolaryngol Clin N Am 45 (2012) 1109–1126
http://dx.doi.org/10.1016/j.otc.2012.06.012
0030-6665/12/$ – see front matter © 2012 Elsevier Inc. All rights reserved.

vocal folds or be an early sign of laryngeal cancer. Patients with mild or self-limited hoarseness may never seek evaluation before resolution of symptoms; persistent hoarseness often leads patients to seek evaluation. The role of the otolaryngologist is generally to diagnose the underlying cause of the symptom of hoarseness and subsequently to manage that condition.

Hoarseness is a common complaint, with an overall prevalence of nearly 30.0% in adults, nearly 50.0% in elderly patients, and 3.9% to 23.0% in children.[1–7] It is slightly more common in women,[1,8,9] and is considerably more common among certain professions, such as telemarketers, aerobics instructors, and teachers, where the prevalence may approach 60%.[1–12] Regardless of the underlying diagnosis, patients with hoarseness may suffer social isolation, depression, and reduction in quality of life.[1,13–16] Hoarseness and the conditions that cause it are a common cause of time lost from work,[1,9,12] and has been estimated to cost approximately $2.5 billion in lost wages.[17]

Although patients frequently complain of hoarseness, it is a nonspecific term for a symptom and not a diagnosis. Clinical evaluation frequently reveals that patients have dysphonia, which is an alteration in voice quality that negatively affects the patient's social or professional communication.

Furthermore, dysphonia may be the presenting symptom of a serious underlying condition necessitating urgent or emergent management. The first task of the otolaryngologist is to determine if the dysphonia reflects a life-threatening condition or if it causes a decrement in quality of life or an impediment to professional function. Non–life-threatening causes of dysphonia still represent a significant health care burden, as stated previously, and can have a major impact on a patient's life. Accordingly, optimal management of these patients represents a large quality-improvement opportunity. A recently published clinical practice guideline was produced by the American Academy of Otolaryngology to address these issues.[18]

This article is not a clinical practice guideline. It reviews the evidence related to the evaluation of a patient with dysphonia and to the evidence for management of some of the common underlying problems that lead to the condition. Specifically, we review the evidence for some common diagnostic studies used in the evaluation of patients presenting with hoarseness (laryngoscopy/stroboscopy, imaging, and electromyographic testing). With regard to management, the myriad diagnoses that can produce dysphonia preclude a comprehensive discussion of the management of each etiology. Clearly, an evidence-based review of the management of laryngeal cancer is beyond the scope of this article. Accordingly, we selectively review the evidence behind interventions for several leading causes of dysphonia.

EVIDENCE-BASED CLINICAL ASSESSMENT

In evaluating dysphonia, a thorough history and head and neck examination allow the clinician to assess the degree of morbidity, to determine possible etiologies, and to target the remainder of the evaluation and planning of appropriate management. Despite the essential role of performing a thorough history and head and neck examination, there is a paucity of validated studies to lend evidentiary support for the importance of their role in the diagnosis and management of the underlying etiologies for dysphonia, excepting visualization of the larynx, which is addressed next. Nonetheless, all of the interventions discussed in this article are based on a clinical assessment of the severity of the suspected underlying etiology (eg, impending airway obstruction, malignancy) and the implications of impairment (eg, occupational impact for those patients who use their voices professionally). This article defers further discussion of these aspects of the clinical assessment of dysphonia to the body of expert opinion already published on this topic.

The remainder of this section focuses on the evidence regarding adjunctive measures beyond the history and general head and neck examination. This section divides these options into (1) visualization of the vocal folds, (2) diagnostic testing, and (3) measurements of the degree of dysphonia.

Visualization of the Larynx

Laryngoscopy

Visualization of the larynx is critical in any assessment of a patient with dysphonia.[19] Laryngoscopy uses optics and light to allow the clinician to visualize the laryngeal structures.[19,20] Traditionally, the larynx has been visualized in the awake clinic patient indirectly using a laryngeal mirror. Although the view may be adequate with a laryngeal mirror, functional examination can be limited, and full visualization may be limited. With the development of optics and associated technologies, laryngoscopy can be performed with a variety of endoscopes: rigid angled laryngoscopes, flexible fiberoptic laryngoscopes, and flexible distal chip laryngoscopes. Video cameras can also be added for further magnification and recording.

More than 20 years ago, a prospective, nonrandomized trial performed by Barker and Dort[21] evaluated the ability to complete either a mirror or rigid endoscopic examination. In the patients who went on to have direct laryngoscopy, Barker and Dort[21] evaluated the accuracy of findings between the 2 techniques. Among the 100 patients they tested, nearly half of patients could not tolerate mirror evaluation. More than 80% tolerated a rigid endoscopic examination. Fewer than 30% underwent direct laryngoscopy, and among them, both examination techniques proved largely accurate, with rigid endoscopic techniques having zero false-negative evaluations.[21] With the significant advances made in endoscopic technology since that report, a 2009 study of 43 patients similarly compared rigid laryngoscopy using a 30° endoscope to mirror examination and showed statistically significant improvements in patient comfort with less gagging (80% preferred rigid endoscopy), improved visualization of laryngeal structures by physicians, and the ability to display results of endoscopic evaluation for patients to see simultaneously.[22] By comparison, a single study has suggested that flexible fiberoptic visualization offers decreased patient discomfort relative to rigid endoscopy (evidenced by cardiovascular response to direct vs fiberoptic laryngoscopy in patients emerging from anesthesia following thyroidectomy) and improved visualization.[23]

Uncontrolled, observational studies, and anecdotal and expert opinion suggest that the use of fiberoptic visualization often affords the ability to palpate the glottis and supraglottis for assessment of sensory function, allows for improved dynamic assessments, and may provide some improved visualization of the subglottic region.[24–28] This must be weighed against good evidence that suggests image quality is improved with the use of rigid endoscopes, however. A randomized case-controlled direct comparison among the 3 most frequently used methods (flexible fiberoptic endoscopes, distal chip flexible endoscopes, and rigid angled endoscopes) in 2008 showed that although flexible fiberoptic endoscopes provide the most cost-effective option for visualizing the larynx, they provided less information than rigid visualization in nearly one-quarter of patients, most notably during stroboscopy.[25]

Although both rigid and flexible endoscopes have specific strengths and weakness, one of the chief advantages of either method over mirror laryngoscopy is the simultaneous use of magnification, video recording, and stroboscopy.

Laryngostroboscopy

Although laryngoscopy alone can visualize anatomic abnormalities, such as masses and impaired mobility of the vocal folds, it cannot provide visualization of the mucosal vibration (the source of the voice). Under constant illumination, the vocal folds vibrate at a much higher frequency than the human eye can discern. Addition of a strobo-scopic light source allows the viewer to discriminate the motion of the vibratory edge of the vocal folds in "slow motion."[29]

In comparison with laryngoscopy alone, stroboscopy improves diagnostic yield, as demonstrated in several observational studies over the past 30 years. In 1991, Sataloff and colleagues[30] reported the largest of these studies, assessing nearly 1900 patients over a 4-year period. Additional diagnoses were discovered in 29% of patients, and the prestrobe diagnoses were found to be inaccurate in 18% of patients.[30] Subse-quent publication of 292 prospectively identified patients who underwent a similar protocol involving initial laryngoscopy followed by stroboscopy showed similar re-sults, with stroboscopy altering the diagnosis and treatment outcome in 14% of the patients.[31] A small (40 patients) retrospective review of stroboscopy use in the setting of laryngeal trauma found that even after computed tomography (CT) and laryngos-copy, stroboscopic evaluation replaced the need for direct laryngoscopy to evaluate mucosal integrity and vocal fold function in several patients. Avoidance of secondary trauma of operative direct laryngoscopy led to earlier discharge for matched grades of laryngeal injury.[32]

A 2010 retrospective review of pediatric patients with unresolved dysphonia after prior endoscopy and treatment found the addition of stroboscopy (both rigid and flex-ible) identified a new diagnosis that resulted in additional therapy in nearly all patients.[33]

Other Techniques to Visualize Vocal Fold Vibration

In addition to stroboscopy, there are several newer technologies, such as videoky-mography, photoglottography, and high-speed digital imaging (HDSI), that have been developed but are not as widely available. A 252-patient prospective trial comparing stroboscopy, in particular, to HDSI (which offers the advantage of evalu-ating the full mucosal wave with increased capture rates and slowed playback for more complete evaluation of the vibratory cycle) showed that a definitive diagnosis was made in all patients in whom a diagnosis was unclear using stroboscopy alone (63% of total).[34] Although these developing technologies may provide increased diag-nostic ability, they are as yet unproven and costly.[34–37]

Direct laryngoscopy

Operative direct laryngoscopy (with or without magnification) as a diagnostic tool may assist in establishing a diagnosis for dysphonia in patients with certain laryngoscopic findings (eg, a mass lesion). It may also be indicated in patients in whom awake visu-alization of the larynx cannot be achieved. Operative direct laryngoscopy offers the additional benefit of palpation of the cricoarytenoid joint and the mucosa of the vocal folds, as well as the opportunity for diagnostic biopsy. Phonomicrosurgical interven-tion can also be done concurrently with diagnosis in selected circumstances.

Although dynamic evaluation in the sedated patient is limited, multiple retrospective reviews suggest that the improved visualization provided by operative positioning, palpation, magnification, and improved depth perception of binocular microscopy results in alternate or additional diagnoses. Poels and colleagues[38] found that, despite preoperative stroboscopy, alternate diagnoses were made in 36% of the 221 patients who underwent direct laryngoscopy. An additional 31% of patients had additional lesions (largely intracordal) discovered at the time of surgery.[8] A more recent review of 100 patients at another tertiary care center identified additional lesions (often bilateral) in 9% of patients. Nearly half of these patients had a change in treatment plans after the altered diagnosis.[39]

Diagnostic Testing for Dysphonia

Although history, physical examination, and visualizing of the larynx are generally adequate to evaluate a patient with dysphonia, further diagnostic testing is indicated in selected patients.

Laryngeal electromyography

Laryngeal electromyography (LEMG) assesses the electrical activity and the functional status of the innervation to the targeted laryngeal muscles (typically cricothyroid, thyroarytenoid, and often posterior cricoarytenoid muscles).

A 2005 study of the practices of laryngologists who belong to the American Broncho-Esphogological Association indicated that among respondents, 75% used LEMG to confirm or diagnose unilateral vocal fold immobility.[40] Evidence to support its use in a purely diagnostic capacity is largely of a nonrandomized, retrospective nature, however. To address this issue specifically, the Neurolaryngology Study Group convened a multidisciplinary panel to examine the evidence for LEMG in diagnosis and prognosis. The diagnostic accuracy was based on multiple small studies and one large unblinded retrospective study, which confirmed the neurologic basis of vocal fold paresis or paralysis in 83% to 92% of cases and was able to contrast neurologic impairment with cricoarytenoid motion disorders in the remaining patients (2%–12%).[41] One of the larger studies reviewed reported that LEMG led to a change in the type of imaging performed in 11% of patients and altered the timing or type of surgical intervention in another 40% of patients.[42]

Meyer and Hillel[43] published an updated review of the literature in 2009 of primarily level IV evidence. They identified a blinded study from Philadelphia[44] that reported increased sensitivity for identification of a paretic nerve from 64% to 86%. Another reviewed study reported that LEMG altered the timing or choice of therapy in nearly 50% of patients.[45] More recent studies (level III evidence) compared the efficacy of LEMG to laryngoscopy for diagnosis of neurologic impairment.[46–48] Sataloff and colleagues[46] reported that LEMG results corroborated laryngoscopic diagnosis in 95% of patients (661 of 689), and identified neurologic abnormality in 22% (14 of 62) without a prior diagnosis. Importantly, Gavazzoni and colleagues[48] caution that no single electrophysiologic parameter alone confers a high sensitivity (although nearly all carried greater than 90% specificity) and adds that duration since onset of impairment decreases the diagnostic certainty.

Hydman and colleagues[49] studied LEMG as a prognostic indicator in recurrent laryngeal nerve injury in 15 patients with vocal fold paresis 2 to 3 weeks after iatrogenic injury but anatomically intact recurrent laryngeal nerves. Patients with axonal injury based on LEMG findings had 50% significantly worsened functional and videostroboscopic outcomes.

Radiographic imaging

Although most patients with dysphonia do not require imaging, abnormalities in structure of the larynx or mobility of the vocal folds may prompt additional investigation with radiographic imaging. Imaging may be useful in assessing the extent of mass lesions. In malignancy, imaging allows assessment of regional lymphatic involvement, as well as defining the extent of the mass. CT or magnetic resonance imaging (MRI) can be used to assess for invasion of the laryngeal cartilage, which offers prognostic information for staging of laryngeal and hypopharyngeal cancer.[50–52] MRI is highly sensitive for identifying cartilage invasion, but it is less specific than CT owing to increased signal patterns often caused by inflammation.

Imaging is also indicated if initial workup of dysphonia reveals a paralyzed vocal fold without a known cause.[52] Historically, a chest radiograph and/or a neck CT with contrast was used to identify vascular anomalies or mass lesions.[50–53] In recent years, radiographs have become extraneous, as both positive and negative results lead to CT imaging.[52,53] In a recent prospective study by El Badawey and colleagues[53] of 86 patients presenting with vocal cord palsy, 36% had positive CT findings, which correlated with the cause for immobility. Most of these were suspicious for malignancy in the lungs or mediastinum.

Skull-base imaging with MRI is indicated in vocal fold paresis with other cranial nerve palsies. Principally, expert opinion supports its use in diagnosing skull base or jugular foramen neoplasm (glomus tumors, schwannomas, and so forth) or metastatic disease responsible for multiple lower cranial nerve palsies.[51,52,55] Two studies of skull base invasion in nasopharyngeal carcinoma found MRI to be more sensitive than CT for identifying bony invasion.[56,57] Several investigators have found that MRI does not add additional sensitivity to CT in terms of identifying the presence of malignancy.[54,55,58]

Dysphonia, and specifically vocal fold paresis, can result from intracranial processes as well. MRI and CT may be warranted if signs or symptoms concerning for stroke warrant intracranial imaging to evaluate for ischemic or hemorrhagic sources. Clearly, for patients with pacemakers or metallic implants, MRI may be contraindicated.[58] In children with vocal fold palsy, one must balance the risk of radiation exposure with CT to the possible need for sedation with MRI.[59] The actual dose of radiation received by the thyroid and its long-term effect are still uncertain.[59,60] The risk of MRI is an approximately 5% chance of an episode of hypoxia during the required sedation.[61–63] In patients with intravenous contrast allergies, gadolinium-enhanced MRI is likely the safer study.

Measurements of Degree of Dysphonia

An additional component of assessing dysphonia is the perceptual component, from either the patient perspective or the clinician perspective. Both attempt to quantify the severity of the voice impairment.

Self-rated assessments

Several commonly used perceptual rating systems are intended to better characterize dysphonia and to assess the negative impact of voice disturbance on a patient's quality of life. The more widely known among them are the 30-question Voice Handicap Index (VHI),[64] with its revised, streamlined 10-question version (VHI-10),[16] and the Voice-Related Quality of Life survey (V-RQOL).[65] In severe voice disorders, patient ratings of severity and quality of life impact were highly correlated on each of the 3 instruments.[65,66,67] Recent studies suggest this correlation persists even in mild to moderately severe dysphonia.[67]

Although scores may be sensitive to change within each individual subject, the scores may be poorly correlated with the morbidity of the underlying disease process or objective measures of voice disorder. Studies validating use in other languages find that spasmodic dysphonia and functional disorders tend to produce worse ratings than nonbenign pathologies.[68,69] A cross-sectional case-controlled survey of patients who underwent total laryngectomy showed a distribution of scores generally equivalent to or better than Chinese patients with benign voice disorders (39–48 vs 38–70).[68,70–72] Additionally, a recent study of almost 500 public school teachers in Brazil using the VHI-10 showed little correlation between teacher ratings of impairment and quality of life and objectively identified voice disorders.[72]

Clinician-rated measures

Two clinician-rated scales are commonly used to assess the acoustic quality and severity of voice disorders. The GRBAS (overall grade [G], roughness [R], breathiness [B], asthenia-weakness [A], and strain [S]) is a clinician-based 0-point to 3-point graded assessment of quality and severity of voice disorder.[69] Although seemingly valid, some concerns exist about the use of this measure.[73]

The Consensus Auditory-Perceptual Evaluation of Voice (CAPE-V) is another provider-rated system developed by the American Speech-Language-Hearing Association.[74,75] It is a standardized measure of roughness, breathiness, strain, pitch, and loudness. Although it may have slightly better interrater reliability than the GRBAS, it is still subject to the experience of the rater[76] and may be biased by lack of blinding of the assessor.[77]

Although these tools allow for an objective quantification of the severity of voice disorders, no evidence has demonstrated that they influence the diagnosis or treatment of patients who present with dysphonia. Without data to suggest additional diagnostic or treatment benefit, these tools may be useful for research purposes and communication among clinicians, but use in clinical practice is at the discretion of the treating clinician.

EVIDENCE-BASED MANAGEMENT OF DYSPHONIA

Management of dysphonia is entirely dependent on its underlying cause. A complete discussion regarding management of all underlying etiologies for dysphonia is beyond the scope of this article. Specifically, dysphonia resulting from external laryngeal trauma, post–endotracheal intubation trauma, postlaryngeal surgery, and laryngeal cancer is not addressed. Additionally, patients with associated airway compromise clearly need urgent management of the airway, which is a topic in itself. This section addresses management of dysphonia associated with laryngeal inflammation, reduced vocal fold mobility, benign vocal fold lesions, and functional voice disorders. Categories of treatment can be divided into voice therapy, medical therapy, and surgical therapy. Oftentimes, a combination of treatment methods is necessary.

Voice Therapy

The approaches for voice therapy are often divided into 3 main categories: hygienic (improving behaviors that can lead to injury of the vocal folds), symptomatic (targeting treatment of abnormal voice quality in the resulting phonated voice), and physiologic (optimizing voice production). Thomas and Stemple conducted a systematic review of the efficacy of voice therapy that revealed the best support for physiologic approaches (randomized and other controlled trials), mixed support in hygienic approaches (controlled trials), and less strong data for symptomatic approaches (observational studies).[77] These approaches are used in the management of voice disorders discussed in the following sections.

Laryngeal inflammation

Laryngeal inflammation can occur as a result of infectious, irritant (allergies, reflux, airborne irritants), or traumatic (phonotrauma and iatrogenic) etiologies. Medical management of the irritants (such as infection, allergens, and reflux) is necessary to resolve the medical component of the inflammation. Voice therapy is used to improve vocal hygiene to prevent further phonotrauma, to allow healing, and to prevent recurrence.[77]

Benign lesions

When an anatomic abnormality (such as vocal fold nodules, cysts, or polyps) interferes with vocal fold vibration, voice therapy has 2 roles:

1. Training on voice production in the presence of the lesion may allow the patient to meet voice needs without other interventions.
2. Voice therapy may help to reduce vocal behaviors that caused the lesion and consequently avoid worsening or recurrence of the lesion.

Voice therapy also plays a role perioperatively in cases in which voice therapy alone cannot meet the patient's voice demands.

The most studied benign lesions in the efficacy of voice therapy are vocal fold nodules.[78] A retrospective review of 26 patients over 6 years revealed either elimination and/or reduction of vocal fold nodules in more than 70% of the patients.[79] More than 80% of patients in this study had either normal voice or mild dysphonia after therapy. Voice therapy is generally accepted as the primary modality of treatment in patients with vocal fold nodules. A survey of members of the American Academy of Otolaryngology–Head and Neck Surgery revealed that 91% of respondents used voice therapy first in vocal fold nodules. In other lesions, no statistical difference existed between the use of voice therapy, medical therapy, or surgical intervention.[80]

Other than vocal fold nodules, very little literature is available that directly assesses the management outcome of voice therapy in benign vocal fold lesions. One retrospective chart review of 57 patients with vocal fold polyps or cysts found complete symptom resolution with voice therapy alone in nearly half of patients under study.[81]

Glottic insufficiency

Voice therapy is commonly used as an adjunct to surgical intervention for glottic insufficiency. The results have been mixed when used alone. Two prospective[82,83] and 1 retrospective,[84] uncontrolled study correlated early involvement of a speech therapist with recovery of vocal fold mobility in cases of paralysis. Perceptual improvement (from the patient's perspective as well as blinded listeners) has been seen in patients who have undergone voice therapy even when more objective measurements (maximum phonation times, acoustic measures, and laryngeal images) do not reveal significant improvement.[85] On the other hand, a retrospective review of 275 patients with vocal fold atrophy showed that treatment success with voice therapy was poor to moderately poor based on patient perception of outcome measures by the VHI-10.[86]

Dysphonia in the setting of normal laryngeal tissue and mobility

Functional voice disorders (dysphonia in the absence of anatomic or physiologic abnormalities of the laryngeal structures) often result from excess muscle tension of intrinsic and extrinsic laryngeal muscles. Psychological and/or personality factors, vocal misuse and abuse, and compensation for underlying disease can all lead to this condition.[87] Voice therapy may help these patients, but organic problems leading to muscle tension dysphonia will still require concomitant medical or surgical management.[87]

Medical Therapy

Steroids

Inflammation of the vocal fold mucosa may produce dysphonia by impairing normal vibration. Oral steroids have been used to counteract this inflammation and, theoretically, allow the vocal fold mucosa to return to its normal vibratory state. Although this may be fairly common in practice, no studies evaluating the role of empiric steroid use for dysphonia were found in the literature. Very low quality evidence does support their effectiveness for dysphonia associated with specific diagnoses (case reports and case series):

- Croup[88]
- Allergies[89,90]
- Lichen planus[91]
- Autoimmune disorders, such as sarcoidosis,[92,93] systemic lupus erythematosus,[94] pemphigus,[95] and relapsing polychondritis[96]

Oral steroids are also commonly used in the setting of dysphonia with airway compromise and in professional voice patients with acute laryngitis and professional performance demands. Although these may be extreme circumstances justifying the use of steroids, no evidence supporting their use in either of these settings was found in the literature.

Steroids can also be delivered through direct injection to the laryngeal structures. One prospective multicenter study of 115 patients evaluated the efficacy of percutaneous vocal fold injections in cases of benign vocal fold lesions[97]; 35% of patients had complete resolution of symptoms, whereas 50% had partial improvement as measured by objective and subjective parameters. No severe complications (including vocal fold atrophy) were observed. Additional very low quality evidence in the form of case reports and case series support steroid injections for the following conditions: laryngeal relapsing polychondritis,[98] laryngeal sarcoidosis,[99,100] Reinke edema,[101] vocal nodules or polyps,[100,102,103] and vocal fold postoperative scar.[100]

Antibiotics

Antibiotics are an important therapeutic modality when a bacterial infection is present and requires treatment. They are not effective in cases of viral laryngitis or upper respiratory tract infections. A Cochrane review in 2007 found no benefit for the use of antibiotics in acute laryngitis (only 2 studies met inclusion criteria).[104] When a bacterial infection causing dysphonia is identified, then directed antibiotic therapy would be appropriate.

Antireflux therapy

Laryngopharyngeal reflux can cause dysphonia when gastric reflux results in inflammation of the laryngeal structures.[105] Since Koufman's research findings, medical treatment with proton pump inhibitors has become commonplace in managing dysphonia. Controversy remains regarding the appropriate use of antireflux medications, as side effects are better understood and efficacy has not been conclusively demonstrated. A 2006 Cochrane systematic review of 302 studies did not find any high-quality trials meeting the inclusion criteria to assess the effectiveness of antireflux therapy for dysphonia.[106]

A few higher-quality studies have demonstrated effectiveness in treating reflux symptoms and improving laryngeal inflammation. A randomized double-blind, placebo-controlled trial with esomeprazole 20 mg twice a day for 3 months in patients with laryngopharyngeal reflux found significant improvement in both symptoms and laryngeal examination.[107] Another prospective, double-blind study assessed the empiric use of pantoprazole as a diagnostic tool for laryngopharyngeal reflux.[108] In this study, all patients were tested with 24-hour, double-probe pH monitors before starting pantoprazole 40 mg twice a day. The study found that response to pantoprazole correlates with pH probe findings of reflux.[109] The benefit of empiric anti-reflux therapy for dysphonia in the absence of laryngeal findings and other clinical symptoms of laryngopharyngeal reflux has not been proven.

Surgical Therapy

Benign laryngeal lesions

Lesions on the true vocal folds interfere with the vibratory mucosa and impair phonation. Voice therapy is used initially, as described previously. Surgical intervention is considered when voice therapy does not result in satisfactory voice production. In 2004, Johns and colleagues[110] assessed the quality-of-life changes in 42 patients who underwent endoscopic laryngeal microsurgery for true vocal fold cysts, polyps, and scarring. VHI scores significantly decreased at 3 months after surgery (49.6 ± 21 to 26.8 ± 21, $P<.001$); the difference was most significant for vocal fold polyps and cysts. No statistically significant improvement was found for patients who underwent surgery for vocal fold scar.

Glottic incompetence

Glottic incompetence refers to incomplete closure of the vocal folds during phonation, which results in a breathy, asthenic voice. Impaired glottic closure can occur with reduced or absent mobility of the true vocal folds (vocal fold paresis and paralysis), as well as from reduced vocal fold tissue bulk (vocal fold atrophy). Although voice therapy is often used as first-line treatment, inadequate response to therapy may be an indication for surgical intervention to medialize the vocal fold and improve glottic closure.

Currently, no therapies restore active movement of the vocal folds. Passive, static medialization occurs with a bulking agent, either by injection laryngoplasty or external framework surgery. Two retrospective studies of selected patients from the same institution (2007 and 2010) compared injection versus medialization laryngoplasty for unilateral vocal fold paralysis. The initial study assessed 19 patients at an average of 3 months postoperatively (range 1–9 months); the subsequent study assessed those plus 15 additional patients at an average of 6.4 months postoperatively (range 1–24 months). These studies found voice improvements with both techniques with no significant difference between groups.[109,111]

Although often considered a temporary fix while awaiting spontaneous improvement in vocal fold mobility, injection laryngoplasty may be adequate treatment. A single-institution, retrospective chart review over 4 years revealed that in 42 patients with potentially recoverable unilateral vocal fold paralysis who underwent injection laryngoplasty, 29% required more definitive management. Seventy-one percent did not need further intervention; they either recovered mobility or compensated adequately. These patients had been followed for a median of 10.5 months (range 6–44 months).[112] In a retrospective chart review of 54 patients, those who had temporary injection medialization were less likely to undergo permanent medialization than patients who opted for observation or voice therapy (5/19 vs 23/35).[113]

A variety of materials have been used for injection laryngoplasty with varying expected durations of benefit. Studies of individual injectables have shown that injection laryngoplasty is effective in improving the voice in patients with glottic insufficiency. Several retrospective chart reviews and prospective case series of individual materials have shown effectiveness of many different injectables:

- Calcium hydroxylapatite[114,115]
- Hyaluronic acid[116]
- Micronized dermis[117–121]

- Autologous fascia[122]
- Autologous fat[123,124]
- Polyacrylamide hydrogel[125]

Few studies compare materials directly. One prospective, randomized controlled study of injection laryngoplasty with 2-year follow-up compared hyaluronic acid gel to collagen.[126] No significant difference was found between them, with both groups achieving improved voice without long-term side effects. The choice of material should be based on the clinical context (ie, short-term or long-term paralysis) and the desired characteristics of the material.

These injections are being done in increasing numbers in the clinic setting. A large, retrospective, multicenter study demonstrated a shift to more injections being performed in the clinic setting with equally high success rates (99% vs 97%) and minimal complications.[127]

Arytenoid adduction rotates the vocal process of the arytenoids medially to improve posterior glottic closure. An evidence-based review in 2003 yielded only 3 studies comparing medialization thyroplasty alone to medialization thyroplasty with arytenoid adduction. No clear benefit was identified with the addition of arytenoid adduction.[128] A more recent retrospective study using 3 blinded reviewers found no significant difference in posterior glottic closure with the addition of arytenoid adduction to thyroplasty.[129]

Reinnervation is another surgical option for paralyzed vocal folds. With reinnervation, patients gain tone within the intrinsic musculature, but not necessarily active mobility. A multicenter, prospective, randomized clinical trial compared medialization laryngoplasty to laryngeal reinnervation for unilateral vocal fold paralysis with 12-month follow-up.[130] Each group showed significant improvement in voice (gauged by untrained listeners, blinded speech pathologists, and patient report [by voice-related quality of life]), but no significant between-group differences were found. A subgroup analysis showed that patients younger than 52 years had more favorable results with reinnervation procedures.

WHAT DOES THE EVIDENCE TELLS US (THE BOTTOM LINE)

In patients presenting with dysphonia, visualization of the larynx is critical to establishing the underlying cause of symptoms. Flexible fiberoptic laryngoscopy is well tolerated and allows a diagnosis in most patients. Rigid angled laryngoscopy, especially with the addition of a stroboscopic light source, improves visualization and may allow for diagnosis when not established by fiberoptic laryngoscopy. For more subtle findings, laryngostroboscopy may alter the diagnosis. Operative laryngoscopy should be reserved for patients in whom a biopsy is needed or a diagnosis was still not established by the less invasive methods. LEMG is not routinely helpful as a first-line diagnostic test for dysphonia, but may offer additional diagnostic or prognostic information in vocal fold paresis or paralysis. CT or MRI imaging can be useful in assessing the extent of a mass lesion or identifying a cause of vocal fold paralysis if history and physical examination are unrevealing, but imaging is not useful in the initial workup of dysphonia. The data do not conclusively recommend one study over another.

Management of dysphonia is entirely dependent on the underlying cause and many of the subtleties of managing this myriad of complex conditions is beyond the scope of this article. In brief, voice therapy can be effective as first-line therapy for some benign lesions of the vocal folds (nodules in particular) and as an adjunct to medical or surgical management if primary therapy is unsuccessful or an organic pathology is at play. Regarding medical therapy, the evidence does not support the routine use of oral steroids for dysphonia, but expert opinion argues for their usefulness in certain circumstances. Antibiotics similarly are not useful to treat dysphonia excepting rare bacterial infections that may respond. Antireflux therapy is supported for patients with symptoms of reflux or laryngeal changes associated with reflux but remains unproven for empiric treatment of dysphonia in the absence of other symptoms or physical findings (diagnostic therapy excepted). Low-quality data support the use of surgery to manage several of the underlying conditions that can lead to dysphonia (glottic insufficiency and certain benign lesions of the vocal folds).

CRITICAL POINTS

- The otolaryngologist must rule out malignancy in patients with persistent dysphonia [Level 5]
- Fiberoptic laryngoscopy allows for a diagnosis in many patients, but angled rigid endoscopy, although not as well tolerated, enhances diagnostic yield [Level 4]
- The addition of a stroboscopic light source increases the diagnostic accuracy and sensitivity of laryngoscopy [Level 4]
- LEMG offers diagnostic and prognostic information in vocal fold paralysis/ paresis [Level 3a]
- Some benign causes of dysphonia will respond to voice therapy (laryngeal inflammation, vocal fold nodules) [Level 3]
- Oral steroids have a limited role in managing routine dysphonia [Level 4/5]
- Antibiotics are not useful for dysphonia, excepting specific bacterial infections of the airway [Level 1a]
- Targeted use of antireflux medications can be beneficial to control laryngeal inflammation and reflux symptoms [Level 1b-], but remains unproven as empiric therapy for isolated dysphonia
- Surgical therapy can improve voice outcomes in glottic insufficiency and selected benign vocal fold lesions not resolving after voice therapy [Level 4]

ACKNOWLEDGMENTS

The authors thank Al Merati, MD, for his review of the manuscript.

REFERENCES

1. Roy N, Merrill RM, Gray SD, et al. Voice disorders in the general population: prevalence, risk factors, and occupational impact. Laryngoscope 2005;115(11): 1988–95.
2. Roy N, Merrill RM, Thibeault S, et al. Prevalence of voice disorders in teachers and the general population. J Speech Lang Hear Res 2004;47(2):281–93.
3. Duff MC, Proctor A, Yairi E. Prevalence of voice disorders in African American and European American preschoolers. J Voice 2004;18(3):348–53.
4. Carding PN, Roulstone S, Northstone K, et al. The prevalence of childhood dysphonia: a cross-sectional study. J Voice 2006;20(4):623–30.
5. Silverman EM. Incidence of chronic hoarseness among school-age children. J Speech Hear Disord 1975;40(2):211–5.
6. Roy N, Stemple J, Merrill RM, et al. Epidemiology of voice disorders in the elderly: preliminary findings. Laryngoscope 2007;117:628–33.
7. Golub JS, Chen PH, Otto KJ, et al. Prevalence of perceived dysphonia in a geriatric population. J Am Geriatr Soc 2006;54(11):1736–9.

8. Coyle SM, Weinrich BD, Stemple JC. Shifts in relative prevalence of laryngeal pathology in a treatment-seeking population. J Voice 2001;15(3):424–40.

9. Titze IR, Lemke J, Montequin D. Populations in the US workforce who rely on voice as a primary tool of trade: a preliminary report. J Voice 1997;11(3):254–9.

10. Jones K, Sigmon J, Hock L, et al. Prevalence and risk factors for voice problems among telemarketers. Arch Otolaryngol Head Neck Surg 2002;128(5):571–7.

11. Long J, Williford HN, Olson MS, et al. Voice problems and risk factors among aerobics instructors. J Voice 1998;12(2):197–207.

12. Smith E, Kirchner HL, Taylor M, et al. Voice problems among teachers: differences by gender and teaching characteristics. J Voice 1998;12(3):328–34.

13. Cohen SM, Dupont WD, Courey MS. Quality-of-life impact of nonneoplastic voice disorders: a meta-analysis. Ann Otol Rhinol Laryngol 2006;115(2):128–34.

14. Benninger MS, Ahuja AS, Gardner G, et al. Assessing outcomes for dysphonic patients. J Voice 1998;12(4):540–50.

15. Mirza N, Ruiz C, Baum ED, et al. The prevalence of major psychiatric pathologies in patients with voice disorders. Ear Nose Throat J 2003;82(10):808–10, 812, 814.

16. Rosen CA, Lee AS, Osborne J, et al. Development and validation of the voice handicap index-10. Laryngoscope 2004;114(9):1549–56.

17. Ramig LO, Verdolini K. Treatment efficacy: voice disorders. J Speech Lang Hear Res 1998;41(1):S101–16.

18. Schwartz SR, Cohen SM, Dailey SH, et al. Clinical practice guideline: hoarseness (dysphonia). Otolaryngol Head Neck Surg 2009;141(3 Suppl 2):S1–31.

19. Johnson JT, Newman RK, Olson JE. Persistent hoarseness: an aggressive approach for early detection of laryngeal cancer. Postgrad Med 1980;67(5): 122–6.

20. Klein HC. Light up the larynx. JAMA 1976;236(9):1017.

21. Barker M, Dort JC. Laryngeal examination: a comparison of mirror examination with a rigid lens system. J Otolaryngol 1991;20(2):100–3.

22. Dunklebarger J, Rhee D, Kim S, et al. Video rigid laryngeal endoscopy compared to laryngeal mirror examination: an assessment of patient comfort and clinical visualization. Laryngoscope 2009;119(2):269–71.

23. Lacoste L, Karayan J, Lehuede MS. A comparison of direct, indirect, and fiberoptic laryngoscopy to evaluate vocal cord paralysis after thyroid surgery. Thyroid 1996;6(1):17–21.

24. Merati AL, Rieder AA. Normal endoscopic anatomy of the pharynx and larynx. Am J Med 2003;115(Suppl 3A):10S–4S.

25. Eller R, Ginsburg M, Lurie D, et al. Flexible laryngoscopy: a comparison of fiber optic and distal chip technologies. Part 1: vocal fold masses. J Voice 2008; 22(6):746–50.

26. Feierabend RH, Shahram MN. Hoarseness in adults. Am Fam Physician 2009; 80(4):363–70.

27. Hammer MJ, Barlow SM. Laryngeal somatosensory deficits in Parkinson's disease: implications for speech respiratory and phonatory control. Exp Brain Res 2010;201(3):401–9.

28. Mau T. Diagnostic evaluation and management of hoarseness. Med Clin North Am 2010;94(5):945–60.

29. Sataloff RT, Hawkshaw MJ, Divi V, et al. Physical examination of voice professionals. Otolaryngol Clin North Am 2007;40(5):953–69, v–vi.

30. Sataloff RT, Spiegel JR, Hawkshaw MJ. Strobovideolaryngoscopy: results and clinical value. Ann Otol Rhinol Laryngol 1991;100(9 Pt 1):725–7.

31. Casiano RR, Zaveri V, Lundy DS. Efficacy of videostroboscopy in the diagnosis of voice disorders. Otolaryngol Head Neck Surg 1992;107(1):95–100.
32. Kennedy TL, Gilroy PA, Millman B. Strobovideolaryngoscopy in the management of acute laryngeal trauma. J Voice 2004;18(1):130–7.
33. Mortensen M, Schaberg M, Woo P. Diagnostic contributions of videolaryngostroboscopy in the pediatric population. Arch Otolaryngol Head Neck Surg 2010; 136(1):75–9.
34. Patel R, Dailey S, Bless D. Comparison of high-speed digital imaging with stroboscopy for laryngeal imaging of glottal disorders. Ann Otol Rhinol Laryngol 2008;117(6):413–24.
35. Kaszuba SM, Garrett CG. Strobovideolaryngoscopy and laboratory voice evaluation. Otolaryngol Clin North Am 2011;40(5):991–1001, vi.
36. Deliyski DD, Hillman RE. State of the art laryngeal imaging: research and clinical implications. Curr Opin Otolaryngol Head Neck Surg 2010;18(3):147–52.
37. Krausert CR, Olszewski AE, Taylor LN, et al. Mucosal wave measurements and visualization techniques. J Voice 2011;25(4):395–405.
38. Poels PJ, de Jong FI, Schutte HK. Consistency of the preoperative and intraoperative diagnosis of benign vocal fold lesions. J Voice 2003;17(3):425–33.
39. Dailey SH, Spanou K, Zeitels SM. The evaluation of benign glottis lesions: rigid telescopic stroboscopy versus suspension microlaryngoscopy. J Voice 2007; 21(1):112–8.
40. Halum SL, Patel N, Smith TL, et al. Laryngeal electromyography for adult unilateral vocal fold immobility: a survey of the American Broncho-Esophagological Association. Ann Otol Rhinol Laryngol 2005;114(6):425–8.
41. Blitzer A, Crumley RL, Dailey SH, et al. Recommendations of the Neurolaryngology Study Group on laryngeal electromyography. Otolaryngol Head Neck Surg 2009;140(6):782–93.
42. Koufman JA, Postma GN, Whang CS. Diagnostic laryngeal electromyography: the Wake Forest experience 1995-1999. Otolaryngol Head Neck Surg 2001; 124(6):603–6.
43. Meyer TK, Hillel AD. Is laryngeal electromyography useful in the diagnosis and management of vocal fold paresis/paralysis? Laryngoscope 2011;121(2):234–5.
44. Heman-Ackah YD, Barr A. The value of laryngeal electromyography in the evaluation of laryngeal motion abnormalities. J Voice 2006;20(3):452–60.
45. Simpson CB, Cheung EJ, Jackson CJ. Vocal fold paresis: clinical and electrophysiologic features in a tertiary laryngology practice. J Voice 2009;23(3): 396–8.
46. Sataloff RT, Praneetvatakul P, Heuer RJ, et al. Laryngeal electromyography: clinical application. J Voice 2010;24(2):228–34.
47. Stager SV, Bielamowicz SA. Using laryngeal electromyography to differentiate presbylarynges from paresis. J Speech Lang Hear Res 2010;53(1):100–13.
48. Gavazzoni FB, Scola RH, Lorenzoni PJ, et al. The clinical value of laryngeal electromyography in laryngeal immobility. J Clin Neurosci 2011;18(4):524–7.
49. Hydman J, Bjorck G, Persson JK, et al. Diagnosis and prognosis of iatrogenic injury of the recurrent laryngeal nerve. Ann Otol Rhinol Laryngol 2009;118(7): 506–11.
50. Merati AL, Halum SL, Smith TL. Diagnostic testing for vocal fold paralysis: survey of practice and evidence-based medicine review. Laryngoscope 2006; 116(9):1539–52.
51. Glastonbury CM. Non-oncologic imaging of the larynx. Otolaryngol Clin North Am 2008;41(1):139–56, vi.

52. Pretorius PM, Milford CA. Investigating the hoarse voice. BMJ 2008;337:a1726.
53. El Badawey MR, Punekar S, Zammit-Maempel I. Prospective study to assess vocal cord palsy investigations. Otolaryngol Head Neck Surg 2008;138(6): 788–90.
54. Wippold FJ 2nd. Head and neck imaging: the role of CT and MRI. J Magn Reson Imaging 2007;25(3):453–65.
55. Ng SH, Chang TC, Ko SF. Nasopharyngeal carcinoma: MRI and CT assessment. Neuroradiology 1997;39(10):741–6.
56. Xie CM, Liang BL, Wu PH, et al. Spiral computed tomography (CT) and magnetic resonance imaging (MRI) in assessment of the skull base encroachment in nasopharyngeal carcinoma. Ai Zheng 2003;22(7):729–33 [in Chinese].
57. Liu AY, Yousem DM, Chalian AA. Economic consequences of diagnostic imaging for vocal cord paralysis. Acad Radiol 2001;8(2):137–48.
58. Stecco A, Sapanaro A, Carriero A. Patient safety issues in magnetic resonance imaging: state of the art. Radiol Med 2007;112(4):491–508.
59. Jaffurs D, Denny A. Diagnostic pediatric computed tomographic scans of the head: actual dosage versus estimated risk. Plast Reconstr Surg 2009;124(4): 1254–60.
60. Mazonakis MA, Tzedakis A, Damilakis J, et al. Thyroid dose from common head and neck CT examinations in children: is there an excess risk for thyroid cancer induction? Eur Radiol 2007;17(5):1352–7.
61. Serafini G, Zadra N. Anaesthesia for MRI in the paediatric patient. Curr Opin Anaesthesiol 2008;21(4):499–503.
62. Kannikeswaran N, Mahajan PV, Sethuraman U, et al. Sedation medications received and adverse events related to sedation for brain MRI in children with and without developmental disabilities. Paediatr Anaesth 2009;19(3): 250–6.
63. Metzner J, Domino KB. Risks of anesthesia or sedation outside the operating room: the role of the anesthesia care provider. Curr Opin Anaesthesiol 2010; 23(4):523–31.
64. Maertens K, de Jong FI. The voice handicap index as a tool for assessment of the biopsychosocial impact of voice problems. B-ENT 2007;3(2):61–6.
65. Morzaria S, Damrose EJ. A comparison of the VHI, VHI-10, and V-RQOL for measuring the effect of botox therapy in adductor spasmodic dysphonia. J Voice 2010;26(3):378–80. [Epub ahead of print].
66. Murry T, Medrado R, Hogikyan ND. The relationship between ratings of voice quality and quality of life measures. J Voice 2004;18(2):183–92.
67. Kasper C, Schuster M, Psychogios G, et al. Voice handicap index and voice-related quality of life in small laryngeal carcinoma. Eur Arch Otorhinolaryngol 2011;268(3):401–4.
68. Xu W, Han D, Li H. Application of the mandarin Chinese version of the voice handicap index. J Voice 2010;24(6):702–7.
69. Yamaguchi H, Shrivastav R, Andrews ML, et al. A comparison of voice quality ratings made by Japanese and American listeners using the GRBAS scale. Folia Phoniatr Logop 2003;55(3):147–57.
70. Kazi R, De Cordova J, Singh A. Voice-related quality of life in laryngectomees: assessment using the VHI and V-RQOL symptom scales. J Voice 2007;21(6): 728–34.
71. Lundstrom E, Hambarberg B, Munck-Wikland E. Voice handicap and health-related quality of life in laryngectomees: assessments with the use of VHI and EORTC questionnaires. Folia Phoniatr Logop 2009;61(2):83–91.

72. da Costa de Ceballos AG, Carvalho FM, de Araujo TM, et al. Diagnostic validity of Voice Handicap Index-10 (VHI-10) compared with perceptive-auditory and acoustic speech pathology evaluations of the voice. J Voice 2010;24(6): 715–8.

73. Kempster GB, Garratt BR, Verdolini Abbott K, et al. Consensus auditory-perceptual evaluation of voice: development of a standardized clinical protocol. Am J Speech Lang Pathol 2009;18(2):124–32.

74. Zraick RI, Kempster GB, Conner NP. Establishing validity of the Consensus Auditory-Perceptual Evaluation of Voice (CAPE-V). Am J Speech Lang Pathol 2011;20(1):14–22.

75. Thomas LB, Stemple JC. Voice therapy: does science support the art? Commun Dis Rev 2007;1(1):49–77.

76. Helou LB, Solomon NP, Henry LR, et al. The role of listener experience on Consensus Auditory-Perceptual Evaluation of Voice (CAPE-V) ratings of post-thyroidectomy voice. Am J Speech Lang Pathol 2010;19(3):248–58.

77. Solomon NP, Helou LB, Stojadinovic A. Clinical versus laboratory ratings of voice using the CAPE-V. J Voice 2011;25(1):e7–14.

78. Leonard R. Voice therapy and vocal nodules in adults. Curr Opin Otolaryngol Head Neck Surg 2009;17(6):453–7.

79. McCrory E. Voice therapy outcomes in vocal fold nodules: a retrospective audit. Int J Lang Commun Disord 2001;36(Suppl):19–24.

80. Sulica L, Behrman A. Management of benign vocal fold lesions: a survey of current opinion and practice. Ann Otol Rhinol Laryngol 2003;112(10): 827–33.

81. Cohen SM, Garrett CG. Utility of voice therapy in the management of vocal fold polyps and cysts. Otolaryngol Head Neck Surg 2007;136(5):742–6.

82. D'Alatri L, Galla S, Rigante M, et al. Role of early voice therapy in patients affected by unilateral vocal fold paralysis. J Laryngol Otol 2008;122(9):936–41.

83. Mattioli F, Bergamini G, Alicandri-Ciufelli M, et al. The role of early voice therapy in the incidence of motility recovery in unilateral vocal fold paralysis. Logoped Phoniatr Vocol 2011;36(1):40–7.

84. Schindler A, Bottero A, Capaccio P, et al. Vocal improvement after voice therapy in unilateral vocal fold paralysis. J Voice 2008;22(1):113–8.

85. Sauder C, Roy N, Tanner K, et al. Vocal function exercises for presbylaryngis: a multidimensional assessment of treatment outcomes. Ann Otol Rhinol Laryngol 2010;119(7):460–7.

86. Gartner-Schmidt J, Rosen C. Treatment success for age-related vocal fold atrophy. Laryngoscope 2011;121(3):585–9.

87. Van Houtte E, Van Lierde K, Claeys S. Pathophysiology and treatment of muscle tension dysphonia: a review of the current knowledge. J Voice 2011;25(2): 202–7.

88. Leung AK, Kellner JD, Johnson DW. Viral croup: a current perspective. J Pediatr Health Care 2004;18(6):297–301.

89. Jackson-Menaldi CA, Dzul AI, Holland RW. Allergies and vocal fold edema: a preliminary report. J Voice 1999;13(1):113–22.

90. Jackson-Menaldi CA, Dzul AI, Holland RW. Hidden respiratory allergies in voice users: treatment strategies. Logoped Phoniatr Vocol 2002;27(2):74–9.

91. Rennie CE, Dwivedi RC, Khan AS, et al. Lichen planus of the larynx. J Laryngol Otol 2011;125(4):432–5.

92. Dean CM, Sataloff RT, Hawkshaw MJ, et al. Laryngeal sarcoidosis. J Voice 2002; 16(2):283–8.

93. Mayerhoff RM, Pitman MJ. Atypical and disparate presentations of laryngeal sarcoidosis. Ann Otol Rhinol Laryngol 2010;119(10):667–71.
94. Ozcan KM, Bahar S, Ozcan I, et al. Laryngeal involvement in systemic lupus erythematosus: report of two cases. J Clin Rheumatol 2007;13(5):278–9.
95. Vasiliou A, Nikolopoulos TP, Manolopoulos L, et al. Laryngeal pemphigus without skin manifestations and review of the literature. Eur Arch Otorhinolaryngol 2007; 264(5):509–12.
96. Eng J, Sabanathan S. Airway complications in relapsing polychondritis. Ann Thorac Surg 1991;51(4):686–92.
97. Woo JH, Kim DY, Kim JW, et al. Efficacy of percutaneous vocal fold injections for benign laryngeal lesions: prospective multicenter study. Acta Otolaryngol 2011; 131(12):1326–32.
98. Woodbury K, Smith LJ. Relapsing polychondritis: a rare etiology of dysphonia and novel approach to treatment. Laryngoscope 2011;121(5):1006–8.
99. Krespi YP, Mitrani M, Husain S, et al. Treatment of laryngeal sarcoidosis with intralesional steroid injection. Ann Otol Rhinol Laryngol 1987;96(6):713–5.
100. Mortensen M, Woo P. Office steroid injections of the larynx. Laryngoscope 2006; 116(10):1735–9.
101. Tateya I, Omori K, Kojima H, et al. Steroid injection for Reinke's edema using fiberoptic laryngeal surgery. Acta Otolaryngol 2003;123(3):417–20.
102. Lee SH, Yeo JO, Choi JI, et al. Local steroid injection via the cricothryoid membrane in patients with a vocal nodule. Arch Otolaryngol Head Neck Surg 2011;137(10):1011–6.
103. Tateya I, Omori K, Kojima H, et al. Steroid injection to vocal nodules using fiberoptic laryngeal surgery under topical anesthesia. Eur Arch Otorhinolaryngol 2004;261(9):489–92.
104. Reveiz L, Cardona AF, Ospina EG. Antibiotics for acute laryngitis in adults. Cochrane Database Syst Rev 2007;(2):CD004783. http://dx.doi.org/10.1002/ 14651858.CD004783.pub3.
105. Koufman JA. The otolaryngologic manifestations of gastroesophageal reflux disease (GERD): a clinical investigation of 225 patients using ambulatory 24-hour pH monitoring and an experimental investigation of the role of acid and pepsin in the development of laryngeal injury. Laryngoscope 1991;101(4 Pt 2 Suppl 53):1–78.
106. Hopkins C, Yousaf U, Pedersen M. Acid reflux treatment for hoarseness. Cochrane Database Syst Rev 2006;(1):CD005054. http://dx.doi.org/10.1002/ 14651858.CD005054.pub2.
107. Reichel O, Dressel H, Wiederanders K, et al. Double-blind, placebo-controlled trial with esomeprazole for symptoms and signs associated with laryngopharyngeal reflux. Otolaryngol Head Neck Surg 2008;139(3):414–20.
108. Masaany M, Marina MB, Sharifa Ezat WP, et al. Empirical treatment with pantoprazole as a diagnostic tool for symptomatic adult laryngopharyngeal reflux. J Laryngol Otol 2011;125(5):502–8.
109. Vinson KN, Zraick RI, Raglan FJ. Injection versus medialization laryngoplasty for the treatment of unilateral vocal fold paralysis: follow-up at six months. Laryngoscope 2010;120(9):1802–7.
110. Johns MM, Garrett CG, Hwang J, et al. Quality-of-life outcomes following laryngeal endoscopic surgery for non-neoplastic vocal fold lesions. Ann Otol Rhinol Laryngol 2004;113(8):597–601.
111. Morgan JE, Zraick RI, Griffin AW, et al. Injection versus medialization laryngoplasty for the treatment of unilateral vocal fold paralysis. Laryngoscope 2007; 117(11):2068–74.

112. Arviso LC, Johns MM 3rd, Mathison CC, et al. Long-term outcomes of injection laryngoplasty in patients with potentially recoverable vocal fold paralysis. Laryngoscope 2010;120(11):2237–40.
113. Yung KC, Likhterov I, Courey MS. Effect of temporary vocal fold injection medialization on the rate of permanent medialization laryngoplasty in unilateral vocal fold paralysis patients. Laryngoscope 2011;121(10):2191–4.
114. Rosen CA, Gartner-Schmidt J, Casiano R, et al. Vocal fold augmentation with calcium hydroxylapatite: twelve-month report. Laryngoscope 2009;119(5): 1033–41.
115. Carroll TL, Rosen CA. Long-term results of calcium hydroxylapatite for vocal fold augmentation. Laryngoscope 2011;121(2):313–9.
116. Song PC, Sung CK, Franco RA Jr. Voice outcomes after endoscopic injection laryngoplasty with hyaluronic acid stabilized gel. Laryngoscope 2010; 120(Suppl 4):S199.
117. Karpenko AN, Dworkin JP, Meleca RJ, et al. Cymetra injection for unilateral vocal fold paralysis. Ann Otol Rhinol Laryngol 2003;112(11):927–34.
118. Milstein CF, Akst LM, Hicks MD, et al. Long-term effects of micronized Alloderm injection for unilateral vocal fold paralysis. Laryngoscope 2005;115(9):1691–6.
119. Remacle M, Lawson G, Jamart J, et al. Treatment of vocal fold immobility by injectable homologous collagen: short-term results. Eur Arch Otorhinolaryngol 2006;263(3):205–9.
120. Kimura M, Nito T, Sakakibara K, et al. Clinical experience with collagen injection of the vocal fold: a study of 155 patients. Auris Nasus Larynx 2008;35(1):67–75.
121. Tan M, Woo P. Injection laryngoplasty with micronized dermis: a 10-year experience with 381 injections in 344 patients. Laryngoscope 2010;120(12):2460–6.
122. Reijonen P, Tervonen H, Harinen K, et al. Long-term results of autologous fascia in unilateral vocal fold paralysis. Eur Arch Otorhinolaryngol 2009; 266(8):1273–8.
123. Cantarella G, Mazzola RF, Domenichini E, et al. Vocal fold augmentation by autologous fat injection with lipostructure procedure. Otolaryngol Head Neck Surg 2005;132(2):239–43.
124. Hsiung MW, Pai L. Autogenous fat injection for glottic insufficiency: analysis of 101 cases and correlation with patients' self-assessment. Acta Otolaryngol 2006;126(2):191–6.
125. Lee SW, Son YI, Kim CH, et al. Voice outcomes of polyacrylamide hydrogel injection laryngoplasty. Laryngoscope 2007;117(10):1871–5.
126. Hertegård S, Hallén L, Laurent C, et al. Cross-linked hyaluronan versus collagen for injection treatment of glottal insufficiency: 2-year follow-up. Acta Otolaryngol 2004;124(10):1208–14.
127. Sulica L, Rosen CA, Postma GN, et al. Current practice in injection augmentation of the vocal folds: indications, treatment principles, techniques, and complications. Laryngoscope 2010;120(2):319–25.
128. Chester MW, Stewart MG. Arytenoid adduction combined with medialization thyroplasty: an evidence-based review. Otolaryngol Head Neck Surg 2003;129(4): 305–10.
129. Li AJ, Johns MM, Jackson-Menaldi C, et al. Glottic closure patterns: type I thyroplasty versus type I thyroplasty with arytenoids adduction. J Voice 2011;25(3): 259–64.
130. Paniello RC, Edgar JD, Kallogjeri D, et al. Medialization versus reinnervation for unilateral vocal fold paralysis: a multicenter randomized clinical trial. Laryngoscope 2011;121(10):2172–9.

Evidence-Based Practice
Endoscopic Skull Base Resection for Malignancy

Rounak B. Rawal[a], Mitchell R. Gore[a], Richard J. Harvey[b],
Adam M. Zanation, MD[a,*]

KEYWORDS

- Evidence-based otolaryngology • Malignant cancer • Head and neck cancer
- Endoscopic resection • Skull base

KEY POINTS

The following points list the level of evidence based on Oxford Center for Evidence-Based Medicine guidelines.

- Esthesioneuroblastoma—Endoscopic approaches may provide higher survival rates compared with traditional craniofacial open surgery. Level 2A.
- Sinonasal melanoma—Traditional craniofacial resection remains the gold standard, but endoscopic methods may provide similar rates of long-term survival for patients. Level 4.
- Nasopharyngeal carcinoma—Endoscopic approaches may provide optimistic results, but evidence comparing outcomes with traditional craniofacial resection is lacking. Level 4.
- Sinonasal adenocarcinoma (SNAC)—Endoscopic approaches may provide optimistic results, but evidence comparing outcomes with traditional craniofacial resection is lacking. Level 4.
- Sinonasal undifferentiated carcinoma (SNUC)—Two-year survival rates for endoscopic approaches are encouraging, but further prospective comparative data are necessary. Level 4.

OVERVIEW OF SINONASAL AND SKULL BASE CANCER

Initial interest in endonasal skull base surgery was first described by Caton and Paul in the late 19th century. Since that time, advances in anatomic knowledge, technology, and level of comfort with endoscopic techniques have allowed the use of combined and wholly endoscopic surgery for various sinonasal malignancies. Endoscopy of

Financial disclosures: RBR gratefully acknowledges support from the Doris Duke Charitable Foundation to University of North Carolina for support of the Clinical Research Fellowship. The authors have no other funding, financial relationships, or conflicts of interest to disclose related to this article.
[a] Department of Otolaryngology-Head and Neck Surgery, University of North Carolina at Chapel Hill, 170 Manning Drive, CB 7070, Chapel Hill, NC 27599-7070, USA; [b] Department of Otolaryngology/Skull Base Surgery, St Vincent's Hospital, 390 Victoria Street, Darlinghurst, Sydney, New South Wales 2010, Australia
* Corresponding author.
E-mail address: adam_zanation@med.unc.edu

Otolaryngol Clin N Am 45 (2012) 1127–1142
http://dx.doi.org/10.1016/j.otc.2012.06.013
0030-6665/12/$ – see front matter © 2012 Elsevier Inc. All rights reserved.

benign tumors allowed for decreased complication rates, reduction in brain retraction, and minimization of neurologic morbidity. Once surgeons were comfortable with resection of sinonasal and skull base benign tumors, attention shifted toward the use of endoscopic methods for sinonasal malignancy.[1,2]

Although there has been a shift in interest away from traditional craniofacial resection (tCFR), use of endoscopy has not changed the principles of oncologic surgery. The primary goal is still complete resection of tumor with negative margins and minimization of morbidity.[3] The use of endoscopy assists by providing superior visualization, higher magnification of vital structures, assurance of appropriate margins, avoidance of cosmetic deformity, and preservation of normal anatomy.[4]

The endoscopic approach has encountered its own criticisms. Resection of the tumor often requires a piecemeal approach and may theoretically increase the chance of tumor seeding.[5] Achievement of hemostasis, adequate visualization, and ability to perform reconstruction are additional barriers facing endoscopic approaches. Early results tend to be encouraging, however. A recent literature review found that endoscopy offers better quality of life outcomes than tCFR,[6] and a second study found a decrease in morbidity when using the endoscopic approach compared with open tCFR.[7] Although these studies are encouraging, further research is necessary when evaluating the endoscopic resection of malignant tumors.

Malignancies of the sinonasal tract and skull base encompass a heterogeneous, diverse group with respect to etiology, epidemiology, and histology, as classified by the World Health Organization.[8] As such, treatment of disease must be specifically tailored to each disease process. Reporting on homogeneous skull base outcomes becomes difficult, especially because sinonasal malignancies are rare and thus outcomes often cannot be reported with sufficient power. Because squamous cell carcinoma is so heterogeneous in presentation and outcome, it has been excluded from this review.

INCIDENCE AND EPIDEMIOLOGY OF SINONASAL AND SKULL BASE CANCER
Esthesioneuroblastoma

- Esthesioneuroblastoma, also known as olfactory neuroblastoma, is a rare tumor, constituting only 3% to 4% of all intranasal tumors.[9,10]
- Esthesioneuroblastoma has a bimodal distribution, with peaks between ages 11 and 20 years and then ages 51 and 60 years.[11,12]

The precise cause of esthesioneuroblastoma remains unclear, although the cell of origin is believed to be the specialized sensory neuroepithelial olfactory cells normally found in the upper part of the nasal cavity, which includes the superior nasal concha, the upper part of the septum, the roof of the nose, and the cribriform plate of the ethmoid.[13]

Sinonasal Melanoma

- Mucosal melanoma accounted for only 1.3% of 85,000 cases of patients with melanoma during a 10-year period as reported by the National Cancer Data Base.[14]
- The incidence of mucosal melanoma differs between geographic and racial boundaries, being particularly common in Japan.[15]
- Of those patients with mucosal melanoma, 55% of lesions were found in the head and neck.
- Mucosal melanoma of the head and neck region has a peak incidence in patients aged 60 to 80 years, with a mean age of presentation of 64.3 years.[16]

The prognosis of patients with sinonasal melanoma is poor. Five-year survival rates range from 14% to 45%.[17-20] The nasal cavity is the most common site of origin, followed by maxillary and ethmoid sinuses.[21] Most patients with mucosal melanoma are asymptomatic, allowing for insidious growth before discovery. Although most patients present without metastasis, one-third of all patients will eventually develop regional or distant metastasis; median time to death after distant metastasis is 3 months.[22]

Nasopharyngeal Carcinoma (NPC)

- In the United States, nasopharyngeal carcinoma (NPC) is rare, with an incidence of less than 1 per 100,000 person-years.[23]
- NPC has a distinct geographic and ethnic variation, being highly endemic to the Cantonese living in the central region of Guangdong Province in southern China.[24]
- The male-to-female ratio is 2:1.
- NPC has a bimodal age distribution, with the first peak occurring in late childhood and a second peak occurring between people aged 50 to 60 years.[25]
- Risk factors for NPC include high levels of Epstein-Barr virus (EBV) antibody titers, family history of NPC, consumption of salt-preserved fish, cigarette smoking, and occupational exposure to formaldehyde and wood dust.

Other than dietary modification, however, no definitive preventative measures have been published.[23] NPC is thought to arise from the epithelial lining of the nasopharynx. The World Health Organization classifies NPC into 3 different types based on degree of differentiation on histopathology (**Table 1**).[8]

Sinonasal Adenocarcinoma (SNAC)

Sinonasal adenocarcinoma (SNAC) comprises 11.4% of all sinonasal tumors[26] and refers to one of several types of tumors. SNAC may be further subdivided into intestinal-type adenocarcinoma (ITAC) and non–intestinal-type adenocarcinoma (non-ITAC), which can be further subdivided into low- and high-grade types (**Fig. 1**).[27,28]

Sinonasal ITAC

Sinonasal ITAC actually consists of a heterogeneous mix of tumors that may be further classified, as published by Barnes (**Table 2**).[29] Each subtype has its own epidemiology, outcomes, and clinically significant differences that are beyond the scope of this article. In general, the prognosis of SNAC is poor, with a 5-year survival between 20% and 50%.[30]

- ITAC has been closely related to occupational exposure to wood and leather dust in many countries, sometimes presenting up to 40 years after exposure.[31]
- Workers in the wood furniture–making industries have up to 500 times the risk of developing ITAC as those in the general population.[32] This occupational exposure may also be the reason why ITAC affects males up to 3 times more often than females, with a mean age of presentation at 65 years old.[33]

Table 1	
World Health Organization classification of NPC	
Stage	**Histopathology**
I	Keratinizing squamous cell carcinoma
II	Nonkeratinizing carcinoma
III	Basaloid squamous cell carcinoma

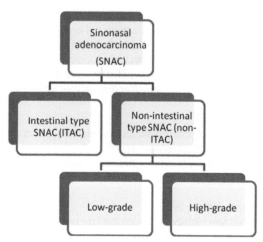

Fig. 1. World Health Organization classification of SNACs.

The theory that ITAC is caused by particulate matter is further corroborated by evidence that the middle and lower turbinates are most affected.[34] Definitive carcinogenic cause for ITAC, however, remains to be discovered.

Sinonasal Non-ITAC

Sinonasal non-ITAC is further subdivided into low-grade and high-grade subtypes, with distinguishing characteristics for each. High-grade non-ITACs are usually marked by increased cytologic atypia, necrosis of adjacent tissue, and higher degrees of mitotic activity.[8]

- High-grade non-ITACs have a more rapid course, with a 3-year survival of 20%,[35] whereas low-grade tumors have excellent prognosis, with 5-year survival of up to 85%.[36]
- Anatomic location of non-ITAC also differs, with high-grade tumors mainly presenting in the maxillary sinus,[36] whereas low-grade ITAC present most commonly in the nasal cavity, followed by the ethmoid and maxillary sinuses.[28]

Table 2
Classification of and survival for intestinal-type SNACs

Barnes	Klesinsasser and Schroede	3-Year Cumulative Survival
Papillary	PTCC - I	82%
Colonic	PTCC - II	54%
Solid	PTCC - III	36%
Mucinous	Alveolar goblet	48%
	Signet ring	0%
Mixed	Transitional	71%

Abbreviation: PTCC, papillary tubular cylinder cell.
Data from Barnes L. Intestinal-type adenocarcinoma of the nasal cavity and paranasal sinuses. Am J Surg Pathol 1986;10(3):192–202; and Kleinsasser O, Schroeder HG. Adenocarcinomas of the inner nose after exposure to wood dust. Morphological findings and relationships between histopathology and clinical behavior in 79 cases. Arch Otorhinolaryngol 1988;245:1–15.

Sinonasal Undifferentiated Carcinoma (SNUC)

Sinonasal undifferentiated carcinoma (SNUC) is a recently recognized, rapidly progressive pathologic entity.

- First described in 1986, its median survival time was first reported at 4 months at the time of diagnosis.[37] Since then, survival time has advanced to a still-dismal 1 year from the time of diagnosis.[38]
- The cause of SNUC remains unknown, especially because SNUC has no association with the EBV.[39]
- Median age of SNUC at diagnosis has been reported to be 50 to 57 years, with an age range of 20 to 84 years.[40]
- Poor prognostic factors include dural invasion and orbital involvement at the time of diagnosis.[41]

EVIDENCE-BASED CLINICAL ASSESSMENT AND DIAGNOSTIC TESTING
Esthesioneuroblastoma Staging

There is no current consensus on the most accurate staging method of esthesioneuroblastoma. Staging was first proposed in 1976 by Kadish and colleagues[42] and has since been modified by Morita and colleagues[12] to divide the malignancy into 4 subtypes based on metastasis (**Table 3**). Other staging methods requiring various procedures have been previously described. Biller and colleagues proposed a staging system that required craniotomy,[43] Dulguerov and Calcaterra described a staging system that required imaging (**Table 4**),[44] and Hyams described a staging system requiring histopathologic specimens.[45] Other authors have argued that combining 1 or more of these staging systems can yield better predictions for patient outcomes than any one of those staging systems alone.[46]

Although PET imaging has been used for occasional case reports,[47,48] no current guidelines exist for its role in the newly diagnosed esthesioneuroblastoma. Dissemination to the cervical lymph nodes is the most common location for metastasis, with an overall rate of metastasis between 20% and 25% of all esthesioneuroblastomas.[49,50] A recent meta-analysis by Zanation and colleagues[51] shows that if clinical, radiographic, or cytologic evidence of esthesioneuroblastoma is apparent, treatment with neck dissection followed by radiotherapy should be instituted. Very limited data exist regarding whether elective treatment of the neck would improve prognosis.

Sinonasal Melanoma Staging

Many staging systems for sinonasal melanoma have been published and no system has been accepted as the gold standard. Thompson and colleagues[52] proposed a

Table 3
Modified Kadish staging for esthesioneuroblastoma

Stage	Extension
A	Tumor limited to the nasal cavity
B	Tumor involving the nasal and paranasal sinuses
C	Tumor extending beyond the nasal and paranasal sinuses, including involvement of the cribriform plate, base of the skull, orbit cavity, or intracranial cavity
D	Tumor with metastasis to cervical nodes or distant sites

Data from Morita A, Ebersold MJ, Olsen KD, et al. Esthesioneuroblastoma: prognosis and management. Neurosurgery 1993;32(5):706–14 [discussion: 714–5]; and Kadish S, Goodman M, Wang CC. Olfactory neuroblastoma. A clinical analysis of 17 cases. Cancer 1976;37(3):1571–6.

Table 4
Dulguerov and Calcaterra staging for esthesioneuroblastoma

Type	Extension
T1	Tumor involving the nasal cavity and/or paranasal sinuses (excluding the sphenoid sinus), sparing the most superior ethmoidal cells
T2	Tumor involving the nasal cavity and/or paranasal sinuses (including the sphenoid sinus) with extension to, or erosion of, the cribriform plate
T3	Tumor extending into the orbit or protruding into the anterior cranial fossa, without dural invasion
T4	Tumor involving the brain

From Dulguerov P, Calcaterra T. Esthesioneuroblastoma: the UCLA experience 1970–1990. Laryngoscope 1992;102(8):843–9; with permission.

combined staging system for sinonasal melanoma that parallels the TNM staging concept, combining classifications that incorporate features of size (Clark level and Breslow thickness), sites of anatomic involvement (T category, Kadish and colleagues[12] and Freedman and colleagues[53]), and the importance of distant spread (Ballantyne[54] and Chang and colleagues[14]) (**Table 5**).

A recent study by Gal and colleagues[21] evaluated staging of sinonasal melanoma according to both the American Joint Committee on Cancer (AJCC) 6th edition site-specific staging classification[55] and the newer AJCC 7th edition site-specific staging classification (**Table 6**).[56] Gal and colleagues[21] found that the newer staging system is

Table 5
Thompson staging system for sinonasal tract and nasopharynx mucosal malignant melanoma

Nasal cavity, paranasal sinuses, and nasopharynx histopathology staging	
Primary tumor	
T1	Single anatomic site
T2	Two or more anatomic sites
Regional lymph node	
N1	Any lymph node metastasis
Distant metastasis	
M1	Distant metastasis
Stage grouping	
Stage I	T1, N0, M0
Stage II	T2, N0, M0
Stage III	Any T, any N, M1
Stage IV	Any T, any N, M

T1, tumor limited to a single anatomic site. A single anatomic site is defined as 1 of the following: nasal cavity, maxillary sinus, frontal sinus, ethmoid sinus, sphenoid sinus, or nasopharynx. Subsites, such as septum, lateral wall, turbinate, nasal floor, or nasal vestibule, are not separately considered.

T2, tumor involving more than 1 anatomic site. More than 1 anatomic site is defined by tumor involvement of more than 1 anatomic site (although not subsite) as cited for T1, including any extension into subcutaneous tissues, skin, palate, pterygoid plate, floor, wall, or apex of the orbit, cribriform plate, infratemporal fossa, dura, brain, middle cranial fossa, cranial nerves, clivus.

From Thompson LD, Wieneke JA, Miettinen M. Sinonasal tract and nasopharyngeal melanomas: a clinicopathologic study of 115 cases with a proposed staging system. Am J Surg Pathol 2003;27(5):594–611; with permission.

Table 6
Staging of mucosal melanoma of the head and neck, AJCC guidelines, 7th edition

Primary tumor (T)	
T3	Mucosal disease
T4a	Moderately advanced disease; tumor involving deep soft tissue, cartilage, bone, or overlying skin
T4b	Very advanced disease; tumor involving brain, dura, skull base, lower cranial nerves (IX, X, XI, XII), masticator space, carotid artery, prevertebral space, or mediastinal structures
Regional lymph nodes (N)	
NX	Regional lymph nodes cannot be assessed
N0	No regional lymph node metastases
N1	Regional lymph node metastases present
Distant metastasis (M)	
M0	No distant metastasis
M1	Distant metastasis present
Staging	
Stage III	T3, N0, M0
Stage IVA	T4a, N0, M0 T3–T4a, N1, M0
Stage IVB	T4B, any N, M0
Stage IVC	Any T, any N, M1

From Edge SE, Byrd DR, Compton CC, et al. AJCC cancer staging manual. 7th edition. New York: Springer, 2009; with permission.

more efficient; it has eliminated T1 and T2 classifications and increased precision in the staging of advanced tumors with regard to survival rates. Overall, 5-year survival rates, however, remained at 24.2% between the 2 staging systems.

Goerres and colleagues retrospectively examined the use of whole body PET with ^{18}F-fluorodeoxyglucose (FDG) during initial staging of patients with sinonasal melanoma.[57] Ten patients were screened with FDG-PET to search for local or distant metastasis. No patients were found to have metastatic spread either preoperatively or postoperatively. Prospective studies in the cutaneous melanoma population have allowed FDG-PET to become the gold standard imaging method for those patients,[58] but further studies are required to extend this conclusion for patients with sinonasal melanoma.

Nasopharyngeal Carcinoma (NPC) Staging

Staging of NPC is done via the AJCC tumor node metastasis (TNM) system **(Table 7)**.[56] Diagnosis of NPC is made definitively with biopsy. Evaluation via imaging is made with computed tomography (CT) scanning or magnetic resonance (MR) imaging, with MR imaging preferred to CT. MR imaging provides a clearer picture of deep tumor infiltration into soft tissue and may cause dramatic changes in the TNM staging of the tumor.[59] Additional imaging may be considered for those patients with advanced tumor staging, such as N3 and higher. Pooled results of a meta-analysis by Xu and colleagues[60] showed that of 1276 eligible patients, 174 (13.7%) patients eventually had distant metastases or secondary primary cancers. The authors conclude that PET/CT scanning could provide a high level of diagnostic performance in detecting these additional metastases if used as a screening tool at the patient's

Table 7
Staging system for cancer of the nasopharynx, AJCC guidelines, 7th edition

Primary tumor (T)	
TX	Primary tumor cannot be assessed
T0	No evidence of primary tumor
Tis	Carcinoma in situ
T1	Tumor confined to the nasopharynx, or tumor extends to oropharynx and/or nasal cavity without parapharyngeal extension[a]
T2	Tumor with parapharyngeal extension[a]
T3	Tumor involves bony structures of skull base and/or paranasal sinuses
T4	Tumor with intracranial extension and/or involvement of cranial nerves, hypopharynx, orbit, or with extension to the infratemporal fossa/masticator space
Regional lymph nodes (N)[b]	
NX	Regional lymph nodes cannot be assessed
N0	No regional lymph node metastasis
N1	Unilateral metastasis in cervical lymph node(s), 6 cm or less in greatest dimension, above the supraclavicular fossa, and/or unilateral or bilateral, retropharyngeal lymph nodes, 6 cm or less, in greatest dimension[c]
N2	Bilateral metastasis in cervical lymph node(s), 6 cm or less in greatest dimension, above the supraclavicular fossa[c]
N3	Metastasis in a lymph node(s) >6 cm and/or to supraclavicular fossa
N3a	Greater than 6 cm in dimension
N3b	Extension to the supraclavicular fossa[d]
Distant metastasis (M)	
M0	No distant metastasis
M1	Distant metastasis

[a] Parapharyngeal extension denotes posterolateral infiltration of tumor.
[b] The distribution and the prognostic impact of regional lymph node spread from nasopharynx cancer, particularly of the undifferentiated type, are different from those of other head and neck mucosal cancers and justify the use of a different N classification scheme.
[c] Midline nodes are considered ipsilateral nodes.
[d] Supraclavicular zone or fossa is relevant to the staging of nasopharyngeal carcinoma. It is defined by 3 points: (1) the superior margin of the sternal end of the clavicle, (2) the superior margin of the lateral end of the clavicle, and (3) the point where the neck meets the shoulder. Note that this would include caudal portions of levels IV and VB. All cases with lymph nodes (whole or part) in the fossa are considered N3b.
From Edge SE, Byrd DR, Compton CC, et al. AJCC cancer staging manual. New York: Springer; 2009; with permission.

initial evaluation. In addition to imaging evaluation, patients with NPC should also have titers of EBV antibody assayed. Plasma EBV titers may allow for better pretreatment risk categorization, initial treatment response, and collection of a baseline level should relapse occur.[61,62]

Sinonasal Adenocarcinoma (SNAC) Staging

All SNACs must undergo biopsy to distinguish between the various types of salivary, intestinal, and nonintestinal SNACs. Most ITACs are clinically advanced (T3 and T4) on presentation; therefore, staging via the TMN staging system has little prognostic significance.[63] Because of the possibility of local spread from salivary gland–type SNAC, it is essential for SNACs to be imaged properly for diagnosis, with MR imaging being preferred to CT.[64] Even so, salivary gland–type adenocarcinomas tend to be underestimated on radiology because of undetected perineural spread.[65] Imaging or endoscopic studies of the gastrointestinal tract, with or without assays of carcinoembryonic antigen, are necessary to rule out metastasis for ITAC.[66,67]

Sinonasal Undifferentiated Carcinoma (SNUC) Staging

SNUC is staged either using the Kadish staging system (see **Table 3**)[12,43] or according to the AJCC staging system for the nasal cavity and ethmoid sinus (see **Table 7**).[57] Although imaging will not be able to provide a distinguishing diagnosis from other nasopharyngeal neoplasms, it is required for SNUC,[68] with MR imaging being the preferred medium. CT scanning may demonstrate regional lymphadenopathy, and distant metastasis can also be excluded with a chest CT scan.[41] Bone scans are appropriate if bone symptoms are present.

EVIDENCE-BASED ENDOSCOPIC SURGICAL MANAGEMENT OF SINONASAL AND SKULL BASE CANCER
Esthesioneuroblastoma Surgery

Goals for the surgical treatment of esthesioneuroblastoma include resection of the entire cribriform plate and crista galli.[69] Numerous articles detail results from endoscopic resection of the tumor versus traditional craniofacial approaches. A meta-analysis published by Devaiah and Andreoli in 2009 compiled results from a total of 1170 cases of esthesioneuroblastoma published in 49 journal articles between 1992 and 2008.[70] Log-rank tests showed a greater survival rate for endoscopic surgery compared with open surgery, even when stratifying for publication year ($P = .0018$). The study was likely confounded by the high number of open surgery techniques used on Kadish C and D staged tumors, whereas endoscopic and endoscopic-assisted techniques were more likely to be used on Kadish A and B staged tumors.

Because of a long and chronic natural history, previous studies show that rigorous monitoring of patients with esthesioneuroblastoma up to 15 to 20 years is necessary.[71] In addition, monitoring of patients who have had endoscopically resected tumors required at least 10 years of follow-up to assess clinical efficacy.[72] Although less than a 10-year follow-up was used, Folbe and colleagues[73] described 23 patients who were treated endoscopically and had a mean follow-up time of 45.2 months (11–152 months). Folbe and colleagues confirmed the results of other smaller studies that even patients with Kadish stage C disease can be effectively treated using solely endoscopic techniques followed by radiation without sacrificing local control.[12,74]

Sinonasal Melanoma Surgery

The use of purely endoscopic methods for malignant mucosal melanoma is relatively new[75] and limited outcomes and patient selection data exist. In addition, a lack of a standardized staging method decreases the ease for homogeneous reporting for sinonasal melanoma. Regardless, surgery remains the mainstay of therapy for sinonasal melanoma. In regard to endoscopic approaches versus traditional craniofacial resection, there is no evidence for or against the use of one approach. Most published studies report on a small number of patients or case reports. Long-term results for endoscopic management of sinonasal melanoma are promising. With a cohort of 11 patients treated endoscopically, Lund and colleagues[76] reported an 80% overall survival at 5 years and 36% disease-free survival. The results of this study are outstanding for this aggressive tumor and likely represent a selection bias that cannot be applied across all sinonasal melanomas.

Limiting factors for the use of endoscopy in sinonasal melanoma include its proclivity for recurrence, late stage at diagnosis, and rarity of occurrence. Because of its poor prognosis, some authors have gone so far as stating that surgical cure may not be possible for sinonasal melanoma and endoscopic surgery should instead be solely used for palliative purposes to improve quality of life and disease-free survival time.[77,78] The major limitation of this disease is the aggressive and early metastasis rate and not necessarily the ability to resect the sinonasal portion of the disease with endoscopic or open techniques.

Nasopharyngeal Carcinoma Surgery

Because of the close proximity to vital neurovascular structures, chemoradiation therapy remains the gold standard treatment of primary NPC. However, salvage surgery is indicated when treating locoregional recurrent NPC. Exclusively endoscopic approaches to NPC were reported by Chen and colleagues[79] in 2007. They published the results of 6 patients who underwent endoscopic nasopharyngectomy in salvaging recurrent T1 to T2A NPC. Results showed no need for conversion to open approaches, no complications during surgery, and only 1 local recurrence in a mean follow-up time of 29 months (16–59 months). Chen and colleagues analyzed a cohort of 37 patients receiving endoscopic salvage nasopharyngectomy in 2009.[80] Short-term results are encouraging, as 35 of 37 patients achieved en bloc extirpation of recurrent tumor with negative surgical margins. No complications were encountered during surgery and no patients required additional postoperative radiation therapy. The 2-year survival rate, local relapse-free survival rate, and progression-free survival rate were 84.2%, 86.3%, and 82.6%, respectively. It is important to remember that both of these retrospective studies had considerable patient selection bias, as all patients (except for 2 T3 staged patients) had early-stage disease (T1 to T2). The literature shows that nasopharyngectomy for patients with high recurrent T stage carries a poor prognosis regardless of surgical method.[81]

Sinonasal Adenocarcinoma (SNAC) Surgery

Assessment of the best surgical treatment of SNAC remains difficult as most studies publish results in combined histologic groups. The choice of whether to use endoscopic, combined endoscopic and open, or traditional craniofacial resection (tCFR) approaches for SNAC remains controversial. Pedunculated or isolated tumors attached to the septum or turbinates can be easily removed with a good margin of normal tissue with either approach. The current gold standard for tumors that abut or transgress the skull base or orbit, however, remains tCFR,[70] and future outcomes must be compared with this.

Nicolai and colleagues[82] found that the 5-year survival rate for adenocarcinoma increased from 60% to 80% when switching from a combined endoscopic and craniofacial resection to a wholly endoscopic approach. It is important to note, however, that selection bias may have confounded these results as patients with more invasive tumors were selected to have combined approaches. Jardeleza and colleagues[83] reported on 12 patients with adenocarcinoma who were treated with wholly endoscopic approaches and found overall disease-free survival and overall survival rates of 91.6% at a median follow-up time of 30 months (10–96 months). A review of the literature performed by Devaiah and Lee in 2010 examined 16 articles (representing 150 retrospective cases) in which either wholly endoscopic or combined endoscopic methods were used.[84] Endoscopic management appears to be a feasible method of surgery with increasingly favorable results, but increased information with better reporting methods (ie, grouping tumors based on histologic subtypes) is required to perform proper meta-analysis.

Sinonasal Undifferentiated Carcinoma (SNUC) Staging

Because of its highly aggressive nature, treatment of SNUC is multimodal, usually including surgical treatment, radiotherapy, and chemotherapy.[85,86] Yet, because of its rarity, no consensus has been achieved regarding optimal surgical methods for treatment. Revenaugh and colleagues[87] recently published the only study using endoscopic methods as a part of multimodal treatment of resection of SNUC. Seven of their patients treated with endoscopic resection and concurrent chemoradiation had a 2-year overall survival rate of 85.7% and a 2-year disease free survival rate of 71.4%. This is slightly better than historical 2-year overall survival rates (42.9–64%) as reported in a review of the literature by Mendenhall and colleagues.[88] Selection bias did not play as large a part in the study by Revenaugh and colleagues because all patients (with an exception of 1 T1-staged patient) had tumors staged at T4 with no nodal metastases.

SUMMARY: ENDOSCOPIC RESECTION OF SINONASAL CANCERS

The preliminary results of endoscopic resection of sinonasal cancers are encouraging; however, the current data must be taken into consideration regarding publication and selection biases:

- There is no single prospective head-to-head comparison with current open surgical gold standard techniques.
- All of the outcome publications come from extremely experienced endoscopic surgeons whose results may not be generalizable to lower-volume practices.
- The full spectrum of skull base and sinonasal cancer surgery must include the gold standard techniques of open craniofacial resection and transfacial/transcranial approaches.

The surgeon and patient must understand the possibility of needing to convert from an endoscopic to open approaches for clearance of margins if needed. The rate of this is often underreported and the importance is understated. The single best determining factor of patient outcomes within the heterogeneous groups of skull base cancers is surgical margin status. This should be the primary oncologic goal regardless of which approach is taken.

BOTTOM LINE: WHAT DOES THE EVIDENCE TELL US?
Esthesioneuroblastoma

Evidence level 2A
Surgical intervention with or without radiation therapy is generally required for all Kadish stages A through D and Dulgeurov stages T1 through T4 of esthesioneuroblastoma. When combined with careful patient selection, endoscopic approaches may provide higher survival rates compared with traditional craniofacial open surgery.

Sinonasal Melanoma

Evidence level 4
Case-series remain the dominant form of reporting for endoscopic techniques of sinonasal malignancy. tCFR remains the predominant gold standard form of therapy, but

with adequate experience, endoscopic methods for extirpation of sinonasal malignancy may provide similar rates of long-term survival for patients.

Nasopharyngeal Carcinoma (NPC)

Evidence level 4

Evidence for endoscopic versus tCFR approaches for salvage surgery of recurrent NPC is lacking. Two studies published encouraging reports of short-term results for endoscopic techniques marked by a decrease in morbidity.[79,80] Endoscopic surgery may result in better outcomes, but further research is required to make this conclusion definitively.

Sinonasal Adenocarcinoma (SNAC)

Evidence level 4

Because of the high degree of heterogeneity in SNAC, a lack of evidence exists in comparing wholly endoscopic versus traditional craniofacial resection versus combined endoscopic and craniofacial resection techniques. When combined with careful patient selection, wholly endoscopic and combined endoscopic approaches do have favorable outcomes.

Sinonasal Undifferentiated Carcinoma (SNUC)

Evidence level 4

Only 1 study examines the use of endoscopic resection of SNUC as a part of a multimodal therapy regimen. There are no studies that compare open versus endoscopic techniques for SNUC.[87] Overall 2-year survival rates are optimistic, however, and further prospective data would help elucidate the role of endoscopy in resection of SNUC.

Evidence grades follow Cochrane evidence-base.

REFERENCES

1. Kim BJ, Kim DW, Kim SW, et al. Endoscopic versus traditional craniofacial resection for patients with sinonasal tumors involving the anterior skull base. Clin Exp Otorhinolaryngol 2008;1(3):148–53. C.
2. Luong A, Citardi MJ, Batra PS. Management of sinonasal malignant neoplasms: defining the role of endoscopy. Am J Rhinol Allergy 2010;24(2):150–5. C.
3. Snyderman CH, Carrau RL, Kassam AB, et al. Endoscopic skull base surgery: principles of endonasal oncological surgery. J Surg Oncol 2008;97(8): 658–64. C.
4. Chen MK. Minimally invasive endoscopic resection of sinonasal malignancies and skull base surgery. Acta Otolaryngol 2006;126(9):981–6. C.
5. Roh HJ, Batra PS, Citardi MJ, et al. Endoscopic resection of sinonasal malignancies: a preliminary report. Am J Rhinol 2004;18(4):239–46. C.
6. de Almeida JR, Witterick IJ, Vescan AD. Functional outcomes for endoscopic and open skull base surgery: an evidence-based review. Otolaryngol Clin North Am 2011;44(5):1185–200. C.
7. Tay HN, Leong JL, Sethi DS. Long-term results of endoscopic resection of nasopharyngeal tumours. Med J Malaysia 2009;64(2):159–62. C.
8. Barnes L, Eveson JW, Reichart P, et al. Pathology and genetics of head and neck tumors. Lyon (France): IARC Press; 2005. B.
9. McCormack LJ, Harris HE. Neurogenic tumors of the nasal fossa. JAMA 1955; 157:318–21. C.

10. Kumar M, Fallon RJ, Hill JS, et al. Esthesioneuroblastoma in children. J Pediatr Hematol Oncol 2002;24:482–7. C.
11. Elkon D, Hightower SI, Lim ML, et al. Esthesioneuroblastoma. Cancer 1979;44: 1087–94. C.
12. Morita A, Ebersold MJ, Olsen KD, et al. Esthesioneuroblastoma: prognosis and management. Neurosurgery 1993;32(5):706–14 [discussion: 714–5]. C.
13. Thompson LD. Olfactory neuroblastoma. Head Neck Pathol 2009;3(3):252–9. C.
14. Chang AE, Karnell LH, Menck HR. The National Cancer Data Base report on cutaneous and noncutaneous melanoma: a summary of 84,836 cases from the past decade. The American College of Surgeons Commission on Cancer and the American Cancer Society. Cancer 1998;83(8):1664–78. B.
15. Papaspyrou G, Garbe C, Schadendorf D, et al. Mucosal melanomas of the head and neck: new aspects of the clinical outcome, molecular pathology, and treatment with c-kit inhibitors. Melanoma Res 2011;21(6):475–82. D.
16. Clifton N, Harrison L, Bradley PJ, et al. Malignant melanoma of nasal cavity and paranasal sinuses: report of 24 patients and literature review. J Laryngol Otol 2011;125(5):479–85. C.
17. Yii NW, Eisen T, Nicolson M, et al. Mucosal malignant melanoma of the head and neck: the Marsden experience over half a century. Clin Oncol (R Coll Radiol) 2003;15(4):199–204. C.
18. Temam S, Mamelle G, Marandas P, et al. Postoperative radiotherapy for primary mucosal melanoma of the head and neck. Cancer 2005;103(2):313–9. C.
19. Manolidis S, Donald PJ. Malignant mucosal melanoma of the head and neck: review of the literature and report of 14 patients. Cancer 1997;80(8):1373–86. C.
20. Owens JM, Roberts DB, Myers JN. The role of postoperative adjuvant radiation therapy in the treatment of mucosal melanomas of the head and neck region. Arch Otolaryngol Head Neck Surg 2003;129(8):864–8. C.
21. Gal TJ, Silver N, Huang B. Demographics and treatment trends in sinonasal mucosal melanoma. Laryngoscope 2011;121(9):2026–33. B.
22. Dauer EH, Lewis JE, Rohlinger AL, et al. Sinonasal melanoma: a clinicopathologic review of 61 cases. Otolaryngol Head Neck Surg 2008;138(3):347–52. C.
23. Chang ET, Adami HO. The enigmatic epidemiology of nasopharyngeal carcinoma. Cancer Epidemiol Biomarkers Prev 2006;15(10):1765–77. B.
24. Yu MC, Yuan JM. Epidemiology of nasopharyngeal carcinoma. Semin Cancer Biol 2002;12(6):421–9. B.
25. Berry MP, Smith CR, Brown TC, et al. Nasopharyngeal carcinoma in the young. Int J Radiat Oncol Biol Phys 1980;6(4):415–21. C.
26. Dulgerov P, Jacobsen MS, Allal AS, et al. Nasal and paranasal sinus carcinoma: are we making progress? A series of 220 patients and a systematic review. Cancer 2002;92:3012–29. B.
27. Bhaijee F, Carron J, Bell D. Low-grade nonintestinal sinonasal adenocarcinoma: a diagnosis of exclusion. Ann Diagn Pathol 2011;15(3):181–4. C.
28. Franchi A, Santucci M, Wenig B. Adenocarcinoma. In: Barnes L, Eveson JW, Reichart P, Sidransky D, editors. World Health Organization classification of tumors. Pathology and genetics of head and neck tumors. Lyon (France): IARC; 2005. p. 20–3. B.
29. Barnes L. Intestinal-type adenocarcinoma of the nasal cavity and paranasal sinuses. Am J Surg Pathol 1986;10(3):192–202. C.
30. Klintenberg C, Olofsson J, Hellquist H, et al. Adenocarcinoma of the ethmoid sinuses. A review of 28 cases with special reference to wood dust exposure. Cancer 1984;54(3):482–8. C.

31. Macbeth R. Malignant disease of the paranasal sinuses. J Laryngol Otol 1965;79: 592–612. D.
32. Acheson ED. Nasal cancer in the furniture and boot and shoe manufacturing industries. Prev Med 1976;5(2):295–315. C.
33. Abecasis J, Viana G, Pissarra C, et al. Adenocarcinomas of the nasal cavity and paranasal sinuses: a clinicopathological and immunohistochemical study of 14 cases. Histopathology 2004;45(3):254–9. C.
34. Thompson LD. Intestinal-type sinonasal adenocarcinoma. Ear Nose Throat J 2010;89(1):16–8. C.
35. Heffner DK, Hyams VJ, Hauck KW, et al. Low-grade adenocarcinoma of the nasal cavity and paranasal sinuses. Cancer 1982;50(2):312–22. C.
36. Knegt PP, Ah-See KW, vd Velden LA, et al. Adenocarcinoma of the ethmoidal sinus complex: surgical debulking and topical fluorouracil may be the optimal treatment. Arch Otolaryngol Head Neck Surg 2001;127(2):141–6. E.
37. Frierson HF, Mills S, Fechner R, et al. Sinonasal undifferentiated carcinoma: an aggressive neoplasm derived from schneiderian epithelium and distinct from olfactory neuroblastoma. Am J Surg Pathol 1986;10:771–9. C.
38. Gorelick J, Ross D, Marentette L, et al. Sinonasal undifferentiated carcinoma: case series and review of the literature. Neurosurgery 2000;47(3):750–4 [discussion: 754–5]. C.
39. Cerilli LA, Holst VA, Brandwein MS, et al. Sinonasal undifferentiated carcinoma: immunohistochemical profile and lack of EBV association. Am J Surg Pathol 2001;25(2):156–63. D.
40. Rischin D, Coleman A. Sinonasal malignancies of neuroendocrine origin. Hematol Oncol Clin North Am 2008;22(6):1297–316 xi. C.
41. O'Reilly AG, Wismayer DJ, Moore EJ. Prognostic factors for patients with sinonasal undifferentiated carcinoma. Laryngoscope 2010;120(Suppl 4):S173. C.
42. Kadish S, Goodman M, Wang CC. Olfactory neuroblastoma. A clinical analysis of 17 cases. Cancer 1976;37(3):1571–6. C.
43. Biller HF, Lawson W, Sachdev VP, et al. Esthesioneuroblastoma: surgical treatment without radiation. Laryngoscope 1990;100:1199–201. B.
44. Dulguerov P, Calcaterra T. Esthesioneuroblastoma: the UCLA experience 1970–1990. Laryngoscope 1992;102(8):843–9. C.
45. Hyams VJ. Tumors of the upper respiratory tract and ear. In: Hyams VJ, Batsakis JG, Michaels L, editors. Atlas of tumor pathology. Second series, fascicle 25. Washington, DC: Armed Forces Institute of Pathology; 1988. p. 240–8. C.
46. Miyamoto RC, Gleich LL, Biddinger PW, et al. Esthesioneuroblastoma and sinonasal undifferentiated carcinoma: impact of histological grading and clinical staging on survival and prognosis. Laryngoscope 2000;110(8):1262–5. C.
47. Nguyen BD, Roarke MC, Nelson KD, et al. F-18 FDG PET/CT staging and posttherapeutic assessment of esthesioneuroblastoma. Clin Nucl Med 2006;31(3):172–4. C.
48. Yu J, Koch CA, Patsalides A, et al. Ectopic Cushing's syndrome caused by an esthesioneuroblastoma. Endocr Pract 2004;10:119–24. C.
49. Gore MR, Zanation AM. Salvage treatment of late neck metastasis in esthesioneuroblastoma: a meta-analysis. Arch Otolaryngol Head Neck Surg 2009;135: 1030–4. B.
50. Davis RE, Weissler MC. Esthesioneuroblastoma and neck metastasis. Head Neck 1992;14:477–82. C.
51. Zanation AM, Ferlito A, Rinaldo A, et al. When, how and why to treat the neck in patients with esthesioneuroblastoma: a review. Eur Arch Otorhinolaryngol 2010; 267(11):1667–71. B.

52. Thompson LD, Wieneke JA, Miettinen M. Sinonasal tract and nasopharyngeal melanomas: a clinicopathologic study of 115 cases with a proposed staging system. Am J Surg Pathol 2003;27(5):594–611. C.
53. Freedman HM, De Santo LW, Devine KD, et al. Malignant melanoma of the nasal cavity and paranasal sinuses. Arch Otolaryngol 1973;97:322–5. C.
54. Ballantyne AJ. Malignant melanoma of the skin of the head and neck. Am J Surg 1970;120(4):425–31. C.
55. Page DL, Fleming ID, Fritz AG. AJCC cancer staging manual. Philadelphia: Lippincott-Raven; 2002. B.
56. Edge SE, Byrd DR, Compton CC, et al. AJCC cancer staging manual. New York: Springer; 2009. B.
57. Goerres GW, Stoeckli SJ, von Schulthess GK, et al. FDG PET for mucosal malignant melanoma of the head and neck. Laryngoscope 2002;112(2): 381–5. C.
58. Rinne D, Baum RP, Hör G, et al. Primary staging and follow-up of high risk melanoma patients with whole-body 18F-fluorodeoxyglucose positron emission tomography. Cancer 1998;82:1664–71. B.
59. Liao XB, Mao YP, Liu LZ, et al. How does magnetic resonance imaging influence staging according to AJCC staging system for nasopharyngeal carcinoma compared with computed tomography? Int J Radiat Oncol Biol Phys 2008; 72(5):1368. C.
60. Xu GZ, Guan DJ, He ZY. (18)FDG-PET/CT for detecting distant metastases and second primary cancers in patients with head and neck cancer. A meta-analysis. Oral Oncol 2011;47(7):560–5 [Epub 2011 May 28]. C.
61. Lin JC, Wang WY, Chen KY, et al. Quantification of plasma Epstein-Barr virus DNA in patients with advanced nasopharyngeal carcinoma. N Engl J Med 2004; 350(24):2461–70. B.
62. Leung SF, Zee B, Ma BB, et al. Plasma Epstein-Barr viral deoxyribonucleic acid quantitation complements tumor-node-metastasis staging prognostication in nasopharyngeal carcinoma. J Clin Oncol 2006;24(34):5414–8. B.
63. Franchi A, Gallo O, Santucci M. Clinical relevance of the histological classification of sinonasal intestinal-type adenocarcinomas. Hum Pathol 1999;30(10): 1140–5. C.
64. Raghavan P, Phillips CD. Magnetic resonance imaging of sinonasal malignancies. Top Magn Reson Imaging 2007;18(4):259–67. D.
65. Ayadi K, Ayadi L, Daoud E, et al. Adenoid cystic carcinoma of the parotid with facial nerve invasion. Tunis Med 2010;88(1):46–8. C.
66. Robles C, Cooper EM. A case of intestinal-type sinonasal adenocarcinoma. J Natl Med Assoc 2004;96(1):117–9. C.
67. McKinney CD, Mills SE, Franquemont DW. Sinonasal intestinal-type adenocarcinoma: immunohistochemical profile and comparison with colonic adenocarcinoma. Mod Pathol 1995;8(4):421–6. C.
68. Phillips CD, Futterer SF, Lipper MH, et al. Sinonasal undifferentiated carcinoma: CT and MR imaging of an uncommon neoplasm of the nasal cavity. Radiology 1997;202(2):477–80. C.
69. Harvey RJ, Winder M, Parmar P, et al. Endoscopic skull base surgery for sinonasal malignancy. Otolaryngol Clin North Am 2011;44(5):1081–140. C.
70. Devaiah AK, Andreoli MT. Treatment of esthesioneuroblastoma: a 16-year meta-analysis of 361 patients. Laryngoscope 2009;119(7):1412–6. B.
71. Bachar G, Goldstein DP, Shah M, et al. Esthesioneuroblastoma: the Princess Margaret Hospital experience. Head Neck 2008;30(12):1607–14. C.

72. de Gabory L, Abdulkhaleq HM, Darrouzet V, et al. Long-term results of 28 esthe-sioneuroblastomas managed over 35 years. Head Neck 2011;33(1):82–6. C.

73. Folbe A, Herzallah I, Duvvuri U, et al. Endoscopic endonasal resection of esthe-sioneuroblastoma: a multicenter study. Am J Rhinol Allergy 2009;23:91–4. C.

74. Gallia GL, Reh DD, Salmasi V, et al. Endonasal endoscopic resection of esthesio-neuroblastoma: the Johns Hopkins Hospital experience and review of the litera-ture. Neurosurg Rev 2011;34(4):465–75. C.

75. Stammberger H, Anderhuber W, Walch C, et al. Possibilities and limitations of endoscopic management of nasal and paranasal sinus malignancies. Acta Oto-rhinolaryngol Belg 1999;53(3):199–205. C.

76. Lund V, Howard DJ, Wei WI. Endoscopic resection of malignant tumors of the nose and sinuses. Am J Rhinol 2007;21(1):89–94. C.

77. Castelnuovo P, Battaglia P, Locatelli D, et al. Endonasal micro-endoscopic treat-ment of malignant tumors of the paranasal sinuses and anterior skull base. Oper-at Tech Otolaryngol Head Neck Surg 2006;17(3):152–67. C.

78. Tabaee A, Nyquist G, Anand VK, et al. Palliative endoscopic surgery in advanced sinonasal and anterior skull base neoplasms. Otolaryngol Head Neck Surg 2010; 142(1):126–8. C.

79. Chen MK, Lai JC, Chang CC, et al. Minimally invasive endoscopic nasopharyng-ectomy in the treatment of recurrent T1-2a nasopharyngeal carcinoma. Laryngo-scope 2007;117(5):894–6. C.

80. Chen MY, Wen WP, Guo X, et al. Endoscopic nasopharyngectomy for locally recurrent nasopharyngeal carcinoma. Laryngoscope 2009;119(3):516–22. C.

81. To EW, Lai EC, Cheng JH, et al. Nasopharyngectomy for recurrent nasopharyn-geal carcinoma: a review of 31 patients and prognostic factors. Laryngoscope 2002;112:1877–82. C.

82. Nicolai P, Battaglia P, Bignami M, et al. Endoscopic surgery for malignant tumors of the sinonasal tract and adjacent skull base: a 10-year experience. Am J Rhinol 2008;22(3):308–16. C.

83. Jardeleza C, Seiberling K, Floreani S, et al. Surgical outcomes of endoscopic management of adenocarcinoma of the sinonasal cavity. Rhinology 2009;47(4): 354–61. C.

84. Devaiah AK, Lee MK. Endoscopic skull base/sinonasal adenocarcinoma surgery: what evidence exists? Am J Rhinol Allergy 2010;24(2):156–60. C.

85. Enepekides DJ. Sinonasal undifferentiated carcinoma: an update. Curr Opin Oto-laryngol Head Neck Surg 2005;13(4):222–5. C.

86. Smullen JL, Amedee RG. Sinonasal undifferentiated carcinoma: a review of the literature. J La State Med Soc 2001;153(10):487–90. C.

87. Revenaugh PC, Seth R, Pavlovich JB, et al. Minimally invasive endoscopic resection of sinonasal undifferentiated carcinoma. Am J Otolaryngol 2011;32(6): 464–9. C.

88. Mendenhall WM, Mendenhall CM, Riggs CE Jr, et al. Sinonasal undifferentiated carcinoma. Am J Clin Oncol 2006;29(1):27–31. C.

GRADES OF RECOMMENDATION

A consistent level 1 studies.
B consistent level 2 or 3 studies *or* extrapolations from level 1 studies.
C level 4 studies *or* extrapolations from level 2 or 3 studies.
D level 5 evidence *or* troublingly inconsistent or inconclusive studies of any level.

Evidence-Based Practice
Management of Glottic Cancer

Dana M. Hartl, MD, PhD*

KEYWORDS

- Larynx • Vocal folds • Squamous cell carcinoma • Surgery • Laser
- Chemoradiation • Radiation therapy

KEY POINTS

The following points list the level of evidence as based on Oxford Center for Evidence-Based Medicine. Additional critical points are provided and points here are expanded at the conclusion of this article.

- Curative treatment for Tis: transoral surgery or radiation therapy. Prefer surgery for younger patients. Save radiotherapy for failure of a surgical approach (level 3).
- Curative treatment for T1a: surgery or radiation therapy (level 3).
- Curative treatment for T1T2 with anterior commissure involvement: surgery provides better initial local control and final laryngeal preservation than radiation therapy (level 3).
- Curative treatment for T2: T2 with normal vocal fold mobility: surgery or radiation therapy (level 3); surgery provides better outcomes for tumors with impaired vocal fold mobility compared with radiation therapy alone (level 3).
- Curative treatment for T3T4: When a nonsurgical organ preservation strategy is chosen, concurrent chemoradiation with cisplatin provides better outcomes than radiation therapy alone or induction chemotherapy with cisplatin and 5-fluorouracil (level 1).

DISEASE OVERVIEW: MAIN ISSUES IN GLOTTIC CARCINOMA

Evidence-based medicine is the "conscientious, explicit and judicious use of current best evidence in making decisions about the care of individual patients," and "integrating experience with the best available data in decision making."[1] Common sense–based medicine tells us that the main goal in treating glottis carcinoma is long-term disease-free survival. Then, if possible, while not compromising oncological outcomes, one should attempt to preserve a functional larynx. For many years, laryngeal squamous cell carcinoma was not thought to be a "chemosensitive" tumor, and surgery and radiation therapy were the only treatment options. For the past 30 years,

Department of Head and Neck Oncology, Institut Gustave Roussy, Villejuif, France
* Institut Gustave Roussy, 114 rue Edouard Vaillant, Villejuif 94805, France.
E-mail address: dana.hartl@igr.fr

Otolaryngol Clin N Am 45 (2012) 1143–1161
http://dx.doi.org/10.1016/j.otc.2012.06.014
0030-6665/12/$ – see front matter © 2012 Elsevier Inc. All rights reserved.
oto.theclinics.com

however, clinical research has shown, with high-level evidence, that these tumors can be cured using combined-modality treatment, the addition of chemotherapy providing high rates of local control, with organ preservation.[2]

For glottic cancer, local control rates best reflect the effects of local treatments. Disease-specific survival for these tumors is related to metastatic disease that may appear years later, and may or may not be affected by the choice of initial therapy. Finally, and contrary to other cancers, in patients with head and neck cancer, overall survival is not always related to the cancer being treated, owing to associated comorbidities that determine a large part of overall survival.

So the question is, how can we optimize locoregional control for glottic cancer, while optimizing preservation of function and quality of life? Can we (and if so, how) optimize disease-free survival through our choice of initial therapies? This article aims at viewing the current evidence available for the management of glottic cancer, at all stages.

EVIDENCE-BASED CLINICAL ASSESSMENT OF GLOTTIC CARCINOMA

The clinical and radiologic workup for glottic carcinoma aims at reconstituting, in the physician's "minds eye," a 3-dimensional image of the tumor. Deep and superficial tumor extensions determine the T stage, but T stage is not the only factor involved in treatment decision making.

Clinical Workup

There is no particular evidence in the medical literature guiding initial clinical evaluation, which thus relies on "common sense–based medicine." The clinical examination is today most often performed using fiberoptic laryngoscopy or a rigid endoscope, but no study has ever prospectively compared mirror laryngoscopy (by experienced physicians) with these technologies. Evaluation under general anesthesia is performed systematically by most teams, but then again, there are no studies to "prove" that this is better than not doing it. Common sense shows that general health and comorbidities should also be thoroughly evaluated.

Laryngeal mobility is a main issue in glottic cancer. Dr Kirchner's[3] seminal study of whole-organ sections has shown that decreased vocal fold motion may be caused simply by a bulky tumor, but also by a tumor invading the paraglottic space. Laryngeal mobility was the only predictor of minor thyroid cartilage invasion by T1 to T3 tumors treated with conservation laryngeal surgery and for early-stage to mid-stage tumors involving the anterior commissure (level 3 evidence).[4–6]

The anterior commissure (AC) must be thoroughly evaluated clinically, as the approach and outcomes differ from tumors without AC involvement (see later in this article). Subglottic extension and proximity of the tumor to the cricoid cartilage must be ascertained in view of organ-preservation surgery, in which a stable cricoid must be preserved.[7]

Radiologic Assessment

Locoregional assessment of glottic cancer relies on computed tomography (CT), magnetic resonance imaging (MRI), and 18-fluorodeoxyglucose positron emission tomography combined with CT scan (PET/CT). CT and MRI have been shown to improve diagnostic accuracy for laryngeal carcinoma as compared with the clinical and endoscopic workup alone (level 2 evidence).[8,9] Using CT, diagnostic accuracy improved from 58% to 80%, and using MRI, accuracy improved from 58% to 88%. The difference between adding CT versus MRI was not significant.

Using pathology as the gold standard, reported sensitivities of CT scan for predicting cartilage invasion by laryngeal carcinoma range from 46% to 67% and can be as low as 10% for early-stage to mid-stage tumors amenable to conservation laryngeal surgery (level 3 evidence).[5] Reported specificities range from 87% to 94% (level 3 evidence).[10] For the diagnosis of cartilage invasion, MRI has been shown to be significantly more sensitive than CT (respective sensitivities of 89% vs 66%) but also significantly less specific than CT (respective specificities of 84% vs 94%) (level 2 evidence).[11] Thus, there is no evidence favoring CT over MRI for the initial staging of laryngeal cancer, and each imaging modality has its limitations and pitfalls.

In the evaluation of the neck, CT, MRI, ultrasound, and PET are clearly more sensitive and specific than neck palpation alone for the diagnosis of metastatic lymphadenopathy (level 2 evidence).[12–14] There does not seem to be a significant difference among these modalities in terms of sensitivity or specificity,[15,16] although one study (level 2 evidence) found that MRI was more accurate for metastatic nodes smaller than 10 mm, but found no difference between MRI or CT for larger nodes.[17] PET/CT is more accurate than PET alone for the staging of the neck (level 2 evidence).[18] One prospective study comparing CT, MRI, ultrasound, and PET/CT using pathology as the gold standard found that PET/CT was significantly the most sensitive and specific imaging modality for detecting metastatic nodes in head and neck cancer (level 2 evidence).[19]

EVIDENCE-BASED MANAGEMENT OF GLOTTIC CARCINOMA

Given the wide range of presentation and tumor extensions, we have approached evidence-based management by attempting to answer several common questions.

What is the Evidence for the Optimum Therapy for In Situ Glottic Carcinoma (Tis)?

Surgery (vocal fold "stripping," transoral laser resection, or open surgery) and radiation therapy have been widely used in the treatment of glottic Tis.

- Initial local control ranges from 56% to 92% with surgery and from 79% to 98% with radiation therapy.
- The final local control after salvage of recurrences ranges from 90% to 100% for both modalities.
- Ultimate laryngeal preservation ranges from 85% to 100% for surgery and 88% to 98% for radiation therapy (level 4 evidence).[20–28]

Retrospective comparative studies have shown that ultimate local control and ultimate laryngeal preservation are not significantly different between these 2 modalities (level 3 evidence).[20,29] Nguyen and colleagues,[29] however, found a significantly higher local recurrence rate after vocal fold stripping, efficiently managed with repeat surgery or radiation therapy. Le and colleagues[20] found that involvement of the AC by the tumor was a significant factor lowering local control, using any treatment modality (level 3 evidence).

Current evidence does not show a difference in terms of ultimate oncological outcomes for Tis, but aspects other than the statistical evidence may be taken into account when treatment planning. Both transoral laser resection and radiation therapy are well tolerated, with low morbidity[21,24,25]; however, local possibilities and expertise play a role in treatment choice. The duration of radiation therapy and the indirect costs also intervene. Finally, radiation therapy is a "one-shot" treatment that cannot be repeated, and some have suggested that it should be used only after other modalities have failed.[25]

What Does the Evidence Say Is the Optimal Treatment for Mid-Vocal Fold T1a Carcinoma?

As for Tis, radiation therapy and surgery, especially transoral laser resection, are widely used in the treatment of T1a glottic carcinoma. Open surgery may be an option in rare selected cases, but has been largely supplanted by transoral laser resection owing to the low morbidity.[30]

- Initial local control rates with both treatment modalities range from 85% to 100% (level 4 evidence). Initial local control, ultimate local control, and survival have not been found to be significantly different (level 3 evidence).[31–33]

Two retrospective studies comparing contemporary cohorts (level 3 evidence) found that ultimate laryngeal preservation rates were higher for tumors initially managed surgically, as compared with initial radiation therapy:

- 96% versus 82% for Stoeckli and colleagues[31]
- 95% versus 77% for Schrijvers and colleagues[32]

However, a relatively recent meta-analysis of 7600 pooled patients found no significant difference in local control or larynx preservation between transoral laser surgery and radiation therapy (level 3 evidence).[34] Thus, if local control and survival are the goal, both therapeutic options are valid, although relatively low-level evidence suggests that the ultimate laryngeal preservation rate is slightly lower for patients initially treated using radiation therapy.

Other factors determining treatment choice are cost, treatment availability, local expertise, and voice quality. Level 3 evidence suggests that transoral laser resection is less costly than radiation therapy.[35–38] Transoral laser resection requires a laser and a surgical team with experience in this type of minimally invasive surgery, however, and may not be available at all sites. Radiation therapy has the "reputation" of better preserving voice quality; however, high-level evidence to prove this is lacking. Current low-level evidence is based on retrospective studies (level 4 evidence) that show conflicting results in terms of voice quality, some showing a better voice after transoral laser resection,[39] others showing a better voice after radiation therapy.[40,41] Ultimate voice quality may be determined by factors other than treatment modality, such as tumor volume or depth of tumor invasion, reflected in the different types of cordectomy in the European Laryngological Association's classification for cordectomies.[42] Depth of invasion may constitute a bias in some studies regarding voice, but also possibly regarding oncological outcomes. Finally, the long-term effects of treatment and the possibility of metachronous second primary head and neck cancer in these patients should be considered. In the study by Holland and colleagues,[43] after a median follow-up of 68 months, 21% of the patients with early laryngeal cancer treated by radiation therapy developed a second primary head and neck cancer (level 4 evidence). The American Broncho-Esophagological Association recommends favoring surgery when possible for younger patients, to "save" radiation therapy as a future treatment option (level 5 evidence).[44]

What Evidence Can Guide Treatment for Tumors T1b or T2 Involving the AC?

AC involvement by early-stage tumors has been shown by level 3 studies to be a factor for decreased local control as compared with tumors without AC invasion, whether treated surgically or with radiation therapy.[28,45–50] Few studies, however, have directly compared these 2 treatment modalities for AC tumors.

- In 2 studies (level 3 evidence), initial local control was better using open surgery than using radiation therapy as first-line treatment,[51,52] although one of these studies found that the subgroup of "purely" AC tumors responded better to radiation therapy initially, but that final local control after salvage was worse as compared with initial surgery.[51]
- A third study also found that surgery (open or transoral laser resection) provided better initial local control and final laryngeal preservation than radiation therapy.[53]

To date, there are no studies directly comparing open surgery for AC tumors with transoral resection for comparable tumors, and thus the choice of surgical approach is not evidence based, although, again, current tendencies are in favor of the transoral approach, because of evidence of lower morbidity as compared with open surgery (level 3 evidence).[47,54]

In conclusion, low-level evidence suggests that one should favor surgery as the initial approach for these tumors; however, other factors may influence treatment choice. Local possibilities and expertise, as well as cost, may be involved. Exposure and tumor visualization are absolutely necessary for transoral laser resection and need to be evaluated before a treatment decision is made. Patient morphology is also a factor for radiation therapy; a low-lying larynx, near the thorax may complicate dosimetry. Finally, precise staging of the cartilage is important, but difficult, given the low sensitivity of CT for early-stage tumors involving the AC (level 3 evidence).[6]

What Does the Evidence Say Is the Best Treatment for T2 Carcinoma?

For T2 tumors with normal vocal fold mobility treated with open conservation surgery, transoral laser resection, or radiation therapy, initial local control rates range from 84% to 95% (level 4 evidence).[28,54–59]

- Four retrospective comparative studies (level 3 evidence) comparing radiation therapy with open or transoral surgery found no significant difference in terms of local control or survival.[31,33,60,61]
- Regarding the surgical approach, one retrospective study found that local control was better with a supracricoid partial laryngectomy as compared with a vertical partial laryngectomy (level 3 evidence).[56]

For T2 tumors with impaired vocal fold mobility, local control rates are lower than for T2 tumors with normal mobility, whether the treatment is radiation therapy, transoral laser resection, or open surgery, with local control rates falling as low as 50%.[7,28,33,53,55,59,62–68] Tumors with impaired vocal fold mobility are at higher risk of minor cartilage invasion (28% histopathological invasion, in one retrospective study), which is often missed on pretherapeutic CT evaluation (level 3 evidence).[6]

Even among tumors with normal vocal fold mobility, not all T2 tumors are the same. For example, Peretti and colleagues[57] divided their group of 109 cT2s into 4 different categories according to the different tumor extensions. They found that

- Tumors with deep extension into the paraglottic space (pT3) had a much lower rate of local control, disease-free survival, and larynx preservation (17% in each case) than more superficial T2 tumors (with respective rates of 69%–100%, level 3 evidence).

- Subglottic extension has implications different from a supraglottic extension for local treatment but also for tumor spread to neck nodes, with a higher risk of paratracheal metastases for tumors with significant subglottic extension.[69]

Thus, there is no high-level evidence to guide treatment choices for T2 tumors. Globally, the use of open surgery has been declining, as transoral resection has taken over as the main surgical approach for conservation laryngeal surgery,[30] but this does not mean that open surgery is not a legitimate option. The evidence shows high rates of local control and preservation of a functional larynx with open surgery, in experienced hands for selected patients.[61,70,71] For tumors with impaired vocal fold mobility, organ-preservation surgery is generally preferable to radiation therapy alone, but there are currently no data comparing surgery with combined modality therapy (concurrent chemoradiation) for these tumors.

What Is the Evidence Regarding the Management of the Neck for Glottic Cancer Staged T1T2cN0?

Without elective treatment of the neck, nodal recurrence rates for early-stage (T1T2) glottic carcinoma are in the range of 4%.[72,73] There is no evidence that elective treatment of the neck improves regional control or disease-free survival.

A recent retrospective cancer registry study analyzed the outcomes of 73 patients with pT2cN0 glottic cancer.[74]

- About half of the patients had undergone elective neck dissection, with occult metastatic nodes found in 10%.
- Multivariate analysis did not find neck dissection or adjuvant treatment to be significantly related to recurrence-free or overall survival, however (level 3 evidence).

Metastatic Delphian nodes were found in 7.5% of patients with T1b or T2 cancers with AC involvement treated with supracricoid partial laryngectomy in a recent study by Wierzbicka and colleagues.[75] Delphian node involvement was a significant prognostic factor for locoregional failure, lower larynx preservation, and lower overall survival (level 3 evidence). This evidence, however, does not confirm the necessity for neck dissection in all patients, but encourages particular vigilance only when treating this specific subtype of cancer, and may be an argument (low-level evidence) in favor of open surgery in these cases. There are currently no guidelines or high-level evidence to guide treatment of the neck for T1T2 glottic tumors, but the low rate of occult disease and regional recurrence would favor the current practice of not treating the neck electively (level 5 evidence).[69]

What Does the Evidence Say Is the Best Treatment for Advanced-Stage Tumors (T3–T4)?

Chemotherapy and radiation therapy

Ever since the seminal study by the Department of Veterans Affairs using induction chemotherapy and radiation therapy for larynx preservation in responders, as opposed to a de facto total laryngectomy, with no adverse effect on survival, nonsurgical organ preservation has become a major goal in the treatment of advanced laryngeal tumors.[2] One must keep in mind, however, that organ-preservation surgery may still be an option for selected tumors staged T3 and T4a. There are no studies directly comparing organ-preservation surgery with nonsurgical organ-preservation protocols for advanced-stage laryngeal tumors, in a prospective manner with comparable patient groups.

Retrospective noncomparative studies (level 4 evidence) show high rates of local control and organ preservation for selected patients treated with open surgery (supracricoid partial laryngectomy)[76,77] or with transoral laser resection.[78,79] As is the case for T1 and T2 tumors, not all T3s or T4s are the same. Vilaseca and colleagues[78] reported a 5-year larynx preservation of 59% for T3 tumors treated with transoral laser resection, citing vocal fold fixation and laryngeal cartilage invasion as significant prognostic factors for lower local control. Thus, organ-preservation surgery remains an option for selected patients in specialized centers.

The highest-level evidence that currently exists for laryngeal cancer is in favor of better locoregional control, organ preservation, and overall survival if concomitant chemoradiation is used as a nonsurgical means of organ preservation, as compared with radiation therapy alone or induction chemotherapy protocols.[80,81] The 3-arm prospective randomized trial conducted by Forastiere and colleagues[80] comparing radiation therapy, induction chemotherapy (cisplatin and 5-fluorouracil) with radiation, and concurrent chemoradiation with cisplatin for advanced laryngeal cancer (level 2 evidence) showed a higher 2-year locoregional control rate for the group treated with concurrent chemoradiation:

- 78% versus 61% for the group treated with induction chemotherapy
- 56% for the group treated with radiation therapy alone

The 2-year laryngeal preservation rate was

- 88% for the chemoradiation arm versus 75% for the induction chemotherapy group
- 70% for the radiation therapy group

In the recent meta-analysis by Blanchard and colleagues[81] of randomized controlled trials (level 1 evidence), overall survival improved from 42.5% to 47.0% in the group of 3216 patients with laryngeal cancer treated with concomitant chemoradiation. The benefit was not significant, however, for adjuvant or neoadjuvant chemotherapy. This study included only randomized controlled trials and compared locoregional treatment alone (radiation therapy ± surgery) with locoregional treatment and chemotherapy. The included studies did not involve taxanes, and the different types of locoregional treatments were not analyzed separately. This evidence would imply, however, that accelerated radiation therapy regimens alone do not provide the survival advantage of concurrent chemoradiation for laryngeal cancer. Current evidence, then, is in favor of concurrent chemoradiation when a nonsurgical organ-preservation strategy is chosen.

This evidence does not imply that this strategy is superior to initial total laryngectomy and radiation therapy in terms of oncological results for all patients. A large database study (level 3 evidence) conducted by Hoffman and colleagues[82] found that radiation therapy alone conferred a lower survival rate on T3N0 glottic cancers, but found no difference in survival when comparing surgery versus concurrent chemoradiation for these tumors. A recent matched-pair analysis of 132 patients, including 59% laryngeal cancers, 50% T3s and 50% T4s, comparing surgery (total or partial laryngectomy) plus radiation therapy (or chemoradation for 51%) versus definitive chemoradiation found no difference in locoregional control, metastasis-free survival or overall survival between the 2 treatment strategies (level 3 evidence).[83]

New chemotherapy drugs

Since these studies were published, new highly efficient drugs have been developed and tested. Adding taxanes (T) to neoadjuvant chemotherapy with cisplatin (P) and

5-fluorouracil (F) significantly improves response rates and organ-preservation rates for laryngeal cancer, as compared with PF alone (level 2 evidence).[84,85] Adding induction TPF to concurrent chemoradiation improved radiologic response rates at 6 to 8 weeks after treatment for stages III to IV head and neck cancers, with no increase in toxicity or compromise in radiation therapy regimens (level 2 evidence).[86] Adding a targeted therapy, cetuximab, to radiation therapy significantly improves survival as compared with radiation therapy alone (level 2 evidence),[87] leading to recent trials of cetuximab plus TPF (C-TPF) or TP (TPE) for induction in advanced head and neck tumors.[88,89] Progress in induction and concurrent chemotherapy and targeted therapies will certainly challenge current evidence favoring concurrent chemoradiation with cisplatin for nonsurgical organ preservation in the near future.

Defining advanced-stage laryngeal cancer
Another question is exactly what does one mean by "advanced" laryngeal cancer. T-stage takes into account the tumor volume and extensions, cartilage invasion, and resectability. Global staging (stages I through IVc) takes into account nodal disease and distant metastases, in addition to T-stage. Prospective randomized trials tend to exclude particularly advanced tumors with extensive invasion of the thyroid cartilage or tongue base, for example.[80] The results of these randomized trials can thus be applied only to these selected patient and tumor subgroups. For extensive stage IV tumors, in fact, current evidence shows an overall survival advantage with a total laryngectomy as compared with definitive chemoradiation. In the database study by Chen and Halpern,[90] 7019 patients with advanced laryngeal cancer (stage III or IV) were evaluated. Those with stage IV cancer treated with total laryngectomy had a significantly better overall survival rate than those treated with chemoradiation, who had a hazard ratio for death of 1.43 (level 3 evidence). Another large retrospective study by Gourin and colleagues[60] included 451 patients, 195 of whom had stage IV laryngeal cancer. Survival was better for patients treated surgically as compared with chemoradiation (hazard ratio 3.5) (level 3 evidence).

Globally, for advanced stage tumors, selected tumors may be amenable to conservation surgery (open or endoscopic) or concurrent chemoradiation with cisplatin. For more advanced tumors, a total laryngectomy should still be considered as an important treatment option. The results of newer protocols with taxanes and cetuximab are encouraging, and eligible patients should be enrolled in these[85] clinical trials when possible.

Is There Sufficient Evidence in Favor of the Use of Exclusive Chemotherapy for Glottic Cancer?

Since the introduction of platinum-based chemotherapy, and more recently with taxane-based treatments, it has become clear that glottic cancer is chemosensitive, with one-fourth to one-third of patients being complete responders and one-half to two-thirds being partial responders.[2,84,91–93] Adding chemotherapy to locoregional treatments (surgery and/or radiation therapy) has been shown to improve overall survival in head and neck cancer.[94,95] Recent level 1 evidence (a meta-analysis of the effects of chemotherapy by tumor site, including 3216 patients with laryngeal cancer) has shown a significant improvement in overall survival with concomitant chemoradiation, for an absolute 5-year survival benefit of 4.5%.[81]

In light of the advantages of chemotherapy, and the high response rates, 7 published studies have investigated using chemotherapy exclusively for treating early-stage, mid-stage, and advanced-stage glottic cancer.[96–102] Five of these studies were retrospective studies of complete responders after 3 cycles of induction chemotherapy (cisplatin and 5-fluorouracil), who then were allowed to decide if they preferred locoregional treatment or to pursue chemotherapy (level 4 evidence).[96–100] Four studies were from the same hospital.[96–99] Four of the studies included only tumors initially considered amenable to conservation laryngeal surgery.[96,98,99,101] In these studies,

- Between 29 and 65 patients were treated with exclusive chemotherapy, for a rate of local control with chemotherapy alone ranging from 54% to 72% and an ultimate larynx preservation rate ranging from 90% to 100%
- Toxicity was acceptable, and no chemotherapy deaths were recorded, but chemotherapy was prematurely stopped in 1% of patients because of toxicity.

To date, only 2 published studies have prospectively treated all complete responders with exclusive chemotherapy (level 3 evidence).[101,102] The study by Holsinger and colleagues[101] included 30 patients with stage II to IVa glottic (n = 14) or supraglottic (n = 16) carcinoma considered amenable to conservation laryngeal surgery:

- Eleven patients, 4 with glottic tumors and 7 with supraglottic tumors, were complete responders after 3 to 4 cycles of chemotherapy (37%), and received 3 more cycles.
- Ten of the 11 patients had no locoregional recurrence after a median follow-up of 5 years, for a local control rate with chemotherapy alone of 91% among the complete responders.

Divi and colleagues[102] prospectively studied 32 patients with stage III to IVb laryngeal and hypopharyngeal tumors, and

- Four patients, 2 with hypopharyngeal cancers and 2 with supraglottic cancers, were complete responders after 1 cycle and received additional chemotherapy.
- All of the patients had recurrences during the additional cycles: 3 in the neck and 1 locally and regionally.

For advanced-stage tumors, exclusive chemotherapy does not provide long-term locoregional control.

Thus, low-level evidence shows that highly selected patients with early-stage glottic cancer may undergo complete remission after exclusive chemotherapy; however, the initial local control rates for these highly selected patients, initially amenable to conservation laryngeal surgery, is not better than other conservation protocols using open surgery, transoral laser resection, or radiation therapy (see earlier in this article). In addition, we currently have no means of preselecting tumors that are more biologically susceptible to respond to chemotherapy, so many patients need to be treated (between 3 and 17[103]) to select the few complete responders (corresponding to 5.8%–33.0% of patients). Higher-level evidence is needed before exclusive chemotherapy can become a standard of care.

What Does the Evidence Say About Follow-up for Patients Treated for Glottic Cancer?

Follow-up aims at early detection of local recurrences, regional recurrences, distant metastases, metachronous second primaries, and complications of treatment, aiming to improve oncologic outcomes by early diagnosis of cancer-related events. Routine follow-up with regular clinical examination is performed in most centers treating laryngeal cancer, and most physicians follow patients for at least 5 years.[104–106] Routine screening using panendoscopy, bronchoscopy, esophagoscopy, ultrasound, CT, and PET are performed less regularly, and there is currently no consensus regarding optimum follow-up, although several guidelines have been published by various professional societies.[105]

- For the diagnosis of recurrence, a prospective study by Boysen and colleagues[107] found that 76% of recurrences (all head and neck sites combined) occurred in the first 2 years following treatment, and another 11% during the third year.
- de Visscher and Manni[108] found that 76% of recurrences, second primaries, or metastases (cancer-related "events") occurred within 3 years of initial treatment (level 3 evidence).
- Similarly, prospectively collected data analyzed by Lester and Wight[109] found that 95% of recurrences or second primaries occurred within 2.7 years for oropharyngeal primaries, 2.3 years for hypopharyngeal primaries, and 4.7 years for laryngeal primaries (level 2 evidence).

Thus, the best evidence implies that follow-up should be the most intense for the first 3 to 5 years if one is to diagnose most of the cancer-related events in this population.

Three published guidelines recommend routine clinical examination at a rate of 19 to 25 visits for the first 5 years (with a skewed distribution toward more frequent examination during the first 2 or 3 years), based primarily on physician surveys.[104,105] This does not answer the question if detection at routine follow-up improves oncologic outcomes. Conflicting level 3 evidence exists regarding the outcome if an event is detected at routine follow-up as compared with events diagnosed in symptomatic patients on self-referral:

- For de Visscher and Manni,[108] survival was better in the group of patients whose event was detected during a routine follow-up visit, whereas
- For Ritoe and colleagues[110] and Boysen and colleagues,[107] no survival difference was found between these 2 types of patients.

In their comprehensive review of the literature, Manikantan and colleagues[105] were unable to find convincing evidence that routine chest radiographs improved detection of second primaries or metastases, often revealed by symptoms (level 3 evidence), or that detection improved survival. They found level 4 evidence that chest CT was more sensitive than chest radiograph. They concluded that "chest CT should be done in symptomatic patients."

For the diagnosis of neck recurrence, ultrasound has been shown to be more sensitive than neck CT, which, in turn, is more sensitive than neck palpation.[105] There is no evidence, however, regarding any improvement in survival or any cost-effectiveness of routine follow-up neck screening using ultrasound or neck CT to detect regional recurrences, as compared with routine clinical follow-up of the neck. Level 3 evidence suggests that routine CT scanning of the neck may provide evidence in favor of recurrence earlier than clinical examination, for a proportion of patients (41% in the study by Hermans and colleagues).[111] This does not imply that earlier detection leads to better outcomes, however.

The high sensitivity (94%), specificity (82%), and negative predictive value (95%) of PET for detecting local recurrence for head and neck cancers treated by radiation therapy or chemoradiation has been confirmed by a large meta-analysis published in 2008 (level 1 evidence).[112] There is currently no evidence showing any improvement in patient outcomes, however, by the routine use of PET. Finally, in the systematic literature review by Manikantan and colleagues,[105] routine follow-up bronchoscopy and esophagoscopy were found to be "not warranted," because of the cost, morbidity, and low rate of second primary tumors diagnosed (2%–6% of patients with laryngeal cancer, level 3 evidence).

Hypothyroidism, symptomatic or subclinical, in patients treated for head and neck cancer has a reported prevalence of 5% to 56%, although the actuarial incidence at 10 years may exceed 90%.[113] There is only one prospective study of hypothyroidism in patients treated for head and neck cancer in which the median time to hypothyroidism was 8 months, and 83% of the cases of hypothyroidism occurred within 1 year of treatment (level 3 evidence).[114] Based on these data, current guidelines recommend thyroid function studies every 6 to 12 months following treatment of head and neck cancers.[115]

BOTTOM LINE: WHAT DOES THE EVIDENCE REALLY SAY ABOUT GLOTTIC CARCINOMA?

We place the highest value on evidence obtained from randomized controlled trials, which provide the best objective, statistically sound evidence to guide decisions for treatment of individual patients. Much has been written, however, about the defects inherent in this approach. Patients enrolled in randomized controlled trials are highly selected in terms of their tumor, but also in terms of comorbidities. Enrolled patients more often tend to be white, educated, insured, health-conscious, and younger than the general population of patients with cancer,[116] and the self-selection of patients for clinical trials may in and of itself constitute a bias toward globally better results than one could expect in the general population.[117]

For glottic carcinoma, we have seen that in the randomized controlled trials comparing different nonsurgical organ preservation strategies, widely invasive tumors with extensive tongue base involvement and/or cartilage invasion were excluded. Thus, we must always be careful when applying the results of these trials to our general patient population, and regularly reevaluate our outcomes in "real life."

Treatment choices for early-stage glottic cancer are currently based on low-level evidence. Conservation surgery (open or transoral laser resection) and radiation therapy are all still valid options for treating Tis, T1, and selected T2 glottic lesions. Subjective selection criteria are still the basis for treatment choice for these lesions. For advanced lesions not amenable to conservation surgery, high-level evidence favors concurrent chemoradiation with cisplatin for nonsurgical organ preservation. With the increasing use of taxanes and cetuximab, however, the optimal combination of chemotherapy, targeted therapy, and radiation therapy is currently unknown. Finally, for large tumors with extensive cartilage and/or tongue base invasion, total laryngectomy followed by radiation therapy is still the treatment of choice for optimization of oncologic outcomes.

In the treatment of glottic carcinoma, the evidence in favor of one type of treatment as opposed to another is globally low level. For now, bias and opinion may still mar our decision making, even in the context of multidisciplinary tumor boards. The opportunities for conservation laryngeal surgery depend on the experience and expertise of the local surgical oncology organ specialists. Guidelines based on expert opinion may be useful, but generally do not provide details on appropriate criteria for patient selection for various treatment modalities (particularly conservation laryngeal surgery). Conservation surgery, and particularly transoral surgery, is often an "à la carte" procedure, and patient heterogeneity can impede coherent evaluation of patient groups. Prospective surgical registries may improve our options for outcomes analysis according to tumor subtypes and "atypical" surgeries.[118]

To optimize patient outcome, current evidence must be combined with experience of the multidisciplinary team managing these patients,[119] along with maintenance of a high regard for the patient-physician relationship, with an honest, open discussion regarding all of the aspects of different treatment options.

CRITICAL POINTS

- Initial workup should include CT and/or MRI of the larynx (level 2 evidence).
- Curative treatment for Tis: transoral surgery or radiation therapy. Prefer surgery for younger patients. Save radiotherapy for failure of a surgical approach (level 3 evidence).
- Curative treatment for T1a: surgery (transoral laser surgery or open surgery) or radiation therapy (level 3).
- Curative treatment for T1T2 with AC involvement: surgery (transoral or open) provides better initial local control and final laryngeal preservation than radiation therapy (level 3).
- Curative treatment for T2: T2 with normal vocal fold mobility may be treated by surgery or radiation therapy (level 3); surgery provides better outcomes for tumors with impaired vocal fold mobility as compared with radiation therapy alone (level 3).
- Curative treatment for T3T4: Conservation laryngeal surgery remains an option for selected tumors (level 4). When a nonsurgical organ preservation strategy is chosen, concurrent chemoradiation with cisplatin provides better outcomes than radiation therapy alone or induction chemotherapy with cisplatin and 5-fluorouracil (level 1). Eligible patients should be referred for inclusion in clinical trials investigating the role of taxanes and cetuximab. For locally advanced tumors, survival is better with initial total laryngectomy followed by radiation therapy (level 3).
- Follow-up should be performed in the clinic for at least 3 to 5 years to detect recurrence, second primary tumors, metastases, and late effects of treatment, although early detection of cancer events has not been sufficiently studied to prove that follow-up improves oncologic outcomes (level 5).

REFERENCES

1. Elstein AS. On the origins and development of evidence-based medicine and medical decision making. Inflamm Res 2004;53(Suppl 2):S184–9.
2. Wolf GT, Waun KH, Gross Fischer S, et al. Induction chemotherapy plus radiation compared with surgery plus radiation in patients with advanced laryngeal cancer. The Department of Veterans Affairs Laryngeal Cancer Study Group. N Engl J Med 1991;324(24):1685–90.
3. Kirchner JA. Fifteenth Daniel C. Baker, Jr, memorial lecture. What have whole organ sections contributed to the treatment of laryngeal cancer? Ann Otol Rhinol Laryngol 1989;98(9):661–7.
4. OCEBM Levels of Evidence Working Group, Howick J, Chalmers I, Glasziou P, et al. The Oxford 2011 levels of evidence. Oxford Centre for Evidence-Based Medicine; 2011. Available at: http://wwwcebmnet/indexaspx?o=5653. Accessed November 28, 2011.
5. Hartl DM, Landry G, Hans S, et al. Organ preservation surgery for laryngeal squamous cell carcinoma: low incidence of thyroid cartilage invasion. Laryngoscope 2010;120(6):1173–6.
6. Hartl DM, Landry G, Hans S, et al. Thyroid cartilage invasion in early-stage squamous cell carcinoma involving the anterior commissure. Head Neck 2011. [Epub ahead of print].

7. Brasnu DF. Supracricoid partial laryngectomy with cricohyoidopexy in the management of laryngeal carcinoma. World J Surg 2003;27(7):817–23.

8. Zbaren P, Becker M, Lang H. Pretherapeutic staging of laryngeal carcinoma. Clinical findings, computed tomography, and magnetic resonance imaging compared with histopathology. Cancer 1996;77(7):1263–73.

9. Zbaren P, Becker M, Lang H. Staging of laryngeal cancer: endoscopy, computed tomography and magnetic resonance versus histopathology. Eur Arch Otorhinolaryngol 1997;254(Suppl 1):S117–22.

10. Becker M, Burkhardt K, Dulguerov P, et al. Imaging of the larynx and hypopharynx. Eur J Radiol 2008;66(3):460–79.

11. Becker M, Zbaren P, Laeng H, et al. Neoplastic invasion of the laryngeal cartilage: comparison of MR imaging and CT with histopathologic correlation. Radiology 1995;194(3):661–9.

12. Hao SP, Ng SH. Magnetic resonance imaging versus clinical palpation in evaluating cervical metastasis from head and neck cancer. Otolaryngol Head Neck Surg 2000;123(3):324–7.

13. King AD, Tse GM, Ahuja AT, et al. Necrosis in metastatic neck nodes: diagnostic accuracy of CT, MR imaging, and US. Radiology 2004;230(3):720–6.

14. Wax MK, Myers LL, Gona JM, et al. The role of positron emission tomography in the evaluation of the N-positive neck. Otolaryngol Head Neck Surg 2003;129(3):163–7.

15. Ashraf M, Biswas J, Jha J, et al. Clinical utility and prospective comparison of ultrasonography and computed tomography imaging in staging of neck metastases in head and neck squamous cell cancer in an Indian setup. Int J Clin Oncol 2011;16(6):686–93.

16. Rumboldt Z, Gordon L, Bonsall R, et al. Imaging in head and neck cancer. Curr Treat Options Oncol 2006;7(1):23–34.

17. Sumi M, Kimura Y, Sumi T, et al. Diagnostic performance of MRI relative to CT for metastatic nodes of head and neck squamous cell carcinomas. J Magn Reson Imaging 2007;26(6):1626–33.

18. Jeong HS, Baek CH, Son YI, et al. Use of integrated 18F-FDG PET/CT to improve the accuracy of initial cervical nodal evaluation in patients with head and neck squamous cell carcinoma. Head Neck 2007;29(3):203–10.

19. Adams S, Baum RP, Stuckensen T, et al. Prospective comparison of 18F-FDG PET with conventional imaging modalities (CT, MRI, US) in lymph node staging of head and neck cancer. Eur J Nucl Med 1998;25(9):1255–60.

20. Le QT, Takamiya R, Shu HK, et al. Treatment results of carcinoma in situ of the glottis: an analysis of 82 cases. Arch Otolaryngol Head Neck Surg 2000; 126(11):1305–12.

21. Garcia-Serra A, Hinerman RW, Amdur RJ, et al. Radiotherapy for carcinoma in situ of the true vocal cords. Head Neck 2002;24(4):390–4.

22. Spayne JA, Warde P, O'Sullivan B, et al. Carcinoma-in-situ of the glottic larynx: results of treatment with radiation therapy. Int J Radiat Oncol Biol Phys 2001; 49(5):1235–8.

23. Damm M, Sittel C, Streppel M, et al. Transoral CO2 laser for surgical management of glottic carcinoma in situ. Laryngoscope 2000;110(7):1215–21.

24. Sengupta N, Morris CG, Kirwan J, et al. Definitive radiotherapy for carcinoma in situ of the true vocal cords. Am J Clin Oncol 2010;33(1):94–5.

25. Fein DA, Mendenhall WM, Parsons JT, et al. Carcinoma in situ of the glottic larynx: the role of radiotherapy. Int J Radiat Oncol Biol Phys 1993;27(2): 379–84.

26. Hartl DM, de Mones E, Hans S, et al. Treatment of early-stage glottic cancer by transoral laser resection. Ann Otol Rhinol Laryngol 2007;116(11):832–6.

27. Peretti G, Nicolai P, Piazza C, et al. Oncological results of endoscopic resections of Tis and T1 glottic carcinomas by carbon dioxide laser. Ann Otol Rhinol Laryngol 2001;110(9):820–6.

28. Smee RI, Meagher NS, Williams JR, et al. Role of radiotherapy in early glottic carcinoma. Head Neck 2010;32(7):850–9.

29. Nguyen C, Naghibzadeh B, Black MJ, et al. Carcinoma in situ of the glottic larynx: excision or irradiation? Head Neck 1996;18(3):225–8.

30. Silver CE, Beitler JJ, Shaha AR, et al. Current trends in initial management of laryngeal cancer: the declining use of open surgery. Eur Arch Otorhinolaryngol 2009;266(9):1333–52.

31. Stoeckli SJ, Schnieper I, Huguenin P, et al. Early glottic carcinoma: treatment according patient's preference? Head Neck 2003;25(12):1051–6.

32. Schrijvers ML, van Riel EL, Langendijk JA, et al. Higher laryngeal preservation rate after CO2 laser surgery compared with radiotherapy in T1a glottic laryngeal carcinoma. Head Neck 2009;31(6):759–64.

33. Jones DA, Mendenhall CM, Kirwan J, et al. Radiation therapy for management of T1-T2 glottic cancer at a private practice. Am J Clin Oncol 2010;33(6):587–90.

34. Higgins KM, Shah MD, Ogaick MJ, et al. Treatment of early-stage glottic cancer: meta-analysis comparison of laser excision versus radiotherapy. J Otolaryngol Head Neck Surg 2009;38(6):603–12.

35. Smith JC, Johnson JT, Cognetti DM, et al. Quality of life, functional outcome, and costs of early glottic cancer. Laryngoscope 2003;113(1):68–76.

36. Goor KM, Peeters AJ, Mahieu HF, et al. Cordectomy by CO2 laser or radiotherapy for small T1a glottic carcinomas: costs, local control, survival, quality of life, and voice quality. Head Neck 2007;29(2):128–36.

37. Cragle SP, Brandenburg JH. Laser cordectomy or radiotherapy: cure rates, communication, and cost. Otolaryngol Head Neck Surg 1993;108(6):648–54.

38. Brandenburg JH. Laser cordotomy versus radiotherapy: an objective cost analysis. Ann Otol Rhinol Laryngol 2001;110(4):312–8.

39. Peeters AJ, van Gogh CD, Goor KM, et al. Health status and voice outcome after treatment for T1a glottic carcinoma. Eur Arch Otorhinolaryngol 2004;261(10):534–40.

40. Krengli M, Policarpo M, Manfredda I, et al. Voice quality after treatment for T1a glottic carcinoma—radiotherapy versus laser cordectomy. Acta Oncol 2004;43(3):284–9.

41. Rydell R, Schalen L, Fex S, et al. Voice evaluation before and after laser excision vs. radiotherapy of T1A glottic carcinoma. Acta Otolaryngol 1995;115(4):560–5.

42. Remacle M, Eckel HE, Antonelli A, et al. Endoscopic cordectomy. A proposal for a classification by the Working Committee, European Laryngological Society. Eur Arch Otorhinolaryngol 2000;257(4):227–31.

43. Holland JM, Arsanjani A, Liem BJ, et al. Second malignancies in early stage laryngeal carcinoma patients treated with radiotherapy. J Laryngol Otol 2002;116(3):190–3.

44. Burns JA, Har-El G, Shapshay S, et al. Endoscopic laser resection of laryngeal cancer: is it oncologically safe? Position statement from the American Broncho-Esophagological Association. Ann Otol Rhinol Laryngol 2009;118(6):399–404.

45. Sachse F, Stoll W, Rudack C. Evaluation of treatment results with regard to initial anterior commissure involvement in early glottic carcinoma treated by external partial surgery or transoral laser microresection. Head Neck 2009;31(4):531–7.

46. Chone CT, Yonehara E, Martins JE, et al. Importance of anterior commissure in recurrence of early glottic cancer after laser endoscopic resection. Arch Otolaryngol Head Neck Surg 2007;133(9):882–7.
47. Bradley PJ, Rinaldo A, Suarez C, et al. Primary treatment of the anterior vocal commissure squamous carcinoma. Eur Arch Otorhinolaryngol 2006;263(10): 879–88.
48. Nozaki M, Furuta M, Murakami Y, et al. Radiation therapy for T1 glottic cancer: involvement of the anterior commissure. Anticancer Res 2000;20(2B):1121–4.
49. Maheshwar AA, Gaffney CC. Radiotherapy for T1 glottic carcinoma: impact of anterior commissure involvement. J Laryngol Otol 2001;115(4):298–301.
50. Rodel RM, Steiner W, Muller RM, et al. Endoscopic laser surgery of early glottic cancer: involvement of the anterior commissure. Head Neck 2009;31(5):583–92.
51. Rucci L, Gallo O, Fini-Storchi O. Glottic cancer involving anterior commissure: surgery vs radiotherapy. Head Neck 1991;13(5):403–10.
52. Zohar Y, Rahima M, Shvili Y, et al. The controversial treatment of anterior commissure carcinoma of the larynx. Laryngoscope 1992;102(1):69–72.
53. Bron LP, Soldati D, Zouhair A, et al. Treatment of early stage squamous-cell carcinoma of the glottic larynx: endoscopic surgery or cricohyoidoepiglottopexy versus radiotherapy. Head Neck 2001;23(10):823–9.
54. Ambrosch P. The role of laser microsurgery in the treatment of laryngeal cancer. Curr Opin Otolaryngol Head Neck Surg 2007;15(2):82–8.
55. Peretti G, Piazza C, Cocco D, et al. Transoral CO(2) laser treatment for T(is)-T(3) glottic cancer: the University of Brescia experience on 595 patients. Head Neck 2010;32(8):977–83.
56. Laccourreye O, Laccourreye L, Garcia D, et al. Vertical partial laryngectomy versus supracricoid partial laryngectomy for selected carcinomas of the true vocal cord classified as T2N0. Ann Otol Rhinol Laryngol 2000;109(10 Pt 1): 965–71.
57. Peretti G, Piazza C, Mensi MC, et al. Endoscopic treatment of cT2 glottic carcinoma: prognostic impact of different pT subcategories. Ann Otol Rhinol Laryngol 2005;114(8):579–86.
58. Peretti G, Piazza C, Bolzoni A, et al. Analysis of recurrences in 322 Tis, T1, or T2 glottic carcinomas treated by carbon dioxide laser. Ann Otol Rhinol Laryngol 2004;113(11):853–8.
59. Mendenhall WM, Amdur RJ, Morris CG, et al. T1–T2N0 squamous cell carcinoma of the glottic larynx treated with radiation therapy. J Clin Oncol 2001; 19(20):4029–36.
60. Gourin CG, Conger BT, Sheils WC, et al. The effect of treatment on survival in patients with advanced laryngeal carcinoma. Laryngoscope 2009;119(7): 1312–7.
61. Marandas P, Hartl DM, Charffedine I, et al. T2 laryngeal carcinoma with impaired mobility: subtypes with therapeutic implications. Eur Arch Otorhinolaryngol 2002;259(2):87–90.
62. Motta G, Esposito E, Motta S, et al. CO(2) laser surgery in the treatment of glottic cancer. Head Neck 2005;27(7):566–73 [discussion: 573–4].
63. Gallo A, de Vincentiis M, Manciocco V, et al. CO2 laser cordectomy for early-stage glottic carcinoma: a long-term follow-up of 156 cases. Laryngoscope 2002;112(2):370–4.
64. Tucker HM, Benninger MS, Roberts JK, et al. Near-total laryngectomy with epiglottic reconstruction. Long-term results. Arch Otolaryngol Head Neck Surg 1989;115(11):1341–4.

65. Dinshaw KA, Sharma V, Agarwal JP, et al. Radiation therapy in T1-T2 glottic carcinoma: influence of various treatment parameters on local control/complications. Int J Radiat Oncol Biol Phys 2000;48(3):723–35.

66. Howell-Burke D, Peters LJ, Goepfert H, et al. T2 glottic cancer. Recurrence, salvage, and survival after definitive radiotherapy. Arch Otolaryngol Head Neck Surg 1990;116(7):830–5.

67. Karim AB, Kralendonk JH, Yap LY, et al. Heterogeneity of stage II glottic carcinoma and its therapeutic implications. Int J Radiat Oncol Biol Phys 1987;13(3): 313–7.

68. Harwood AR, DeBoer G. Prognostic factors in T2 glottic cancer. Cancer 1980; 45(5):991–5.

69. de Bree R, Leemans CR, Silver CE, et al. Paratracheal lymph node dissection in cancer of the larynx, hypopharynx, and cervical esophagus: the need for guidelines. Head Neck 2011;33(6):912–6.

70. Laccourreye O, Diaz EM Jr, Bassot V, et al. A multimodal strategy for the treatment of patients with T2 invasive squamous cell carcinoma of the glottis. Cancer 1999;85(1):40–6.

71. Chevalier D, Laccourreye O, Brasnu D, et al. Cricohyoidoepiglottopexy for glottic carcinoma with fixation or impaired motion of the true vocal cord: 5-year oncologic results with 112 patients. Ann Otol Rhinol Laryngol 1997;106(5):364–9.

72. Smee R, Bridger GP, Williams J, et al. Early glottic carcinoma: results of treatment by radiotherapy. Australas Radiol 2000;44(1):53–9.

73. Chera BS, Amdur RJ, Morris CG, et al. T1N0 to T2N0 squamous cell carcinoma of the glottic larynx treated with definitive radiotherapy. Int J Radiat Oncol Biol Phys 2010;78(2):461–6.

74. Pantel M, Wittekindt C, Altendorf-Hofmann A, et al. Diversity of treatment of T2N0 glottic cancer of the larynx: lessons to learn from epidemiological cancer registry data. Acta Otolaryngol 2011;131(11):1205–13.

75. Wierzbicka M, Leszczynska M, Mlodkowska A, et al. The impact of prelaryngeal node metastases on early glottic cancer treatment results. Eur Arch Otorhinolaryngol 2012;269(1):193–9.

76. Dufour X, Hans S, De Mones E, et al. Local control after supracricoid partial laryngectomy for "advanced" endolaryngeal squamous cell carcinoma classified as T3. Arch Otolaryngol Head Neck Surg 2004;130(9):1092–9.

77. Laccourreye O, Salzer SJ, Brasnu D, et al. Glottic carcinoma with a fixed true vocal cord: outcomes after neoadjuvant chemotherapy and supracricoid partial laryngectomy with cricohyoidoepiglottopexy. Otolaryngol Head Neck Surg 1996;114(3):400–6.

78. Vilaseca I, Bernal-Sprekelsen M, Luis Blanch J. Transoral laser microsurgery for T3 laryngeal tumors: prognostic factors. Head Neck 2010;32(7):929–38.

79. Hinni ML, Salassa JR, Grant DG, et al. Transoral laser microsurgery for advanced laryngeal cancer. Arch Otolaryngol Head Neck Surg 2007;133(12):1198–204.

80. Forastiere AA, Goepfert H, Maor M, et al. Concurrent chemotherapy and radiotherapy for organ preservation in advanced laryngeal cancer. N Engl J Med 2003;349(22):2091–8.

81. Blanchard P, Baujat B, Holostenco V, et al. Meta-analysis of chemotherapy in head and neck cancer (MACH-NC): a comprehensive analysis by tumour site. Radiother Oncol 2011;100(1):33–40.

82. Hoffman HT, Porter K, Karnell LH, et al. Laryngeal cancer in the United States: changes in demographics, patterns of care, and survival. Laryngoscope 2006; 116(9 Pt 2 Suppl 111):1–13.

83. Rades D, Schroeder U, Bajrovic A, et al. Radiochemotherapy versus surgery plus radio(chemo)therapy for stage T3/T4 larynx and hypopharynx cancer: results of a matched-pair analysis. Eur J Cancer 2011;47(18):2729–34.

84. Pointreau Y, Garaud P, Chapet S, et al. Randomized trial of induction chemotherapy with cisplatin and 5-fluorouracil with or without docetaxel for larynx preservation. J Natl Cancer Inst 2009;101(7):498–506.

85. Posner MR, Norris CM, Wirth LJ, et al. Sequential therapy for the locally advanced larynx and hypopharynx cancer subgroup in TAX 324: survival, surgery, and organ preservation. Ann Oncol 2009;20(5):921–7.

86. Paccagnella A, Mastromauro C, D'Amanzo P, et al. Induction chemotherapy before chemoradiotherapy in locally advanced head and neck cancer: the future? Oncologist 2010;15(Suppl 3):8–12.

87. Bonner JA, Harari PM, Giralt J, et al. Radiotherapy plus cetuximab for locoregionally advanced head and neck cancer: 5-year survival data from a phase 3 randomised trial, and relation between cetuximab-induced rash and survival. Lancet Oncol 2010;11(1):21–8.

88. Haddad RI, Tishler RB, Norris C, et al. Phase I study of C-TPF in patients with locally advanced squamous cell carcinoma of the head and neck. J Clin Oncol 2009;27(27):4448–53.

89. Argiris A, Heron DE, Smith RP, et al. Induction docetaxel, cisplatin, and cetuximab followed by concurrent radiotherapy, cisplatin, and cetuximab and maintenance cetuximab in patients with locally advanced head and neck cancer. J Clin Oncol 2010;28(36):5294–300.

90. Chen AY, Halpern M. Factors predictive of survival in advanced laryngeal cancer. Arch Otolaryngol Head Neck Surg 2007;133(12):1270–6.

91. Urba S, Wolf G, Eisbruch A, et al. Single-cycle induction chemotherapy selects patients with advanced laryngeal cancer for combined chemoradiation: a new treatment paradigm. J Clin Oncol 2006;24(4):593–8.

92. Rapidis AD, Trichas M, Stavrinidis E, et al. Induction chemotherapy followed by concurrent chemoradiation in advanced squamous cell carcinoma of the head and neck: final results from a phase II study with docetaxel, cisplatin and 5-fluorouracil with a four-year follow-up. Oral Oncol 2006;42(7):675–84.

93. Vermorken JB. A new look at induction chemotherapy in locally advanced head and neck cancer. Oncologist 2010;15(Suppl 3):1–2.

94. Pignon JP, le Maitre A, Maillard E, et al. Meta-analysis of chemotherapy in head and neck cancer (MACH-NC): an update on 93 randomised trials and 17,346 patients. Radiother Oncol 2009;92(1):4–14.

95. Pignon JP, Bourhis J, Domenge C, et al. Chemotherapy added to locoregional treatment for head and neck squamous-cell carcinoma: three meta-analyses of updated individual data. MACH-NC Collaborative Group. Meta-Analysis of Chemotherapy on Head and Neck Cancer. Lancet 2000;355(9208):949–55.

96. Laccourreye O, Brasnu D, Bassot V, et al. Cisplatin-fluorouracil exclusive chemotherapy for T1-T3N0 glottic squamous cell carcinoma complete clinical responders: five-year results. J Clin Oncol 1996;14(8):2331–6.

97. Laccourreye O, Veivers D, Hans S, et al. Chemotherapy alone with curative intent in patients with invasive squamous cell carcinoma of the pharyngolarynx classified as T1-T4N0M0 complete clinical responders. Cancer 2001;92(6):1504–11.

98. Laccourreye O, Veivers D, Bassot V, et al. Analysis of local recurrence in patients with selected T1-3N0M0 squamous cell carcinoma of the true vocal cord managed with a platinum-based chemotherapy-alone regimen for cure. Ann Otol Rhinol Laryngol 2002;111(4):315–21 [discussion: 321–2].

99. Vachin F, Hans S, Atlan D, et al. Long-term results of exclusive chemotherapy for glottic squamous cell carcinoma complete clinical responders after induction chemotherapy. Ann Otolaryngol Chir Cervicofac 2004;121(3):140–7 [in French].

100. Bonfils P, Trotoux J, Bassot V. Chemotherapy alone in laryngeal squamous cell carcinoma. J Laryngol Otol 2007;121(2):143–8.

101. Holsinger FC, Kies MS, Diaz EM Jr, et al. Durable long-term remission with chemotherapy alone for stage II to IV laryngeal cancer. J Clin Oncol 2009; 27(12):1976–82.

102. Divi V, Worden FP, Prince ME, et al. Chemotherapy alone for organ preservation in advanced laryngeal cancer. Head Neck 2010;32(8):1040–7.

103. Hartl DM, Brasnu DF. Chemotherapy alone for glottic carcinoma: a need for higher-level evidence. Ann Otol Rhinol Laryngol 2009;118(8):543–5.

104. Morton RP, Hay KD, Macann A. On completion of curative treatment of head and neck cancer: why follow up? Curr Opin Otolaryngol Head Neck Surg 2004;12(2): 142–6.

105. Manikantan K, Khode S, Dwivedi RC, et al. Making sense of post-treatment surveillance in head and neck cancer: when and what of follow-up. Cancer Treat Rev 2009;35(8):744–53.

106. Joshi A, Calman F, O'Connell M, et al. Current trends in the follow-up of head and neck cancer patients in the UK. Clin Oncol (R Coll Radiol) 2010;22(2): 114–8.

107. Boysen M, Lovdal O, Tausjo J, et al. The value of follow-up in patients treated for squamous cell carcinoma of the head and neck. Eur J Cancer 1992;28(2–3): 426–30.

108. de Visscher AV, Manni JJ. Routine long-term follow-up in patients treated with curative intent for squamous cell carcinoma of the larynx, pharynx, and oral cavity. Does it make sense? Arch Otolaryngol Head Neck Surg 1994;120(9): 934–9.

109. Lester SE, Wight RG. 'When will I see you again?' Using local recurrence data to develop a regimen for routine surveillance in post-treatment head and neck cancer patients. Clin Otolaryngol 2009;34(6):546–51.

110. Ritoe SC, Krabbe PF, Kaanders JH, et al. Value of routine follow-up for patients cured of laryngeal carcinoma. Cancer 2004;101(6):1382–9.

111. Hermans R, Pameijer FA, Mancuso AA, et al. Laryngeal or hypopharyngeal squamous cell carcinoma: can follow-up CT after definitive radiation therapy be used to detect local failure earlier than clinical examination alone? Radiology 2000;214(3):683–7.

112. Isles MG, McConkey C, Mehanna HM. A systematic review and meta-analysis of the role of positron emission tomography in the follow up of head and neck squamous cell carcinoma following radiotherapy or chemoradiotherapy. Clin Otolaryngol 2008;33(3):210–22.

113. Miller M, Agarwal A. Hypothyroidism in postradiation head and neck cancer patients: incidence, complications, and management. Curr Opin Otolaryngol Head Neck Surg 2009;17(2):1111–5.

114. Sinard R, Tobin E, Mazzaferri E, et al. Hypothyroidism after treatment for nonthyroid head and neck cancer. Arch Otolaryngol 2000;126(5):652–7.

115. Network NCC. NCCN clinical practice guidelines in oncology. Head and neck cancers. NCCNorg; 2011. version 2.2011.

116. Al Refaie W, Vickers S, Zhong W, et al. Cancer trials versus the real world in the United States. Ann Surg 2011;254(3):438–42.

117. Clark A, Lammiman M, Goode K, et al. Is taking part in clinical trials good for your health? A cohort study. Eur J Heart Fail 2009;11(11):1078–83.
118. Korenkov M, Troidl H, Sauerland S. Individualized surgery in the time of evidence-based medicine. Ann Surg 2011. [Epub ahead of print].
119. Marshall J. Surgical decision-making: integrating evidence, inference, and experience. Surg Clin North Am 2006;86(1):201–15.

Management of Well-Differentiated Thyroid Cancer

Selena Liao, MD*, Maisie Shindo, MD

KEYWORDS

- Evidence-based otolaryngology • Well-differentiated thyroid cancer
- Follicular carcinoma • Papillary carcinoma • Neck dissection

KEY POINTS

The following points list the level of evidence as based on grading of the Oxford Centre for Evidence-Based Medicine. Additional critical points are provided, and points here are expanded at the conclusion of this article.

- Clinical staging with appropriate imaging can allow for planning of surgical management and should include preoperative ultrasonography, or alternative methods of computed tomography, magnetic resonance imaging, or positron emission tomography. Evidence level A.
- Suspicious lymph nodes should be assessed for malignancy using ultrasound-guided fine-needle aspiration. Evidence level A.
- Tumors larger than 1 cm should be resected via near-total or total thyroidectomy. Evidence level A.
- Tumors smaller than 1 cm may be initially managed via total lobectomy. Evidence level A.
- All presurgically involved levels of lymph nodes should be resected via compartment resection rather than berry picking. Evidence level A.
- Lateral neck involvement warrants compartment resection of at least levels II-A, III, and IV. Evidence level A.

OVERVIEW

Thyroid cancer is the most common of all endocrine cancers. Well-differentiated thyroid cancer comprises the majority of thyroid cancers, about 90%, and includes both papillary and follicular carcinomas. Most of these, about 85%, are of the papillary subtype. The incidence of thyroid cancer has been reported to be increasing, mostly due to increased detection rates, with one study showing a 2.4-fold increase from 3.6 per 100,000 in 1973 to 8.7 per 100,000 in 2002.[1] Overall mortality in this study was low, at 0.5 deaths per 100,000.

Department of Otolaryngology – Head and Neck Surgery, Oregon Health and Sciences University, 3181 Southwest Sam Jackson Park Road, SJH01, Portland, OR 97239, USA
* Corresponding author.
E-mail address: liao@ohsu.edu

Otolaryngol Clin N Am 45 (2012) 1163–1179
http://dx.doi.org/10.1016/j.otc.2012.06.015
0030-6665/12/$ – see front matter © 2012 Elsevier Inc. All rights reserved.

In 2006, a task force within the American Thyroid Association (ATA) developed a set of guidelines for the management of thyroid nodules and differentiated thyroid cancer. These guidelines were most recently revised in 2009.[2] Nevertheless, not all of the recommendations have Grade A evidence and there are still many areas of controversy regarding surgical management.

EVIDENCE-BASED CLINICAL ASSESSMENT FOR THYROID CANCER
Staging

Accurate staging is important in determining the prognosis and tailoring the treatment of patients with differentiated thyroid cancer. Unlike with many other tumor types, the presence of distant metastasis, for example in lungs and bones, does not obviate primary resection (thyroidectomy) because metastatic disease may respond to radioactive iodine therapy (RAI) after surgical removal of neck disease.[3] Surgery comprises removal of all thyroid tissue along with the primary tumor, as well as that of regional nodal disease, and is one of the most important initial treatments. Complete resection of the thyroid gland and locoregional disease is particularly important for facilitating RAI for metastatic disease. Furthermore, patients having 5 or more clinically apparent metastases, a metastasis greater than 3 cm, or extranodal tumor extension were found to have a more adverse prognosis than those having none of these features.[4] Therefore, it is important to assess the extent of local disease and regional lymph node involvement before surgery.

Imaging: Ultrasonography

Preoperative ultrasonography is the most important imaging modality in the evaluation of thyroid nodules and thyroid cancer. The ATA Surgery Working Group guidelines recommend ultrasonography of the lateral neck to assess for metastatic nodes when thyroid cancer is diagnosed.[2] Ultrasonography identifies suspicious cervical adenopathy in the setting of thyroid malignancy. The sensitivity of detecting metastatic nodes that may alter overall management ranges from 20% to 31%.[5,6] Sonographic features suggestive of metastatic lymph nodes are:

- Cystic change
- Calcifications
- Loss of the fatty hilus
- A rounded rather than oval shape
- Hypoechogenicity
- Increased vascularity

Of these, detection of loss of the fatty hilus is 100% sensitive, but has very low specificity (29%).[7,8] The only criterion with high sensitivity as well as relatively high specificity is peripheral vascularity (86% sensitivity, 82% specificity). All other potential criteria have sensitivity of less than 60%, and are thus inadequate for use as a single criterion for the identification of malignancy.[9]

In a series of 3874 patients, Ito and colleagues[4] investigated the diagnostic accuracy of ultrasonography for lateral node metastasis in patients who underwent therapeutic or prophylactic modified neck dissection, reporting a specificity of 95% and a sensitivity of 43%. The presence of certain features, while low in sensitivity, can be highly specific for metastasis. For example, in a patient with known papillary thyroid cancer, the presence of cystic areas or punctate microcalcifications in a node are virtually diagnostic of metastasis (100% specificity). A lymph node short axis of less than 5 mm is also highly specific for metastasis (96%). Thus, an ultrasound scan can potentially alter the surgical approach in as many as 20% of patients.[10,11]

Imaging: Computed Tomography, Magnetic Resonance Imaging, Positron Emission Tomography

The limitations of ultrasonography are that evaluation is uniquely operator dependent, and it cannot easily visualize retropharyngeal, deep paraesophageal, or mediastinal nodes. Therefore, alternative imaging procedures, such as computed tomography (CT), magnetic resonance imaging (MRI), or positron emission tomography (PET), may be preferable in some clinical settings.[12,13] However, the sensitivities of these studies for the detection of cervical lymph node metastases are all relatively low (30%–40%).[14,15] Of the 3 modalities, CT with contrast is probably the most sensitive. The disadvantage of obtaining a contrast CT is that the iodine load necessitates a delay in any planned subsequent RAI, often beyond 3 months postoperatively. Nevertheless, these alternative imaging modalities are necessary for assessing the presence of deep cervical nodes that ultrasonography cannot detect, as well as the extent of invasive tumors, such as with invasion of the trachea, involvement of esophagus, and encasement or invasion of major vessels.

Laryngoscopy, Esophagoscopy, and Tracheoscopy

In addition, laryngoscopy, esophagoscopy, and tracheoscopy may also be necessary in the assessment of large, rapidly growing, retrosternal, or invasive tumors to determine the possibility of involvement of extrathyroidal tissues.

Biopsy

When a suspicious lymph node is identified, malignancy should be confirmed by ultrasound-guided fine-needle aspiration (FNA) if it will change the extent of the operative procedure. If the node is very small or cystic, it may be difficult to attain a sufficient sample for cytologic analysis, in which case the needle washout from the aspirate can also be sent for a thyroglobulin level. Elevated thyroglobulin from an FNA washout, even in a noncellular or hypocellular nondiagnostic aspirate, can confirm metastasis. This FNA measurement of thyroglobulin is valid even in patients with circulating thyroglobulin autoantibodies.[16,17]

EVIDENCE-BASED SURGICAL TECHNIQUE FOR THYROID CANCER
Extent of Resection

Once the diagnosis of well-differentiated thyroid cancer has been established, the primary treatment modality is surgical resection. The current ATA guidelines recommend near-total or total thyroidectomy for all tumor sizes greater than 1 cm.[2] Regarding less extensive surgery, studies have shown increased recurrence and decreased survival rates in the patient population who undergo subtotal thyroidectomy.[18,19]

One argument for total thyroidectomy over lobectomy is the risk of thyroid cancer in the contralateral lobe. Several studies have demonstrated that of patients who originally underwent hemithyroidectomy and then subsequent completion thyroidectomy, the incidence of papillary thyroid cancer in the remaining lobe was found to be between 35% and 55%.[20–24] Even more compelling is evidence that patients with larger tumors who undergo lobectomy rather than total thyroidectomy fare worse in terms of recurrence and survival. A retrospective study by Hay and colleagues[25] that examined 2444 cases over 60 years showed that the recurrence and death rate was higher during the initial decade, in which the majority of surgical resections were lobectomies rather than total thyroidectomies, implying that lobectomy alone may be insufficient. Furthermore, an even larger study by Bilimoria and colleagues[26] in 2007 of 52,173 patients in the National Cancer database demonstrated higher recurrence rates and lower survival rates in those patients with tumors larger than 1 cm who underwent lobectomy only. This finding was maintained even in the subset of patients whose tumors ranged in size from 1 to 2 cm.

Microcarcinoma Versus Macrocarcinoma

For tumors less than 1 cm in size at diagnosis, however, many studies have indicated that lobectomy alone may have equivalent outcomes to more extensive resection, and may therefore be the initial surgery of choice.[27] In another study, Hay's group[28] reexamined nearly the same patient population over a 60-year period, focusing on those with tumors less than 1 cm in size, and found no significant difference in recurrence and survival rates between those undergoing lobectomy versus total thyroidectomy. Even the Bilimoria study did not find a difference in recurrence or survival rates in those patients undergoing either lobectomy or total thyroidectomy with tumors smaller than 1 cm.[26]

A more recent study by Ogilvie and colleagues,[29] however, raises the question of whether the "less than 1 cm" category of microcarcinoma should be further subdivided. These investigators retrospectively reviewed 130 records of node-negative patients with tumors smaller than 1 cm and found that when subdivided into a 6- to 10-mm group and a less than 6-mm group, a larger tumor size was still significantly associated with higher rates of adverse pathologic features and central node positivity. Nevertheless, there remains a lack of evidence to show whether lobectomy only in the 6- to 10-mm group results in any increase in recurrence or mortality rates in comparison with total thyroidectomy.

Tumor Involvement of the Recurrent Laryngeal Nerve

Invasive well-differentiated thyroid carcinoma is uncommon, but does occur in about 16% of patients.[30] Thyroid surgeons strive to avoid damage to the recurrent laryngeal nerves during routine operations; however, in cases where local disease is found to involve the nerve, there is some question as to how aggressively one should resect. The recurrent laryngeal nerve has been found to be involved in 33% to 61% of invasive thyroid cancers and is the most commonly involved nerve in the central compartment.[30–34] Recurrent laryngeal nerve involvement, however, may not predict the same morbidity or mortality as invasion of other structures. Chan and colleagues[35] reported high long-term survival rates in patients with known preoperative vocal cord paralysis and complete nerve transection caused by gross involvement. McCaffrey and colleagues[30] noted that invasion of the recurrent laryngeal nerve did not independently affect survival rates, in contrast to invasion of other structures, such as the trachea and esophagus, which independently decreased survival. McCaffrey's group argues for incomplete excision and treatment of residual disease with adjuvant RAI, as data have not shown complete excision to provide a survival benefit.[36] The development and use of adjunctive RAI has played a large role in allowing more surgical discretion regarding the extent of resection and preservation of vocal cord function despite nerve involvement.

In a previous *Otolaryngologic Clinics* review on the management of invasive thyroid cancer, Urken[37] noted that several factors should play a role in the determination of surgical extent:

- Preoperative preexisting vocal cord paralysis as documented by laryngoscopic examination
- Involvement of the contralateral recurrent laryngeal nerve
- Tumor histology
- Likelihood of disease response to RAI

In most cases, all attempts at nerve preservation should be performed with resection of obvious gross tumor. If the tumor can be dissected off of the nerve, the nerve can be left intact. However, if the tumor encases the nerve and resection is impossible without nerve sacrifice, especially in cases of known ipsilateral preoperative paralysis, the nerve should be resected. In cases of known contralateral preoperative paralysis, however, the potential morbidity from ipsilateral sacrifice and resulting bilateral vocal cord paralysis with possible need for tracheostomy may reasonably cause one to decide against full nerve resection. Also of note are several studies that have shown the possibility of recovery of vocal cord function after tumor resection in cases where nerve involvement was in the form of compression rather than infiltration.[36,38] Chiang and colleagues[39] have shown that extensive dissection of the recurrent laryngeal nerve can be performed with relatively low rates of temporary nerve palsy, and in their particular study, no cases of permanent palsy. Complete resection, however, as shown by Nishida and colleagues,[33] results in a high rate of permanent paralysis, even despite attempts at reanastomosis.

If there is need for recurrent laryngeal nerve sacrifice, rehabilitation procedures such as immediate reinnervation can be performed if sufficient distal stump remains for anastomosis. If direct reanastomosis is not possible because of a large gap, anastomosis of ansa cervicalis or ansa hypoglossi to the distal stump can be performed. Nerve grafting using a portion of the ansa cervicalis is another option. If accidental transection of the recurrent laryngeal nerve occurs during any operation, immediate repair is recommended to preserve muscle tone to laryngeal muscles, which can facilitate improvement in voice rehabilitation therapy.

Central Neck Dissection

The 2009 ATA guidelines provide recommendations regarding central neck dissection as an adjunct operation for thyroid cancer.[2] These guidelines define central neck dissection as "at a minimum... consist[ing of] removal of the prelaryngeal, pretracheal, and paratracheal lymph nodes...[either] unilateral or bilateral."[40] The central neck compartment consists of level VI, and occasionally level VII, as defined by the Memorial Sloan-Kettering system.[40] The superior boundary is the hyoid bone and the lateral boundaries, the carotid arteries. The definition for the inferior border is somewhat variable between the sternal notch or the innominate artery. Level VI is the main zone of lymphatic drainage for the majority of thyroid cancers. Those involving the upper pole, pyramidal lobe, and isthmus may also drain to levels II and III of the lateral neck. The lateral portion of the hemithyroid lobe may drain toward lateral neck levels III and IV.[41]

The ATA guidelines recommend that therapeutic central-compartment dissection of level VI be performed for all patients with known clinical involvement of either the central or lateral neck compartments.[2] However, in patients without evidence of nodal disease, the choice of whether to do an elective central neck dissection at the time of initial cancer resection is controversial. The ATA guidelines give only a C recommendation for elective central neck dissection in "patients with papillary thyroid carcinoma with clinically uninvolved central neck lymph nodes, especially for advanced primary tumors."[2] Likewise, they give a C rating for "thyroidectomy without prophylactic central neck dissection...[in patients with] small (T1–T2), noninvasive, clinically node-negative papillary thyroid carcinoma and most follicular cancer," in recognition that the current evidence is not strong either for or against the procedure, with only expert opinion to guide which groups of patients might benefit the most.

Central Neck Dissection in the Setting of Known Nodal Involvement

The central compartment is the most likely region of nodal recurrence.[42,43] Within the central compartment lymphatic drainage tends to flow to the ipsilateral side, and there is a higher rate of positive nodes found in the ipsilateral central compartment versus the contralateral side or the lateral neck.

It is rare to find patients with clinical evidence of lateral involvement without central involvement, but skip metastases can occur. Lateral node metastasis has been shown to have an independent correlation predicting central metastasis.[44] Roh and colleagues[45] performed a review of 22 patients who presented with lateral neck recurrences, none of whom had had previous central neck dissections with their initial thyroidectomies. At reoperation, elective central neck dissection showed 86% of patients to have central metastases, most frequently in the ipsilateral paratracheal compartment.

A study by Leboulleux and colleagues[46] regarding prognostic factors for persistent or recurrent disease in patients with locally advanced thyroid cancer at the time of diagnosis found that the presence of metastasis, specifically to the central compartment, significantly increased the risk of persistent disease after RAI.

Lymph node positivity has been shown in many studies to affect the rate of recurrence in differentiated thyroid cancer.

- Harwood and colleagues[47] compared the records of well-differentiated thyroid cancer patients, half of whom were N0 at time of diagnosis, and found that there were significantly more recurrences in patients with nodal involvement than in those without.
- Mazzaferri and Jhiang[48] looked at 1355 patients over 40 years and discovered the presence of cervical node metastases to significantly correlate with higher recurrence rates at 30 years, regardless of cancer subtype.
- The long-term study by Hay and colleagues[28] on patients with papillary thyroid microcarcinoma also found that recurrence rates were higher in node-positive patients, with more than 80% of all recurrences localizing to regional neck nodes.

Furthermore, several studies have also indicated lymph node positivity to have an effect on survival. In a large study of 9904 patients in the Surveillance, Epidemiology, and End Results (SEER) database, 77% of whom were node negative on presentation, cervical lymph node metastasis had a risk ratio of 1.34 on overall survival rates and was statistically significant.[49] This study refuted a previous study in 2003 that used the same database and did not find positive cervical nodes to affect mortality.[50]

Yet there are other studies showing that cervical node metastases have an independently significant effect.

- Harwood's group[47] also found that when matching for age, nodal metastasis also resulted in a worse survival prognosis, especially in older populations.
- Another study by Scheumann and colleagues[51] confirmed a decrease in survival for node-positive patients, even when controlling for age, tumor invasion, and distant metastasis.
- In addition, a more recent study by Lundgren and colleagues[52] performed a large population-based study of 5123 patients that showed cervical metastases to have an odds ratio of 2.5 on mortality, even after adjusting for TNM stage.
- Finally, a 2010 study by Grant and colleagues[53] examined 420 patients who underwent thyroidectomy with or without neck dissection based on the 4 recommendations set out by the 2009 ATA guidelines for management of thyroid cancer, and found only a 5% nodal recurrence rate in this group.

The evidence also supports the recommendation for compartment-oriented central compartment dissection of the involved compartments rather than "berry picking" when metastatic disease is identified in the central compartment either radiographically or intraoperatively. A study by Musacchio and colleagues[54] demonstrated increased local recurrence rates in patients whose neck disease was managed only through berry picking of visualized metastases rather than thorough neck dissections.

Role of Prophylactic or Elective Central Neck Dissection

Restaging
Proponents of the procedure point to the high rate of positive nodes found in otherwise clinically node-negative patients, with several studies finding rates between 31% and 64%.[44,55–58] Tumor size does not seem to affect these rates, with percentages remaining high in studies that looked at patients with microcarcinoma, as well as those with tumors greater than 1 cm in size. Finding positive nodes during prophylactic central neck dissection can significantly affect future treatment plans for patients. For example, it has been found to result in a high rate of restaging and adjustment of postsurgical therapy, particularly RAI.

- In one study by Shindo and colleagues,[56] 27% of patients age 45 years or older who underwent the procedure were reclassified from Stage I/II to Stage III.
- Hughes and colleagues[59] found similar results, with upstaging of 28.6% of patients, resulting in an increase in the dose of postsurgical RAI from 30 mCi to 150 mCi.

By contrast, more accurate staging through lymph node status can also decrease the number of patients who undergo RAI, a treatment that carries its own risk of complications and side effects including, for example, abdominal discomfort, neck tenderness, salivary dysfunction, and decreased tear production. A retrospective study from France of elective central neck dissection in clinically N0 patients showed that lymph node status affected 30.5% of cases, with half of them resulting in the decision not to treat with RAI in patients who would have originally qualified because of tumor size, but who were found to have no operative histopathologic evidence of positive nodes.[60]

Thyroglobulin concentrations
Central neck dissection may also reduce the follow-up burden for recurrence surveillance in some patients. There are studies that have shown patients with papillary thyroid cancer who undergo central neck dissection to have lower rates of postoperative thyroglobulin concentrations regardless of original tumor size.

- One Australian study of papillary thyroid carcinoma patients with tumors larger than 1 cm found that those who underwent elective central neck dissection in addition to total thyroidectomy had significantly lower postoperative stimulated serum thyroglobulin levels.[61] These patients also had a higher percentage of undetectable thyroglobulin at 6-month follow-up.
- Another study from Korea, on patients with papillary thyroid microcarcinoma, similarly found a significant reduction in the postoperative stimulated serum thyroglobulin level before RAI treatment.[62]

Complications
On the other hand, opponents of elective central neck dissection state that the rate of complications is higher than when thyroidectomy is performed alone. Furthermore, the procedure has not yet been shown to provide a conclusive long-term reduction in recurrence rates or change in survival rates. In this regard, better data on long-term

outcomes need to be shown before the additional operative time, costs, and potential risks to patients can be justified.

The most common complications associated with central elective neck dissection are identical to thyroidectomy alone:

- Unintentional parathyroid removal
- Hypocalcemia
- Recurrent laryngeal nerve injury
- Chyle leak
- Hematoma

It might be expected that patients undergoing additional neck dissection may have increased rates of parathyroid autotransplantation, resulting from the larger resection area and the parathyroid gland being often difficult to discern from lymph tissue. Indeed, this complication is noted to be significant in several studies.[55,59,61] Not surprisingly, then, many studies have also shown higher rates of transient hypocalcemia, usually defined as symptoms of hypocalcemia or a calcium level under the normal range for less than 6 months, to be increased after central neck dissection is added to thyroidectomy.[58,63,64]

Regarding complications in patients undergoing reoperation for recurrence, studies have shown overall complication rates to be low.

- Chao and colleagues[65] performed a retrospective review of 115 patients and found only a 5.2% rate of transient hypoparathyroidism and a 1.7% rate each of permanent hypoparathyroidism and permanent recurrent laryngeal nerve injury.
- A study by Kim and colleagues[66] also found no new cases of recurrent laryngeal nerve injury in patients undergoing reoperation.

Recurrence

As noted, although studies have shown patients with central neck dissection to have reduced thyroglobulin levels and decreased overall recurrence rates as defined by rising thyroglobulin or positive radioiodine scan, there are currently few studies that show a significant difference in recurrence between patients who receive neck dissection and those who do not.

- The same study by Leboulleux and colleagues[46] showing central neck nodes to be a risk factor for persistent disease did not find them to also be significant for recurrence.
- The study by Mazzaferri and Jhiang[48] that also indicated nodal disease to negatively affect survival only found this to be significant for patients with the follicular subtype and not for other thyroid cancers.
- In a study from Korea by So and colleagues[67] that found a reduction in postoperative thyroglobulin levels with elective central neck dissection, this difference disappeared after RAI therapy and, at 3-year follow-up, no significant difference in locoregional control rates was found.
- Even the study from the Mayo Clinic that showed only a 5% recurrence rate in patients undergoing central neck dissection did not compare this rate with that of those patients who did not have the additional procedure.[53]
- Of note, Leboulleux's group[46] also found overall survival rates in their patients to be high, 99% at 10 years, regardless of having undergone neck dissection or not.

Some surgeons have claimed that their experience in thyroid surgery allows their clinical judgment to decide which patients require central neck dissection, using preoperative and intraoperative information. A study by Shen and colleagues[68] found that a smaller percentage of patients who underwent thyroidectomy alone at their institution developed locoregional nodal recurrences, with more of them having disease-free status, when compared with those who underwent both thyroidectomy and central neck dissection. Their conclusion was that their surgeons were able to correctly identify those patient groups that would not benefit from additional neck dissection, thus avoiding an unnecessary increased risk of operative complications.

Reoperation

In addition, in contrast to other studies that have shown higher rates of surgical complications in patients undergoing reoperation in the neck for recurrence compared with neck dissection done at initial thyroidectomy, Shen and colleagues[69] have also claimed that their rate of reoperative complications is lower than when undertaking concurrent neck dissection. In another study comparing 189 central neck dissections done at time of thyroidectomy with 106 reoperations, they found that transient hypocalcemia occurred significantly more often in the primary operative group, although they did not find any differences between groups in rates of hematoma formation, permanent hypoparathyroidism, or recurrent laryngeal nerve injury.[69]

Paratracheal node dissection: bilateral versus ipsilateral

Another question among those practicing elective neck dissection concerns the utility of performing bilateral versus ipsilateral paratracheal node dissection. Studies have reported very different rates of positivity in contralateral nodes, from 1.4% to 69%, and there are no studies describing long-term recurrence rates for the contralateral neck after a unilateral lobe primary tumor.

- One study described the routine use of bilateral central neck dissection for all thyroid cancer diagnoses, with a 25% rate of contralateral neck node positivity.[70] Unfortunately, this study did not delineate the percentage of patients who were clinically node negative at the time of diagnosis. It did, however, note that there was no significant difference in complication rates regarding recurrent laryngeal nerve injury or permanent hypocalcemia between those undergoing bilateral central neck dissection rather than unilateral or no neck dissection. As in other studies, rates of inadvertent parathyroid removal were higher in the bilateral group, but with no apparent long-term sequelae.
- Shindo and Stern[71] compared complication rates between those undergoing total thyroidectomy with central neck dissection and those without. Their results showed no increase in rate of hypocalcemia in the group who underwent central neck dissection. Of note, most patients in their central neck dissection group underwent ipsilateral paratracheal and pretracheal compartment dissection.
- Another study by Roh and colleagues[72] on patients who did present with unilateral primary papillary carcinoma and without clinical node positivity found that 9.8% of this population had positive contralateral nodes after elective central neck dissection, and that ipsilateral metastases independently predicted contralateral metastases.

It has been noted that rates of metastasis to the ipsilateral lateral neck are higher than to the contralateral central neck. Another Korean study of patients with known lateral neck nodes found that the rate of contralateral central neck positivity was high, at 34.3%, and was associated with metastasis to all lateral neck levels.[73] In this study, other risk factors for contralateral central metastasis included multifocal primary tumors, lymphovascular invasion and, unsurprisingly, positive ipsilateral central nodes.

Lateral Neck Dissection

Metastasis to the lateral neck compartments warrants dissection of the involved compartments, given that positive lymph nodes, as noted previously, increase the risk of recurrence and decrease survival rates. The 2009 ATA guidelines recommend that "therapeutic lateral neck compartmental lymph node dissection should be performed for patients with biopsy-proven metastatic lateral cervical lymphadenopathy."[2] As already noted, lateral neck involvement without central neck involvement is rare, although skip metastases can occur. Chung and colleagues[74] found a 7.7% rate of skip metastases in 7.7% of patients with papillary microcarcinoma who had undergone both central and lateral neck dissections for preoperative evidence of lateral metastasis.

Risk factors for lateral compartment involvement have been found to include[74–78]:

- Younger patient age
- Gender
- Tumor multifocality
- Tumor calcifications
- Upper pole tumor location
- Larger tumor size
- Extrathyroidal extension
- Central node positivity
- Ipsilateral involvement of other lateral neck levels
- Contralateral lateral involvement

Some investigators recommend more aggressive treatment of the lateral compartment if any positive lymph nodes are found in the central compartment.

- Goropoulous and colleagues[79] looked at 39 patients who underwent central and bilateral lateral neck dissections in addition to total thyroidectomy, and found that of the patients who were found to have positivity in the central neck, 80% also had concurrent ipsilateral lateral neck disease and 52% were also positive in the contralateral lateral neck. However, this study included patients with a variety of tumor sizes, with a trend toward lateral positivity with larger tumors.
- Machens and colleagues[80] conducted a retrospective review of patients who underwent both primary and reoperative neck dissections for both papillary and medullary thyroid cancer, and found that the ipsilateral lateral compartment was involved almost as frequently as the central compartment for all groups.
- By contrast, however, a study by Wang and colleagues[81] found that only 3% of N0 necks were found to have lateral disease, and that risk factors for lateral recurrence and decreased survival included older patients and tumor size greater than 4 cm.

Extent of Lateral Neck Dissection

There is also some controversy over whether performing lateral neck dissection requires full clearance of levels II through V, or whether selective dissection may be performed based on clinical data. The most common neck levels involved with lateral metastases are II, III, and IV, with level III having the highest probability of positive nodes in most studies.[75,76,79,82] Ahmadi and colleagues,[83] however, found level IV to be the most commonly involved level in their recent study of 49 patients, with level IV also being the most common site of recurrence.

Some argue that the surgeon's judgment, based on both preoperative clinical data and intraoperative findings, may be sufficient to determine the extent of lateral dissection. Caron and colleagues[84] also found a low rate of recurrence to levels I and V (3% for both levels combined) in a population that had had previous resection rates of 3.9% for level I and 18.6% for level V. Nevertheless, several studies have shown that multiple-level involvement is common in the lateral neck. There is also concern that preoperative assessment may not be very sensitive at finding involved lymph nodes.

- Wu and colleagues[85] showed that of 100 patients who had at least 1 positive lateral neck node, 77% had involvement of multiple lateral neck levels and that the sensitivity of preoperative ultrasonography for the lateral neck was only in the 40% to 60% range per level.
- Kupferman and colleagues[86] also found preoperative ultrasonography to be only 20% sensitive for level V involvement.

Many investigators, however, have advocated thorough lateral neck dissection for any known lateral involvement.

- Kupferman and colleagues[75] found a relatively high rate of involvement of level V metastases, of 21%. This study, however, involved a variety of patient and tumor characteristics.
- Farrag and colleagues[82] also found a high rate of level V metastases, with 40% of patients who underwent lateral neck dissection for clinically proven involvement of at least one lateral level. This study further differentiated within level V, finding that all of the level V metastases were in V-B, with 0% involvement of V-A. Differentiation within level II showed a 60% overall involvement of level II, with only an 8.5% involvement of II-B; however, all positive level II-B were also positive in II-A.
- Ahmadi and colleagues[83] noted equal rates of level V involvement for both primary resections and lateral neck dissection for recurrence.
- In another retrospective review of recurrence in the lateral neck after initial lateral neck dissection, one group found a relatively high rate of level II recurrence, of 19% to 21%, whether or not the patient had undergone previous dissection of that level.[84]

THE BOTTOM LINE: WHAT DOES THE EVIDENCE TELL US?

A thorough clinical assessment of the extent of local disease and regional lymph node metastasis is necessary for staging accurately, determining prognosis, and tailoring appropriate treatments in thyroid cancer. This assessment includes preoperative ultrasonography or alternative imaging techniques such as CT, MRI, and PET. Malignancy should be confirmed in any suspicious lymph node using ultrasound-guided FNA if it will change the extent of the planned operative procedure. Near-total or total thyroidectomy should be performed in well-differentiated thyroid cancer with tumor size of greater than 1 cm. For low-risk tumors without nodal metastases of size less than 1 cm, total lobectomy may be sufficient for locoregional control; however, the current evidence cautions against using tumor size alone as a criteria for reducing the extent of surgical resection. Invasive thyroid cancer is relatively uncommon, but when it occurs there is a significant rate of recurrent laryngeal nerve involvement. Current evidence suggests that conservative surgical technique with nerve preservation can be performed in the majority of cases without adversely affecting survival rates; however, management should be performed on a case-by-case basis. There are options for nerve salvage, but complete resection often results in significant patient morbidity. Central neck and lateral neck dissection in the case of known positive nodes is certainly recommended, as node positivity has been linked to increased rates of recurrence and mortality.

There is controversy, however, regarding the role of prophylactic central neck dissection in the case of preoperatively node-negative patients. Evidence shows a high rate of occult central node metastasis with tumors of all sizes, the finding of which can affect staging and decision-making for postoperative adjuvant therapy and follow-up. Rates of permanent complications have not been shown to be significantly increased when node dissection is performed by experienced hands, although there is evidence for a higher rate of transient hypocalcemia. Thus far, however, there is little evidence to definitively demonstrate improvement in recurrence or survival rates for patients undergoing prophylactic central neck dissection, because of the difficulty in obtaining a sufficient number of patients to power such a study.[87] Controversy also exists regarding the performance of lateral neck dissection. Some evidence suggests that prophylactic lateral neck dissection should be performed in cases of central node positivity, and there is also evidence that this is less likely to occur in younger patients and with smaller tumor sizes. Even when the lateral neck has known involvement, the necessary extent of dissection has been debated. Most investigators agree that levels II, III, and IV are the most commonly involved and should likely be included in all lateral neck dissections. Level I has also been found by most investigators to have a low level of involvement, and its inclusion in routine dissection has been suggested to be unnecessary unless preoperative evidence suggests metastasis specifically to that level. There seems to be disagreement, however, on the routine inclusion of level V. Overall, the existing set of ATA management guidelines provide a reasonable methodology for decision-making regarding surgical treatment of thyroid cancer; however, there are still many areas where continued research will help us to better define an optimal plan of action for patients.

CRITICAL POINTS

- Clinical staging with appropriate imaging can allow for appropriate planning of surgical management and should include preoperative ultrasonography, or alternative methods such as CT, MRI, or PET. Evidence level A.
- Suspicious lymph nodes should be assessed for malignancy using ultrasound-guided FNA. Evidence level A.
- Tumors greater than 1 cm in size should be resected via near-total or total thyroidectomy. Evidence level A.
- Tumors less than 1 cm in size may be initially managed via total lobectomy; Evidence level A
- Attempts at preservation of the recurrent laryngeal nerve should be made when possible, but resection is reasonable in cases of gross involvement with tumor. Evidence level B.
- All presurgically involved levels of lymph nodes should be resected via compartment resection rather than "berry picking." Evidence level A.
- Elective central neck dissection may improve staging accuracy, affect future treatment plans, and reduce surveillance burden with minimal complications when performed by experienced hands. Evidence level B.
- Lateral neck involvement warrants compartment resection of at least levels II-A, III, and IV. Evidence level A.

REFERENCES

1. Davies L, Welch HG. Increasing incidence of thyroid cancer in the United States, 1973-2002. JAMA 2006;295(18):2164–7.

2. American Thyroid Association (ATA) Guidelines Taskforce on Thyroid Nodules and Differentiated Thyroid Cancer, Cooper D, Doherty G, Haugen B, et al. Revised American Thyroid Association management guidelines for patients with thyroid nodules and differentiated thyroid cancer. Thyroid 2009;19(11): 1167–214.

3. Stephenson BM, Wheeler MH, Clark OH. The role of total thyroidectomy in the management of differentiated thyroid cancer. Curr Opin Gen Surg 1994;53–9.

4. Ito Y, Fukushima M, Tomoda C, et al. Prognosis of patients with papillary carcinoma having clinically apparent metastasis to the lateral compartment. Endocr J 2009;56(6):759–66.

5. Solorzano CC, Carneiro DM, Ramirez M, et al. Surgeon-performed ultrasound in the management of thyroid malignancy. Am Surg 2004;70(7):576–80.

6. Ito Y, Miyauchi A. Lateral lymph node dissection guided by preoperative and intra-operative findings in differentiated thyroid carcinoma. World J Surg 2008; 32(5):729–39.

7. Frasoldati A, Valcavi R. Challenges in neck ultrasonography: lymphadenopathy and parathyroid glands. Endocr Pract 2004;10(3):261–8.

8. Kuna SK, Bracic I, Tesic V, et al. Ultrasonographic differentiation of benign from malignant neck lymphadenopathy in thyroid cancer. J Ultrasound Med 2006; 25(12):1531–7.

9. Leboulleux S, Girard E, Rose M, et al. Ultrasound criteria of malignancy for cervical lymph nodes in patients followed up for differentiated thyroid cancer. J Clin Endocrinol Metab 2007;92(9):3590–4.

10. Stulak JM, Grant CS, Farley DR, et al. Value of preoperative ultrasonography in the surgical management of initial and reoperative papillary thyroid cancer. Arch Surg 2006;141(5):489–94.

11. Kouvaraki MA, Shapiro SE, Fornage BD, et al. Role of preoperative ultrasonography in the surgical management of patients with thyroid cancer. Surgery 2003;134(6):946–54.

12. Kresnik E, Gallowitsch HJ, Mikosch P, et al. Fluorine-18-fluorodeoxyglucose positron emission tomography in the preoperative assessment of thyroid nodules in an endemic goiter area. Surgery 2003;133(3):294–9.

13. Zbaren P, Becker M, Lang H. Pretherapeutic staging of hypopharyngeal carcinoma. Clinical findings, computed tomography, and magnetic resonance imaging compared with histopathologic evaluation. Arch Otolaryngol Head Neck Surg 1997;124(2):908–13.

14. Jeong HS, Baek CH, Son YI, et al. Integrated ^{18}F-FDG PET-CT for the initial evaluation of cervical node level of patients with papillary thyroid carcinoma: comparison with ultrasound and contrast-enhanced CT. Clin Endocrinol 2006;65(3):402–7.

15. Kim E, Park JS, Son KR, et al. Preoperative diagnosis of cervical metastatic lymph nodes in papillary thyroid carcinoma: comparison of ultrasound, computed tomography, and combined ultrasound with computed tomography. Thyroid 2009;18(4):411–8.

16. Uruno T, Miyauchi A, Shimizu K, et al. Usefulness of thyroglobulin measurement in fine-needle aspiration biopsy specimens for diagnosing cervical lymph node metastasis in patients with papillary thyroid cancer. World J Surg 2005;29(4): 483–5.

17. Boi F, Baghino G, Atzeni F, et al. The diagnostic value for differentiated thyroid carcinoma metastases of thyroglobulin (Tg) measurement in washout fluid from fine-needle aspiration biopsy of neck lymph nodes is maintained in the presence of circulating anti-Tg antibodies. J Clin Endocrinol Metab 2006;91(4):1364–9.

18. Shaha AR, Shah JP, Loree TR. Low-risk differentiated thyroid cancer: the need for selective treatment. Ann Surg Oncol 1996;4(4):328–33.

19. Duren M, Yavuz N, Bukey Y, et al. Impact of initial surgical treatment on survival of patients with differentiated thyroid cancer: experience of an endocrine surgery center in an iodine-deficient region. World J Surg 2000;24(11):1290–4.

20. Kim ES, Kim TY, Koh JM, et al. Completion thyroidectomy in patients with thyroid cancer who initially underwent unilateral operation. Clin Endocrinol 2004;61(1): 145–8.

21. Kupferman ME, Mandel SJ, DiDonato L, et al. Safety of completion thyroidectomy following unilateral lobectomy for well-differentiated thyroid cancer. Laryngoscopy 2002;112(7 Pt 1):1209–12.

22. Pacini F, Elisei R, Capezzone M, et al. Contralateral papillary thyroid cancer is frequent at completion thyroidectomy with no difference in low-and high-risk patients. Thyroid 2001;11(9):877–81.

23. Pasieka JL, Thompson NW, McLeod MK, et al. The incidence of bilateral well-differentiated thyroid cancer found a completion thyroidectomy. World J Surg 1992;16(4):711–6.

24. Erdem E, Gülçelik MA, Kuru B, et al. Comparison of completion thyroidectomy and primary surgery for differentiated thyroid carcinoma. Eur J Surg Oncol 2003;29(9):747–9.

25. Hay ID, Thompson GB, Grant CS, et al. Papillary thyroid carcinoma managed at the mayo clinic during six decades (1940-1999): temporal trends in initial therapy and long-term outcome in 2444 consecutively treated patients. World J Surg 2002;25:879–85.

26. Bilimoria KY, Bentrem DJ, Ko CY, et al. Extent of surgery affects survival for papillary thyroid cancer. Ann Surg 2007;246(3):375–84.

27. Nixon IJ, Ganly I, Patel SG, et al. Thyroid lobectomy for treatment of well differentiated intrathyroid malignancy. Surgery 2012;151(4):571–9.

28. Hay ID, Hutchinson ME, Gonzalez-Losada T, et al. Papillary thyroid microcarcinoma: a study of 900 cases observed in a 60-year period. Surgery 2008;144:980–8.

29. Ogilvie JB, Patel KN, Heller KS. Impact of the 2009 American Thyroid Association guidelines on the choice of operation for well-differentiated thyroid microcarcinoma. Surgery 2010;148(6):1222–6.

30. McCaffrey TV, Bergstralh EJ, Hay ID. Locally invasive papillary thyroid carcinoma: 1940-1990. Head Neck 1994;16(2):165–72.

31. Breaux GP, Guillamondequi OM. Treatment of locally invasive carcinoma of the thyroid: how radical? Am J Surg 1980;140(4):514–7.

32. Nakao K, Kurozumi K, Fukushima S, et al. Merits and demerits of operative procedure to the trachea in patients with differentiated thyroid cancer. World J Surg 2001;25(6):723–7.

33. Nishida T, Nakao K, Hamaji M, et al. Preservation of recurrent laryngeal nerve invaded by differentiated thyroid cancer. Ann Surg 1997;226(1):85–91.

34. Kowalski LP, Filho JG. Results of the treatment of locally invasive thyroid carcinoma. Head Neck 2002;24(4):340–4.

35. Chan WF, Lo CY, Lam KY, et al. Recurrent laryngeal nerve palsy in well-differentiated thyroid carcinoma: clinicopathologic features and outcome study. World J Surg 2004;28(11):1093–8.

36. Falk SA, McCaffrey TV. Management of the recurrent laryngeal nerve in suspected and proven thyroid cancer. Otolaryngol Head Neck Surg 1995;113(1):42–8.

37. Urken M. Prognosis and management of invasive well-differentiated thyroid cancer. Otolaryngol Clin North Am 2010;43(2):301–28.

38. Chiang FY, Lin JC, Lee KW, et al. Thyroid tumors with preoperative recurrent laryngeal nerve palsy: clinicopathologic features and treatment outcome. Surgery 2006;140(3):413–7.

39. Chiang FY, Lu IC, Tsai CJ, et al. Does extensive dissection of recurrent laryngeal nerve during thyroid operation increase the risk of nerve injury? Evidence from the application of intraoperative neuromonitoring. Am J Otol 2011;32(6):499–503.

40. American Thyroid Association Surgery Working Group, American Association of Endocrine Surgeons, American Academy of Otolaryngology-Head and Neck Surgery, Carty S, Cooper D, Doherty G, et al. Consensus statement on the terminology and classification of central neck dissection for thyroid cancer. Thyroid 2009;19(11):1153–8.

41. Grodski S, Cornford L, Sywak M, et al. Routine level VI lymph node dissection for papillary thyroid cancer: surgical technique. ANZ J Surg 2007;77(4):203–8.

42. Qubain S, Nakano S, Baba M, et al. Distribution of lymph node micrometastases in pN0 well-differentiated thyroid carcinoma. Surgery 2002;131(3):249–56.

43. Roh JL, Kim JM, Park CI. Central compartment reoperation for recurrent/persistent differentiated thyroid cancer: patterns of recurrence, morbidity, and prediction of postoperative hypocalcemia. Ann Surg Oncol 2011;18(5):1312–8.

44. Lee SH, Lee SS, Jin SM, et al. Predictive factors for central compartment lymph node metastasis in thyroid papillary microcarcinoma. Laryngoscope 2008;118(4): 659–62.

45. Roh JL, Park JY, Rha K, et al. Is central neck dissection necessary for the treatment of lateral cervical nodal recurrence of papillary thyroid carcinoma? Head Neck 2007;29(10):901–5.

46. Leboulleux S, Rubino C, Baudin E, et al. Prognostic factors for persistent or recurrent disease of papillary thyroid carcinoma with neck lymph node metastases and/or tumor extension beyond the thyroid capsule at initial diagnosis. J Clin Endocrinol Metab 2005;90(10):5723–9.

47. Harwood J, Clark O, Dunphy J. Significance of lymph node metastasis in differentiated thyroid cancer. Am J Surg 1978;136(1):107–12.

48. Mazzaferri E, Jhiang S. Long-term impact of initial surgical and medical therapy on papillary and follicular thyroid cancer. Am J Med 1994;97(5):418–28.

49. Podnos Y, Smith D, Wagman L, et al. The implication of lymph node metastasis on survival in patients with well-differentiated thyroid cancer. Am Surg 2005;71(9):731–4.

50. Bhattacharyya N. A population-based analysis of survival factors in differentiated and medullary thyroid carcinoma. Otolaryngol Head Neck Surg 2003;128(1):115–23.

51. Scheumann G, Gimm O, Wegener G, et al. Prognostic significance and surgical management of locoregional lymph node metastases in papillary thyroid cancer. World J Surg 1994;18(4):559–67.

52. Lundgren C, Hall P, Dickman P, et al. Clinically significant prognostic factors for differentiated thyroid carcinoma: a population-based, nested case-control study. Cancer 2006;106(3):524–31.

53. Grant C, Stulak J, Thompson G, et al. Risks and adequacy of an optimized surgical approach to the primary surgical management of papillary thyroid carcinoma treated during 1999-2006. World J Surg 2010;34(6):1239–46.

54. Musacchio MJ, Kim AW, Vijungco JD, et al. Greater local recurrence occurs with "berry picking" than neck dissection in thyroid cancer. Am Surg 2003;69(3): 191–7.

55. Moo TA, McGill J, Allendorf J, et al. Impact of prophylactic central neck lymph node dissection on early recurrence in papillary thyroid carcinoma. World J Surg 2010;34(6):1187–91.

56. Shindo M, Wu J, Park E, et al. The importance of central compartment elective lymph node excision in the staging and treatment of papillary thyroid cancer. Arch Otolaryngol Head Neck Surg 2006;132(6):650–4.

57. Wada N, Duh QY, Sugino K, et al. Lymph node metastasis from 259 papillary thyroid microcarcinomas. Ann Surg 2003;237(3):399–407.

58. Roh JL, Kim JM, Park C. Central cervical nodal metastasis from papillary thyroid microcarcinoma: pattern and factors predictive of nodal metastasis. Ann Surg Oncol 2008;15(9):2482–6.

59. Hughes D, White M, Miller B, et al. Influence of prophylactic central lymph node dissection on postoperative thyroglobulin levels and radioiodine treatment in papillary thyroid cancer. Surgery 2010;148(6):1100–6.

60. Bonnet S, Hartl D, Leboulleux S, et al. Prophylactic lymph node dissection for papillary thyroid cancer less than 2 cm: implications for radioiodine treatment. J Clin Endocrinol Metab 2009;94(4):1162–7.

61. Sywak M, Cornford L, Roach P, et al. Routine ipsilateral level VI lymphadenectomy reduces postoperative thyroglobulin levels in papillary thyroid cancer. Surgery 2006;140(6):1000–5.

62. So Y, Seo M, Son YI. Prophylactic central lymph node dissection for clinically node-negative papillary thyroid microcarcinoma: influence on serum thyroglobulin level, recurrence rate, and postoperative complications. Surgery 2012; 151(2):192–8.

63. Henry J, Gramatica L, Denizot A, et al. Morbidity of prophylactic lymph node dissection in the central neck area in patients with papillary thyroid carcinoma. Langenbecks Arch Surg 1998;383(2):167–9.

64. Zetoune T, Keutgen X, Buitrago D, et al. Prophylactic central neck dissection and local recurrence in papillary thyroid cancer: a meta-analysis. Ann Surg Oncol 2010;17(12):3287–93.

65. Chao TC, Jeng LB, Lin JD, et al. Reoperative thyroid surgery. World J Surg 1997; 21(6):644–7.

66. Kim M, Mandel S, Baloch Z, et al. Morbidity following central compartment reoperation for recurrent or persistent thyroid cancer. Arch Otolaryngol Head Neck Surg 2004;130(10):1214–6.

67. So Y, Son Y, Hong S, et al. Subclinical lymph node metastasis in papillary thyroid microcarcinoma: a study of 551 resections. Surgery 2010;148(3): 526–31.

68. Shen W, Ogawa L, Ruan D, et al. Central neck lymph node dissection for papillary thyroid cancer: the reliability of surgeon judgment in predicting which patients will benefit. Surgery 2010;148(2):398–403.

69. Shen W, Ogawa L, Ruan D, et al. Central neck lymph node dissection for papillary thyroid cancer: comparison of complication and recurrence rates in 295 initial dissections and reoperations. Arch Surg 2010;145(3):272–5.

70. Sadowski B, Snyder S, Lairmore T. Routine bilateral central lymph node clearance for papillary thyroid cancer. Surgery 2009;146(4):696–703.

71. Shindo ML, Stern A. Total thyroidectomy with and without selective neck dissection. Arch Otolaryngol Head Neck Surg 2010;136:584–7.

72. Roh JL, Kim JM, Park C. Central lymph node metastasis of unilateral papillary thyroid carcinoma: patterns and factors predictive of nodal metastasis, morbidity, and recurrence. Ann Surg Oncol 2011;18(8):2245–50.

73. Koo B, Choi E, Park YH, et al. Occult contralateral central lymph node metastases in papillary thyroid carcinoma with unilateral lymph node metastasis in the lateral neck. J Am Coll Surg 2010;210(6):895–900.

74. Chung YS, Kim JY, Bae JS, et al. Lateral lymph node metastasis in papillary thyroid carcinoma: results of therapeutic lymph node dissection. Thyroid 2009; 19(3):241–6.
75. Kupferman ME, Patterson M, Mandel SJ, et al. Patterns of lateral neck metastasis in papillary thyroid carcinoma. Arch Otolaryngol Head Neck Surg 2004;130(7): 857–60.
76. Lim YS, Lee JC, Lee YS, et al. Lateral cervical lymph node metastases from papillary thyroid carcinoma: predictive factors of nodal metastasis. Surgery 2011; 150(1):116–21.
77. Jeong JJ, Lee YS, Lee SC, et al. A scoring system for prediction of lateral neck node metastasis from papillary thyroid cancer. J Korean Med Sci 2011;26(8): 996–1000.
78. Kwak JY, Kim EK, Kim MJ, et al. Papillary microcarcinoma of the thyroid: predicting factors of lateral neck node metastasis. Ann Surg Oncol 2009;16(5): 1348–55.
79. Goropoulous A, Karamoshos K, Christodoulou A, et al. Value of the cervical compartments in the surgical treatment of papillary thyroid carcinoma. World J Surg 2004;28(12):1275–81.
80. Machens A, Hinze R, Thomusch O, et al. Pattern of nodal metastasis for primary and reoperative thyroid cancer. World J Surg 2001;26:22–8.
81. Wang TS, Dubner S, Sznyter LA, et al. Incidence of metastatic well-differentiated thyroid cancer in cervical lymph nodes. Arch Otolaryngol Head Neck Surg 2004; 130(1):110–3.
82. Farrag T, Lin F, Brownlee N, et al. Is routine dissection of level II-B and V-A necessary in patients with papillary thyroid cancer undergoing lateral neck dissection for FNA-confirmed metastases in other levels. World J Surg 2009; 33(8):1680–3.
83. Ahmadi N, Grewal A, Davidson BJ. Patterns of cervical lymph node metastasis in primary and recurrent papillary thyroid cancer. J Oncol 2011;2011:735678 [Epub 2011 Nov 17].
84. Caron NR, Tan YY, Ogilvie JB, et al. Selective modified radical neck dissection for papillary thyroid cancer—is level I, II and V dissection always necessary? World J Surg 2006;30:833–40.
85. Wu G, Fraser S, Pai SI, et al. Determining the extent of lateral neck dissection necessary to establish regional disease control and avoid reoperation after previous total thyroidectomy and radioactive iodine for papillary thyroid cancer. Head Neck 2011 Nov 3. [Epub ahead of print]. http://dx.doi.org/10.1002/hed.21937.
86. Kupferman ME, Weinstock YE, Santillan AA, et al. Predictors of level V metastasis in well-differentiated thyroid cancer. Head Neck 2008;30(11):1469–74.
87. American Thyroid Association, Carling T, Carty SE, Ciarleglio MM, et al. Design and feasibility of a prospective randomized controlled trial of prophylactic central lymph node dissection for papillary thyroid carcinoma. Thyroid 2012;22(3): 237–44.

Evidence-Based Practice
Management of the Clinical Node-Negative Neck in Early-Stage Oral Cavity Squamous Cell Carcinoma

Marcus M. Monroe, MD, Neil D. Gross, MD*

KEYWORDS

- Evidence-based otolaryngology • N0 neck • Squamous cell carcinoma • Oral cavity

KEY POINTS

The following points list the level of evidence as based on Oxford Center for Evidence-Based Medicine. Additional critical points are provided and points here are expanded at the conclusion of this article.

- The presence of lymph node metastases in oral cavity squamous cell carcinoma (OCSCC) continues to be one of the most important prognostic factors. In clinical node-negative (cN0) early-stage OCSCC, the prevalence of occult nodal disease ranges from 18% to 30% for T1 lesions and 24% to 53% for T2 tumors.
- Preoperative factors, including characteristics of the primary tumor, histopathologic features, and preoperative imaging, can help adjust the estimated risk of nodal disease.
- The most appropriate management strategy for dealing with the cN0 neck remains controversial, with observation, elective neck dissection, and sentinel lymph node biopsy reported as potential management strategies. There is insufficient evidence to recommend any single management strategy over another (level of evidence 1a-; grade D).
- The current literature is hampered by inadequately powered studies regarding the role of elective neck dissection in early-stage clinically node-negative OCSCC.

OVERVIEW

Spread to the cervical lymphatics continues to be one of the most important prognostic factors in patients with oral cavity squamous cell carcinoma (OCSCC), with a reduction in survival of at least 30%.[1] As such, the presence of lymphatic spread is an integral consideration when deciding on the use of adjuvant therapy. In patients with a clinically negative neck (ie, those with no evidence of cervical lymphatic spread by physical examination and imaging studies), there is continued controversy as to the most appropriate management strategy.

None of the authors have conflicts of interest or financial disclosures.
Department of Otolaryngology/Head and Neck Surgery, Oregon Health and Science University, Portland, OR, USA
* Corresponding author. Department of Otolaryngology/Head and Neck Surgery, Oregon Health and Science University, 3181 Sam Jackson Park Road, PV-01, Portland, OR 97239-3098.
E-mail address: grossn@ohsu.edu

Otolaryngol Clin N Am 45 (2012) 1181–1193
http://dx.doi.org/10.1016/j.otc.2012.06.016
0030-6665/12/$ – see front matter Published by Elsevier Inc.

oto.theclinics.com

Elective treatment with neck dissection, sentinel lymph node biopsy, radiation, and observation are proposed strategies for managing the clinically node-negative (cN0) neck. The debate surrounding these management choices has been longstanding, with recent reinvigoration from the increasing interest in transoral surgical approaches and the avoidance of external incisions in the management of early-stage head and neck malignancies.

Despite several decades of intensive debate in the medical literature, the role of elective neck dissection (END) in patients with cN0 OCSCC remains controversial. The conflicting conclusions of a large number of heterogeneous retrospective studies and the lack of large-scale, adequately powered prospective studies contribute to the confusion surrounding this topic. This article provides a critical review of the evidence surrounding the management of the cN0 patient with early-stage OCSCC.

EVIDENCE-BASED CLINICAL ASSESSMENT
Choosing an Appropriate Therapeutic Threshold

Before any clinical assessment of the risk of lymphatic metastases, the physician should establish an appropriate treatment threshold beyond which the potential benefits of treatment outweigh the morbidity. This a priori defined threshold forms the backdrop that frames all management decisions regarding the risk of lymphatic metastases. Although little controversy exists at the extremes of risk, the benefit becomes less clear in cases with intermediate risk of occult nodal disease. Having a defined level at which the potential benefits of elective treatment outweigh the risks provides a rational approach to the application of treatment.

Given the fundamental importance of defining a treatment threshold in interpreting estimates of the risk of occult nodal disease and the subsequent application of treatment, it is surprising that little attention has been paid to this question in the literature. In their often-quoted paper, Weiss and colleagues[2] used a decision tree analysis to derive a treatment threshold of 20%. This analysis was based on the risk of nodal disease, the effectiveness of primary and salvage surgery, and a subjective assignment of the usefulness of treatment outcomes. Based on this analysis, they argued that patients with a risk of nodal metastases greater than 20% would benefit from END. Although many continue to use a 20% risk of nodal metastases as a general guideline for performing END, the clinical data used to generate this threshold are based on historical series that may not reflect contemporary treatment outcomes. More recent publications have recommended treatment thresholds ranging from 17% to 40%.[3,4] Given the lack of high-quality evidence surrounding any of these treatment thresholds, they should be interpreted with caution. Such thresholds should not be interpreted as absolute values that define when treatment is appropriate. Rather, they should serve to emphasize that any interpretation of the risk of nodal metastases needs to be done in the framework of a predefined threshold for action.

Assessing the Risk of Occult Nodal Disease

Assessment of the primary site

Once a threshold for END has been defined, an initial assessment of the risk of nodal disease is based on the site and classification of the primary tumor (T classification). Subsequent evaluation of specific tumor characteristics, including depth of invasion, histologic tumor grade, and presence of perineural and/or lymphovascular invasion, can be used to adjust the probability estimates of occult nodal disease.

Rates of regional metastatic spread differ by oral cavity subsite. Squamous cell carcinoma involving the tongue is the most well-studied subsite of the oral cavity.

Early-stage tongue carcinomas have higher rates of metastatic spread than floor of mouth carcinomas.[5,6] Comparisons with other oral cavity subsites are limited.

The probability of occult nodal disease based on the clinical T classification has been estimated in multiple END studies in early OCSCC (**Table 1**).[5,7,8] Differences in patient populations, subsite distribution, extent of dissection, and methods of histologic node analysis between these studies make comparative estimates of the prevalence of occult nodal disease difficult. In END series in which elective treatment of the neck was applied universally, the prevalence of occult positive nodes ranges from 6% to 25% for T1 OCSCC, whereas the prevalence for T2 OCSCC ranges from 20% to 32%. When the studies comparing observation and neck dissection are included (**Table 2**), the prevalence of occult node disease in early OCSCC can approach 40% to 50%,[4,6–17] although these numbers may be inflated because of selection bias.

Although location and clinical T classification can be obtained from preoperative examination alone, other factors that have been reported to affect the prevalence of occult nodal disease require further diagnostic testing. These factors include histopathologic details such as tumor grade, lymphovascular invasion, perineural spread, and depth of invasion.

The depth of invasion of the primary tumor, particularly for oral tongue squamous cell carcinoma, has been reported to significantly influence the prevalence of occult node positivity. A depth of invasion greater than 4 mm has been associated with an increased risk of occult node metastasis. Asakage and colleagues[9] studied 44 patients with T1 and T2 squamous cell carcinoma of the oral tongue who were treated with partial glossectomy and observation of the neck. At 5 years, 21 of the 44 had developed neck metastases. On multivariate analysis, only the depth of invasion predicted subsequent cervical node metastases with a relative risk ratio of 9.4 (95% confidence interval [CI] 1.5–57.7) for lesions 4 mm or greater in thickness.[9] Additional retrospective studies noted an association between increased tumor thickness and an increased risk of occult node disease.[10,18,19]

The importance of a tumor depth 4 mm or greater has been validated as an important predictor of occult node metastasis in prospective randomized controlled trials evaluating END versus observation for early-stage OSCC.[11,16] In a study comparing hemiglossectomy alone or with elective radical neck dissection for early-stage oral tongue squamous cell carcinoma, Fakih and colleagues[11] showed an increased rate of occult nodal disease (67% vs 8%; $P<.01$) for tumors with a depth of 4 mm or greater in the END arm of the study. In the observation arm, they showed a corresponding increased rate of delayed regional node metastases in tumors with a depth of 4 mm or greater (76% vs 22%; $P<.01$). Similar trends were noted in a prospective study by Kligerman and colleagues[16] that compared resection alone versus resection with selective neck dissection (levels I–III) for early-stage OCSCC. The investigators observed a trend toward an increase in occult node positivity with tumors greater than 4 mm in depth (30% vs 7%; $P = .11$).

Table 1
Representative series showing the range in prevalence of occult nodal metastases by T classification in early OCSCC

Investigators	n	T1 (%)	T2 (%)
Iype et al[35]	172	25.4	29.4
Thiele et al[15]	122	5.9	19.7
Civantos et al[32]	140	25.0	32.0

Table 2
Retrospective series comparing END and observation (Obs) in early-stage OCSCC

Investigators	n	Population	% Occult N+ (END)	% Delayed N+ (Obs)	% Salvaged	% Survival for END, Obs (y)	Recommendation
Ebrahimi et al[36]	153	T1–T2 OC	37	39	21	92, 69 (5)	END
Dias et al[5]	49	T1 OT, FOM	21	28	38	97, 74 (3)	END
Haddadin et al[26]	137	T1–T2 OT	38	41	35	80.5, 53.6 (5)	END
Capote et al[23]	154	T1–T2	0	27	32	92.5, 71.4 (5)	END
Cunningham et al[24]	54	T1–T2 OT, FOM	14	42	56	88, 77 (3)	END
Lydiatt et al[27]	156	T1–T2 OT	20	17	50	55, 33	END
Duvvuri et al[37]	359	T1–T2 OC, OP	23	27	N/A	73, 58	END
Keski-Santti et al[8]	80	T1–T2 OT	34	44	33	82, 77 (5)	END
Franceschi et al[25]	149	T1–T2 OT	41	26	41	62, 63 (5)	Obs
O'Brien et al[18]	162	T1–T4 OC, OP	30	9	80	86, 94 (3)	Obs
Khafif et al[38]	590	T1–T4 OC, OP, L	41	16	49	56, 49	Obs
D'Cruz et al[39]	359	T1–T2, OT	20	47	46	74, 68 (5)	Obs
Layland et al[40]	621	T1–T4 OC	12	N/A	31	54, 58	Obs
Liu et al[41]	131	T1 OT	24	23	N/A	80, 74 (4)	Obs

Abbreviations: FOM, floor of mouth; L, larynx; OC, oral cavity; OP, oropharynx; OT, oral tongue.

Because of these findings, many have recommended END when the depth of invasion exceeds 4 mm. Although the evidence strongly suggests that an increase in the depth of the primary tumor is significantly associated with an increased risk of node positivity, interpretations of the degree to which it influences this risk and the best cutoff value in tumor thickness are clouded by significant heterogeneity in the study populations, extent of node dissection, and techniques for measuring tumor thickness.

Perhaps the greatest limitation to the use of the 4-mm tumor thickness cutoff is the difficulty in obtaining this information before it is needed. Although staged END can be performed after treatment of the primary tumor and pathologic analysis of the specimen, many surgeons prefer to address the primary tumor and regional lymphatics at the same surgical setting. A preoperative biopsy can provide an estimate of tumor thickness but may be subject to sampling error. To overcome these limitations, Taylor and colleagues[12] reported using ultrasound (US) to assess the depth of the primary lesion. In a consecutive series of 21 patients with oral tongue and floor of mouth squamous cell carcinoma, the investigators noted a high concordance between pathologic tumor thickness and preoperative US estimation of thickness.[12] However, the results of this study have yet to be replicated in a large series of patients with OCSCC and therefore should be interpreted with caution.

Other histopathologic parameters, such as lymphovascular invasion, tumor grade, and perineural spread, have less consistent relationships with the risk of cervical node metastases than either clinical tumor classification or thickness. As such, the usefulness of these parameters to adjust predictions regarding the risk of occult node disease is not clear.

Assessment of the neck

The sensitivity of physical examination for the detection of cervical node metastases is reported to range from 60% to 80%,[20] which is less than the useful level for decision making.

Imaging A variety of imaging techniques can provide increased sensitivity and specificity for the detection of regional node metastases. US, magnetic resonance imaging (MRI), computed tomography (CT), photon emission tomography (PET), and PET-CT/MRI fusion have all been examined in the context of the N0 neck, with varying accuracy.

The usefulness of these imaging studies lies, in part, in their ability to shift the probability or risk of nodal metastasis past (either above or below) the predetermined threshold for treatment. The decision to obtain imaging of the neck should consequently be made in light of the estimated probability of occult disease based on the initial examination of the primary lesion. In some patients, the initial risk of nodal metastases may exceed a threshold at which testing for the sake of determining whether END is necessary is unwarranted. For instance, a large, deeply invasive T2 tongue carcinoma may have an estimated risk of nodal metastases that is high enough to warrant END regardless of the findings of any imaging study. In this case, imaging may provide valuable additional information about the primary tumor or potentially the extent of dissection, but would not alter the decision of whether or not treatment is needed.

Several prospective studies have compared the performance of various imaging modalities in the examination of the neck in patients with OCSCC: Stuckensen and colleagues[21] compared the ability of PET, MRI, CT, and US to detect cervical node metastases in 106 patients with OCSCC who underwent END. Using pathologic assessment as the gold standard: PET had the greatest accuracy: sensitivity 70%, specificity 82%; US: 84%, 68%; CT: 66%, 74%; MRI: 64%, 69%. In a study of 463 patients with OCSCC, Liao and colleagues[22] reported that preoperative 18F-fluorodeoxyglucose

(FDG) PET had a sensitivity and specificity of 77.7% and 58.0%, respectively. When examination is restricted to patients with clinically N0 disease, the reported sensitivities and specificities decline markedly. Ng and colleagues[13] prospectively compared the performance of CT, MRI, and PET in 134 patients with OCSCC without palpable adenopathy. Overall, 35 (26.1%) had neck metastases. The best sensitivity and specificity for the detection of occult nodal disease was with PET imaging visually correlated to CT/MRI (57.1% and 96%, respectively) compared with PET alone (51.4% and 91.9%) or CT/MRI alone (31.4% and 91.9%). Based on these data, the posttest probability of occult nodal metastasis with a negative PET correlated with CT/MRI was 3.3% in T1 tumors and 9.2% in T2 tumors.

Kyzas and colleagues[14] performed a meta-analysis examining the diagnostic performance of 18F-FDG PET in patients with head and neck squamous cell carcinoma. For the cN0 subpopulation, the investigators found 10 studies with 311 patients for analysis. For this subpopulation, the sensitivity of PET was only 50% (95% CI 37%–63%), whereas specificity was 87% (95% CI 76%–93%). The positive likelihood ratio was 3.83 (95% CI 1.90–7.75) and the negative likelihood ratio was 0.57 (95% CI 0.43–0.77).

This means that, with an estimated pretest probability of occult nodal metastasis of 20%, the posttest probability with a positive PET scan shifts to 49%. The posttest probability with a negative PET scan is 12%, which is less than the commonly cited threshold of 20% for consideration of END.[2] Therefore, a PET scan may be beneficial in the initial evaluation of the cN0 neck, depending on an individual's treatment threshold.

EVIDENCE-BASED MANAGEMENT
END Versus Observation

A large number of retrospective studies have compared END with observation and have arrived at differing conclusions (**Table 2**).[4,6–8,12,15,18,21–27] These studies generally suffer from inadequate statistical power related to small sample size and significant selection bias that limit interpretation of the results. Furthermore, comparisons between these studies are hampered by differences in surgical technique, such as the extent of neck dissection performed and patient populations (eg, proportion of patients with T1 and T2 classification and differences in distribution of oral cavity subsites).

Only 4 prospective studies have compared END and observation in N0 patients with OCSCC (**Table 3**).[2,15,20,28]

1. In 1980, Vandenbrouk and colleagues[28] compared radical neck dissection with observation in 75 patients with cT1 to T3N0 OCSCC. No significant difference in 3-year disease-free survival (DFS) was noted, with 46% DFS in the END cohort and 58% in the observation cohort.
2. In 1989, Fakih and colleagues[11] reported no significant survival advantage for patients undergoing hemiglossectomy and radical END compared with hemiglossectomy and observation. DFS at 1 year was 63% in the END cohort compared with 52% in those treated with initial observation and therapeutic neck dissection, if required. This difference was not statistically significant.
3. In 1994, Kligerman and colleagues[16] compared selective (levels I–III) END with observation in patients with T1 to T2 oral tongue and floor of mouth squamous cell carcinoma. At 3.5 years, they noted a statistically significant difference in DFS between patients who were managed electively (72%) versus those initially observed (49%; $P = .04$).

Table 3
Prospective studies comparing END with Obs in early-stage OCSCC

Investigators	n	Population	Intervention (Primary, Neck)	% Occult N+ (END)	% Delayed N+ (Obs)	% Salvage	% DFS for END, Obs (y)	Survival Advantage
Vandenbrouk et al[28]	75	T1–T3 OT, FOM	RT, RND	49	53	84	46, 58 (3)	None
Fakih et al[11]	70	T1–T2 OT	RSX, RND	33.3	57	30	63, 52 (1)	None
Kligerman et al[16]	67	T1–T2 OT, FOM	RSX, SND	21	42	27	72, 49 (3)	END
Yuen et al[29]	71	T1–T2 OT	RSX, SND	22	31	100	89, 87 (5)	None

Abbreviations: DFS, disease-free survival; RND, radical neck dissection; RSX, resection; RT, radiation; SND, selective neck dissection.

4. In 2009, Yuen and colleagues[29] compared selective END with observation and noted no significant disease-specific survival advantage in 71 patients with T1 and T2 oral tongue carcinoma (89% at 5 years in the END cohort compared with 87% in the observation arm, $P = .89$).

No prospective study has shown a difference in overall survival.

The success of a strategy of observation relies primarily on the effectiveness of salvage surgery in those patients who develop delayed node metastases. An increase in the nodal disease burden and a higher incidence of extracapsular tumor extension have been reported in patients who undergo therapeutic neck dissection for delayed metastases versus up-front END.[16,26,30] The significantly improved DFS noted by Kligerman and colleagues[16] is, in part, the result of a salvage rate of only 27% in patients who were managed initially with resection and observation. The investigators speculated that a possible reason for poor outcome noted with observation was that their study included many patients of low socioeconomic level who returned for follow-up with advanced neck recurrence. The investigators implied that improved follow-up may have resulted in less advanced disease at the time of salvage surgery, and potentially improved survival. Others have reported much higher salvage rates following initial observation. Given the fundamental importance of the surgical salvage rate in determining the effectiveness of a strategy of observation, and the wide range of salvage rates reported in these 4 studies (27%–100%), the conclusions must be interpreted with care.

However, the most glaring limitation of the studies to date remains the lack of adequate statistical power to detect a meaningful difference in survival. If an 80% 5-year survival is assumed, to detect a 10% difference in survival (power 80%, α 0.05), approximately 300 patients per study arm would be required.[17] Even combined, the total population of the 4 prospective studies to date is much less than this number.

Fasluna and colleagues[7] performed a meta-analysis combining the data from these 4 prospective trials to determine whether there was a survival advantage with END. They noted a significant reduction in the relative risk of disease-specific death in patients treated with END in both a fixed effects (relative risk 0.57; 95% CI 0.36–0.89) and random effects model (relative risk 0.59; 95% CI 0.37–0.96). However, the heterogeneity in the study populations, treatments, and outcomes between these studies raises concern about the validity of such a systematic review. As such, there is currently insufficient evidence to recommend for or against a policy of END in the clinically negative neck in early-stage OCSCC (level of evidence 1a−; grade D).

Therefore, the question of the value of END in N0 patients with OCSCC remains unanswered. A multi-institutional effort will be required to achieve adequate accrual for a properly powered study. However, there is little enthusiasm from cooperative groups to address primarily surgical questions. Even the American College of Surgeons Oncology Group (ACOSOG) no longer supports head and neck clinical trials. In contrast, such fundamental questions are being addressed for patients with melanoma by the Multicenter Selective Lymphadenectomy series of prospective studies. There remains an unmet need for the organization and funding of multicenter head and neck clinical trials to address surgical questions.

Sentinel Lymph Node Biopsy

Increasing evidence has been published in the last decade regarding the effectiveness of sentinel lymph node biopsy (SLNB) for early-stage OCSCC. This subject has been the focus of numerous retrospective and prospective series, primarily from Europe. In 2005, Paleri and colleagues[31] performed a meta-analysis of the available studies on a combined 301 patients with OCSCC and 49 with oropharyngeal squamous cell carcinoma. The sensitivities of SLNB in the series ranged from 0.75 to 1, with a pooled sensitivity using the random effects model of 0.926 (95% CI 0.852–0.964).

Since that time, the ACOSOG multi-institutional trial evaluating the diagnostic accuracy of SLNB in the United States has been reported.[32] The study examined the accuracy of SLNB in 140 patients with early-stage (T1–T2N0) OCSCC. Most of these patients had oral tongue (n = 95) and floor of mouth (n = 26) primaries. With routine hematoxylin and eosin analysis they noted a 94% (95% CI 0.88–0.98) negative predictive value (NPV). With additional sectioning of the sentinel node and immunohistochemical analysis, the NPV improved to 96% (95% CI 0.90–0.98). SLNB performed similarly for floor of mouth and oral tongue primaries. Improved performance was noted for T1 versus T2 lesions (NPV 100% vs 94%) and for surgeons experienced in SLNB compared with novices (NPV 100% vs 95%).

The results of both the ACOSOG trial and earlier experiences are encouraging that SLNB can accurately stage the neck in early-stage OCSCC. The diagnostic accuracy of SLNB, combined with the perception that it is less morbid than a staging selective END, has led to some adopting SLNB as the initial approach to staging the neck in early-stage OCSCC, particularly in Europe where it has become the standard approach for some centers.[10] Although intuitively SLNB should be associated with reduced morbidity compared with END, the data supporting this for OCSCC are sparse.

Murer and colleagues[33] examined subjective impairment, functional shoulder status, and postoperative complications in 62 consecutive patients treated for early-stage OCSCC. Thirty-three of these patients underwent SLNB alone. The remaining 29 underwent a selective (I–III) END for an initial positive sentinel node, 20 of which were performed immediately following positive frozen section analysis of the sentinel node. The remaining 9 cases underwent a staged neck dissection.

The investigators noted a higher incidence of shoulder dysfunction as measured with a modified relative Constant score, longer scar length, and more postoperative complications in the END cohort compared with the SLNB group. However, this study was limited by the comparison groups not being equivalent given the presence of known neck disease in the cohort undergoing neck dissection. It is theoretically possible that prior SLNB may change the risks associated with subsequent neck dissection, either through distortion of anatomy, inflammation in the case of staged neck dissection, or even knowledge of positive neck disease, which may affect the extent of dissection. Furthermore, the investigators make no mention as to whether level 2b was dissected, a factor known to be associated with shoulder dysfunction.

Schiefke and colleagues[34] examined quality of life (QOL) outcomes and functional status in 49 patients undergoing transoral surgical resection for oral and oropharyngeal squamous cell carcinoma. Twenty-four of these patients underwent SNLB. The remaining 25 underwent selective (I–III) END.

QOL measurements included the health-related EORTC QLQ-30, the disease-specific EORTC QLQ-H&N35, and the Hospital Anxiety and Depression Scale. No differences were noted in the EORTC QLQ-30, whereas only the swallowing subset of the EORTC QLQ-H&N35 showed a significant difference between SLNB and END. Patients having SLNB were also more likely to have less fear of disease progression and experienced significantly less impairment from cervical scars, less sensory dysfunction, and better shoulder function as assessed by the Constant Shoulder Score. This study was limited by potential selection bias given the lack of randomization. Furthermore, the END cohort contained 8 patients with oropharyngeal and hypopharyngeal carcinoma, whereas the SLNB cohort comprised only patients with OCSCC.

Overall, the evidence to date suggests that, for experienced clinicians, SLNB is a reliable method for staging the cN0 neck in patients with early-stage OCSCC (level of evidence 1b, grade 1). However, conclusive data showing a reduction in morbidity compared with END is lacking (level of evidence 4, grade C). As with END, evidence showing a clear survival benefit for SLNB compared with observation is also lacking. Furthermore, concerns have been raised about the widespread adoption of SLNB, which is a technically more demanding procedure. Although initial data are encouraging, SLNB should not be considered a replacement for END outside a clinical trial.

WHAT DOES THE EVIDENCE SUGGEST ABOUT OCSCC?

Spread to the lymph nodes is one of the most important prognostic factors in OCSCC. Multiple retrospective and prospective studies place the risk of occult disease in early-stage cN0 OCSCC between 20% and 50% depending on the stage, subsite, and histopathologic features. There remains a lack of conclusive evidence regarding the appropriate risk threshold beyond which END should be undertaken (level of evidence 3b, grade B). Surgeon experience, resources, patient comorbidity and preferences should therefore continue to guide decisions regarding the appropriate threshold for END in cN0 patients with OCSCC. Depending on the therapeutic threshold, PET or PET/CT imaging may offer additional information that can shift the risk of occult nodal disease to more than or less than the defined treatment threshold (level of evidence 1b, grade A).

Management options for the cN0 neck include observation, END, and SLNB. Evidence to show that END is superior to observation for cN0 early-stage OCSCC is lacking. Of the 4 randomized clinical trials to date comparing END with observation for early-stage OCSCC, only 1 showed a significant improvement in DFS. All 4 trials displayed major limitations, most significantly a lack of adequate statistical power to show a meaningful difference in survival. Although the most recent meta-analysis of these studies showed a significant survival benefit in favor of END, there is troublesome heterogeneity in the patient populations, methods of treatment, follow-up, and surgical salvage rates between studies, which makes meta-analyses inconclusive (level of evidence 1a−, grade D). SLNB by experienced surgeons has been shown to adequately stage the neck compared with END (level of evidence 1b, grade A). There is a lack of high-quality data showing a reduction in morbidity between SLNB and END (level of evidence 4, grade C). SLNB should not be considered a standard replacement for END outside a clinical trial at this time.

With a lack of clear evidence to guide treatment, decisions regarding the most appropriate management strategy for the cN0 neck in early-stage OCSCC should be based on provider experience, an individualized assessment of the risk of nodal disease, and a frank discussion with the patient regarding the advantages and disadvantages of each approach. A prospective, multicenter, randomized controlled trial comparing END with observation would be of great value.

CRITICAL POINTS

- The presence of lymph node metastases in OCSCC continues to be one of the most important prognostic factors. In the cN0 early-stage OCSCC, the prevalence of occult nodal disease ranges from 18% to 30% for T1 lesions and 24% to 53% for T2 tumors.
- Many continue to cite a treatment threshold of 20% for END. However, there is a lack of evidence defining the most appropriate treatment threshold (level of evidence 3b, grade B).

- Preoperative factors including characteristics of the primary tumor (subsite and size classification), histopathologic features, and preoperative imaging can help adjust the estimated risk of nodal disease.
- The most appropriate management strategy for dealing with the cN0 neck remains controversial, with observation, END, and SLNB reported as potential management strategies. There is insufficient evidence to recommend one management strategy over another at this time (level of evidence 1a-, grade D).
- The current literature is hampered by inadequately powered studies. Large, multi-institutional clinical trials are needed to properly define the role of END in early-stage squamous cell carcinoma of the oral cavity.

REFERENCES

1. SEER stat fact sheets: oral cavity and pharynx. SEER; 2012. Available at: http://seer.cancer.gov/statfacts/html/oralcav.html. Accessed January 1, 2012.
2. Weiss MH, Harrison LB, Isaacs RS. Use of decision analysis in planning a management strategy for the stage N0 neck. Arch Otolaryngol Head Neck Surg 1994;120(7):699–702.
3. Song T, Bi N, Gui L, et al. Elective neck dissection or "watchful waiting": optimal management strategy for early stage N0 tongue carcinoma using decision analysis techniques. Chin Med J (Engl) 2008;121(17):1646–50.
4. Okura M, Aikawa T, Sawai NY, et al. Decision analysis and treatment threshold in a management for the N0 neck of the oral cavity carcinoma. Oral Oncol 2009;45(10):908–11.
5. Dias FL, Lima RA, Kligerman J, et al. Relevance of skip metastases for squamous cell carcinoma of the oral tongue and the floor of the mouth. Otolaryngol Head Neck Surg 2006;134(3):460–5.
6. Jerjes W, Upile T, Petrie A, et al. Clinicopathological parameters, recurrence, locoregional and distant metastasis in 115 T1-T2 oral squamous cell carcinoma patients. Head Neck Oncol 2010;2:9.
7. Fasunla AJ, Greene BH, Timmesfeld N, et al. A meta-analysis of the randomized controlled trials on elective neck dissection versus therapeutic neck dissection in oral cavity cancers with clinically node-negative neck. Oral Oncol 2011;47(5):320–4.
8. Keski-Santti H, Atula T, Tornwall J, et al. Elective neck treatment versus observation in patients with T1/T2 N0 squamous cell carcinoma of oral tongue. Oral Oncol 2006;42(1):96–101.
9. Asakage T, Yokose T, Mukai K, et al. Tumor thickness predicts cervical metastasis in patients with stage I/II carcinoma of the tongue. Cancer 1998;82(8):1443–8.
10. Po Wing Yuen A, Lam KY, Lam LK, et al. Prognostic factors of clinically stage I and II oral tongue carcinoma–A comparative study of stage, thickness, shape, growth pattern, invasive front malignancy grading, Martinez-Gimeno score, and pathologic features. Head Neck 2002;24(6):513–20.
11. Fakih AR, Rao RS, Borges AM, et al. Elective versus therapeutic neck dissection in early carcinoma of the oral tongue. Am J Surg 1989;158(4):309–13.
12. Taylor SM, Drover C, Maceachern R, et al. Is preoperative ultrasonography accurate in measuring tumor thickness and predicting the incidence of cervical metastasis in oral cancer? Oral Oncol 2010;46(1):38–41.
13. Ng SH, Yen TC, Chang JT, et al. Prospective study of [18F]fluorodeoxyglucose positron emission tomography and computed tomography and magnetic

resonance imaging in oral cavity squamous cell carcinoma with palpably negative neck. J Clin Oncol 2006;24(27):4371–6.

14. Kyzas PA, Evangelou E, Denaxa-Kyza D, et al. 18F-fluorodeoxyglucose positron
emission tomography to evaluate cervical node metastases in patients with head
and neck squamous cell carcinoma: a meta-analysis. J Natl Cancer Inst 2008;
100(10):712–20.

15. Thiele OC, Seeberger R, Flechtenmacher C, et al. The role of elective supraomo-
hyoidal neck dissection in the treatment of early, node-negative oral squamous
cell carcinoma (OSCC): a retrospective analysis of 122 cases. J Craniomaxillofac
Surg 2012;40(1):67–70.

16. Kligerman J, Lima RA, Soares JR, et al. Supraomohyoid neck dissection in the
treatment of T1/T2 squamous cell carcinoma of oral cavity. Am J Surg 1994;
168(5):391–4.

17. Rodrigo JP, Shah JP, Silver CE, et al. Management of the clinically negative neck
in early-stage head and neck cancers after transoral resection. Head Neck 2011;
33(8):1210–9.

18. O'Brien CJ, Traynor SJ, McNeil E, et al. The use of clinical criteria alone in the
management of the clinically negative neck among patients with squamous cell
carcinoma of the oral cavity and oropharynx. Arch Otolaryngol Head Neck
Surg 2000;126(3):360–5.

19. Kurokawa H, Yamashita Y, Takeda S, et al. Risk factors for late cervical lymph
node metastases in patients with stage I or II carcinoma of the tongue. Head
Neck 2002;24(8):731–6.

20. Hao SP, Ng SH. Magnetic resonance imaging versus clinical palpation in evaluating cervical metastasis from head and neck cancer. Otolaryngol Head Neck
Surg 2000;123(3):324–7.

21. Stuckensen T, Kovacs AF, Adams S, et al. Staging of the neck in patients with oral
cavity squamous cell carcinomas: a prospective comparison of PET, ultrasound,
CT and MRI. J Craniomaxillofac Surg 2000;28(6):319–24.

22. Liao CT, Wang HM, Huang SF, et al. PET and PET/CT of the neck lymph nodes
improves risk prediction in patients with squamous cell carcinoma of the oral
cavity. J Nucl Med 2011;52(2):180–7.

23. Capote A, Escorial V, Munoz-Guerra MF, et al. Elective neck dissection in early-
stage oral squamous cell carcinoma–does it influence recurrence and survival?
Head Neck 2007;29(1):3–11.

24. Cunningham MJ, Johnson JT, Myers EN, et al. Cervical lymph node metastasis
after local excision of early squamous cell carcinoma of the oral cavity. Am J
Surg 1986;152(4):361–6.

25. Franceschi D, Gupta R, Spiro RH, et al. Improved survival in the treatment of
squamous carcinoma of the oral tongue. Am J Surg 1993;166(4):360–5.

26. Haddadin KJ, Soutar DS, Oliver RJ, et al. Improved survival for patients with clinically T1/T2, N0 tongue tumors undergoing a prophylactic neck dissection. Head
Neck 1999;21(6):517–25.

27. Lydiatt DD, Robbins KT, Byers RM, et al. Treatment of stage I and II oral tongue
cancer. Head Neck 1993;15(4):308–12.

28. Vandenbrouck C, Sancho-Garnier H, Chassagne D, et al. Elective versus therapeutic radical neck dissection in epidermoid carcinoma of the oral cavity: results
of a randomized clinical trial. Cancer 1980;46(2):386–90.

29. Yuen AP, Ho CM, Chow TL, et al. Prospective randomized study of selective neck
dissection versus observation for N0 neck of early tongue carcinoma. Head Neck
2009;31(6):765–72.

30. Andersen PE, Cambronero E, Shaha AR, et al. The extent of neck disease after regional failure during observation of the N0 neck. Am J Surg 1996;172(6):689–91.

31. Paleri V, Rees G, Arullendran P, et al. Sentinel node biopsy in squamous cell cancer of the oral cavity and oral pharynx: a diagnostic meta-analysis. Head Neck 2005;27(9):739–47.

32. Civantos FJ, Zitsch RP, Schuller DE, et al. Sentinel lymph node biopsy accurately stages the regional lymph nodes for T1-T2 oral squamous cell carcinomas: results of a prospective multi-institutional trial. J Clin Oncol 2010;28(8):1395–400.

33. Murer K, Huber GF, Haile SR, et al. Comparison of morbidity between sentinel node biopsy and elective neck dissection for treatment of the n0 neck in patients with oral squamous cell carcinoma. Head Neck 2011;33(9):1260–4.

34. Schiefke F, Akdemir M, Weber A, et al. Function, postoperative morbidity, and quality of life after cervical sentinel node biopsy and after selective neck dissection. Head Neck 2009;31(4):503–12.

35. Iype EM, Sebastian P, Mathew A, et al. The role of selective neck dissection (I-III) in the treatment of node negative (N0) neck in oral cancer. Oral Oncol 2008; 44(12):1134–8.

36. Ebrahimi A, Moncrieff MD, Clark JR, et al. Predicting the pattern of regional metastases from cutaneous squamous cell carcinoma of the head and neck based on location of the primary. Head Neck 2010;32(10):1288–94.

37. Duvvuri U, Simental AA Jr, D'Angelo G, et al. Elective neck dissection and survival in patients with squamous cell carcinoma of the oral cavity and oropharynx. Laryngoscope 2004;114(12):2228–34.

38. Khafif RA, Gelbfish GA, Tepper P, et al. Elective radical neck dissection in epidermoid cancer of the head and neck. A retrospective analysis of 853 cases of mouth, pharynx, and larynx cancer. Cancer 1991;67(1):67–71.

39. D'Cruz AK, Siddachari RC, Walvekar RR, et al. Elective neck dissection for the management of the N0 neck in early cancer of the oral tongue: need for a randomized controlled trial. Head Neck 2009;31(5):618–24.

40. Layland MK, Sessions DG, Lenox J. The influence of lymph node metastasis in the treatment of squamous cell carcinoma of the oral cavity, oropharynx, larynx, and hypopharynx: N0 versus N+. Laryngoscope 2005;115(4):629–39.

41. Liu TR, Chen FJ, Yang AK, et al. Elective neck dissection in clinical stage I squamous cell carcinoma of the tongue: does it improve regional control or survival time? Oral Oncol 2011;47(2):136–41.

Index

Otolaryngol Clin N Am 45 (2012) 1195–1201
http://dx.doi.org/10.1016/S0030-6665(12)00111-9
0030-6665/12/$ – see front matter © 2012 Elsevier Inc. All rights reserved.

oto.theclinics.com

Moving?

Make sure your subscription moves with you!

To notify us of your new address, find your **Clinics Account Number** (located on your mailing label above your name), and contact customer service at:

Email: journalscustomerservice-usa@elsevier.com

800-654-2452 (subscribers in the U.S. & Canada)
314-447-8871 (subscribers outside of the U.S. & Canada)

Fax number: 314-447-8029

Elsevier Health Sciences Division
Subscription Customer Service
3251 Riverport Lane
Maryland Heights, MO 63043

*To ensure uninterrupted delivery of your subscription, please notify us at least 4 weeks in advance of move.

Printed and bound by CPI Group (UK) Ltd, Croydon, CR0 4YY

03/10/2024

01040458-0009